Primary Care for the Obstetrician and Gynecologist

Primary Care for the Obstetrician and Gynecologist

Yvonne S. Thornton, M.D., M.P.H., F.A.C.O.G., F.A.C.S.
Associate Clinical Professor of Obstetrics and Gynecology
Columbia University College of Physicians and Surgeons
New York, New York

Director, The Perinatal Diagnostic Testing Center
Morristown Memorial Hospital
Morristown, New Jersey

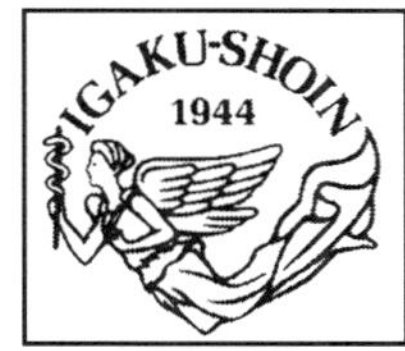

IGAKU-SHOIN New York • Tokyo

Published and distributed by

IGAKU-SHOIN Medical Publishers, Inc.
One Madison Avenue, New York, New York 10010

IGAKU-SHOIN Ltd.,
5–24–3 Hongo, Bunkyo-ku, Tokyo 113–91

Library of Congress Cataloging-in-Publication Data

Primary care for the obstetrician and gynecologist / [edited by]
Yvonne S. Thornton.
p. cm.
Includes bibliographical references and index.
1. Women—Diseases. 2. Women—Medical care. 3. Gynecologists.
I. Thornton, Yvonne S.
[DNLM: 1. Physical Examination—methods. 2. Primary Health Care.
3. Women's Health. WB 200 P952 1996]
RC48.6.P733 1996
616′.0082—dc20
DNLM/DLC 96-31523
for Library of Congress CIP

ISBN: 0–89640–324–6 (New York)
ISBN: 4–260–14324–7 (Tokyo)

Printed and bound in the U.S.A.
10 9 8 7 6 5 4 3 2 1

Preface

The obstetrician-gynecologist is in the unique position of being both a primary care physician *and* a specialist. A recent Gallup poll survey reported that 72% of general medical examinations given to women were performed by an OB/GYN compared to 57% by all other providers. Over seven million women a year will have their general medical examination performed by their gynecologist. Often the obstetrician-gynecologist is the only physician they have known or from whom they would seek primary medical care and advice.

In the past, our patients generally were asked to disrobe only from the waist down. Now, we have become more aware of our responsibility to examine the "whole patient." This book was written to serve as a practical clinical resource for the busy OB/GYN clinician. The purpose of this book is to inform, guide and enlighten practicing obstetricians and gynecologists about the most current concepts of management and to help them recognize pertinent clinical abnormalities that may present during a routine patient visit. Each chapter is geared towards assisting the OB/GYN to properly diagnose and identify disorders, and to develop a basic understanding of routine as well as specific laboratory results peculiar to a certain disease entity. This book is not meant to transform OB/GYN practitioners into specialists in other disciplines.

Until recently, American medicine was predominately focused on specialization rather than primary care. With the rapid emerging prominence of managed care, there has been a reversal of that emphasis back to primary care. Often, the OB/GYN is called upon to initiate the patient's entry into the health care system. With the increased emphasis on primary care, many physicians, OB/GYN and non-OB/GYN, may feel that their present fund of medical knowledge and expertise is inadequate for what will be required to appropriately treat or direct their patients. This text, hopefully, will enhance the knowledge of the OB/GYN as well as the general practitioner in the practice of primary care and preventive medicine for women.

Yvonne S. Thornton, M.D., M.P.H.

Book Dedication

This book is dedicated to the memory of

Roy H. Petrie, M.D., Sc.D.

(1940–1995)

My professor, my mentor, my friend

Acknowledgments

At this time, I want to recognize and applaud the efforts of the American College of Obstetricians and Gynecologists for its success in raising the public consciousness of the need for the OB/GYN to be designated as a primary care physician. Drs. William C. Andrews, Robert C. Cefalo and Vicki L. Seltzer should also be congratulated as pioneers in the primary care area for the obstetrician-gynecologist.

Finally, I want to express my profound gratitude to Richard U. Levine, M.D. who gave me this opportunity to be involved in such a worthwhile undertaking.

Yvonne S. Thornton, M.D., M.P.H.

Foreword

As obstetrician-gynecologists, our mission is to improve the health of our female patients. Patient demands and managed care have changed the landscape of our practice, and this evolution in care has been addressed by ACOG, medical schools, and residency programs.

There is an increasing demand to expand the scope of our practices to include primary care and preventive care. In reality, increasing numbers of women view their obstetrician-gynecologist as their principal source of health care and consider their visit as a general medical exam except when pregnant. This has created a demand for resource material which updates us, so we can continue to provide excellent care.

To respond to this need, Dr. Yvonne Thornton has assembled a series of topics which address the most common problems seen in the office. She has included chapters on cardiac disease, thyroid disease, anemia, hypertension, diabetes, and common neurological disorders. She has also included chapters on HIV and nutrition, which are more recent patient concerns. The chapter on Resuscitation in the Office provides important information on office emergencies.

By Dr. Thornton's select choice of topics, she has made it easier for us to improve our care of women and their health.

Richard U. Levine, M.D.

Contributors

Paul R. Becherer, M.D., M.P.H., FACP
Raleigh Infectious Disease Associates
Raleigh, North Carolina

Elise Belilos, M.D.
Instructor of Medicine
State University of New York at Stony Brook
Division of Rheumatology
Winthrop University Hospital
Mineola, New York

Steven E. Carsons, M.D.
Associate Professor of Medicine
State University of New York at Stony Brook
Division of Rheumatology
Winthrop University Hospital
Mineola, New York

Diego A. Diaz, M.D.
Clinical Fellow
Division of Pulmonary and Critical Care Medicine
The New York Hospital–Cornell Medical Center
New York, New York

Paul E. Fenster, M.D.
Associate Professor of Medicine
University of Arizona College of Medicine
Section of Cardiology
Tucson, Arizona

Connie J. Holladay, M.D.
Fellow, Division of Endocrinology and Metabolism
Department of Medicine
The University of Tennessee
Memphis, Tennessee

James R. Hurley, M.D.
Associate Professor of Medicine
Associate Professor of Radiology
Cornell University Medical College
Division of Endocrinology and Metabolism and Division of Nuclear Medicine
The New York Hospital–Cornell Medical Center
New York, New York

Kathleen M. Kelly, M.D., FACS, FCCM
Assistant Clinical Professor
University of Medicine and Dentistry of New Jersey
Director, Surgical Intensive Care Unit
Morristown Memorial Hospital
Department of Surgery
Morristown, New Jersey

Abbas E. Kitabchi, M.D., Ph.D.
Professor of Medicine and Biochemistry
Director, Division of Endocrinology and Metabolism
University of Tennessee, Memphis, College of Medicine
Memphis, Tennessee

Jeffrey A. Kuller, M.D.
Assistant Professor of Obstetrics and Gynecology
University of North Carolina School of Medicine
Department of Obstetrics and Gynecology
Division of Maternal-Fetal Medicine
Chapel Hill, North Carolina

Maureen A. Murtaugh, Ph.D., R.D.
Assistant Professor
Rush University
Rush-Presbyterian-St. Luke's Medical Center
Department of Clinical Nutrition
Chicago, Illinois

Nancy Nealon, M.D.
Clinical Assistant Professor of Neurology
Cornell University Medical College
New York, New York

Brendan Phibbs, M.D., FACP, FACC
Professor of Clinical Medicine
University of Arizona College of Medicine
Chief of Cardiology, Padre Kino Hospital—Section of Cardiology
University of Arizona Health Sciences Center
Tucson, Arizona

Velvie Pogue, M.D.
Assistant Professor of Clinical Medicine
Columbia University College of Physicians and Surgeons
Director, Hypertension Services
Harlem Hospital Center
Department of Medicine
New York, New York

Abraham Sanders, M.D.
Associate Professor of Clinical Medicine
Cornell University Medical College
Division of Pulmonary Critical Care
The New York Hospital–Cornell Medical Center
New York, New York

Rachelle A. Scott, M.D.
Associate Professor of Medicine
Cornell University Medical College
Department of Dermatology
The New York Hospital–Cornell Medical Center
New York, New York

Jeanne A. Smith, M.D., M.P.H.
Associate Professor of Clinical Medicine
Columbia University College of Physicians and Surgeons
Department of Medicine
Division of Hematology
Harlem Hospital Center
New York, New York

Jonathan D.K. Trager, M.D.
Clinical Fellow
Department of Dermatology
The New York Hospital-Cornell Medical Center
New York, New York

Christine B. Villarino, M.D.
Cardiology Fellow
Department of Medicine
University of Arizona College of Medicine
Tucson, Arizona

Alan D. Weinberg, M.S.
Assistant Clinical Professor
Columbia University School of Public Health
Columbia-Presbyterian Medical Center
Department of Surgery
Division of Cardiothoracic Surgery
New York, New York

Jerome Yankowitz, M.D.
Assistant Professor of Obstetrics and Gynecology
University of Iowa Hospitals and Clinics
Department of Obstretics and Gynecology
Division of Maternal-Fetal Medicine
Iowa City, Iowa

Paul E. Zachary, Jr., M.D.
Assistant Professor of Internal Medicine
St. Louis University School of Medicine
Division of Gastroenterology & Hepatology
St. Louis University Health Sciences Center
St. Louis, Missouri

Contents

Chapter 1

Cardiac Disorders

Paul E. Fenster
Christine B. Villarino

CORONARY HEART DISEASE

Cardiovascular disease is the number one cause of death in both women and men. Coronary heart disease is the major culprit, claiming approximately 236,000 female lives annually.[1] This outnumbers female deaths caused by all cancers combined.[2] Forty percent of all coronary events in women are fatal; 67% of sudden deaths in women occur in individuals without a history of coronary heart disease.[1] Therefore, prevention and treatment of coronary heart disease are very important aspects of the general health care of the female patient.

Prevention of coronary heart disease through risk factor education is a fundamental role of the primary care physician. For many female patients, this physician may well be the obstetrician/gynecologist. In many instances, the patient must be educated about coronary heart disease, since many women believe that cancer is their primary health risk. The patient should be made aware of the fact that death caused by coronary atherosclerosis has an incidence four and six times greater in the white and black female populations, respectively, than death from breast cancer.[1] Coronary heart disease is also a leading cause of disability. Although ischemic heart disease occurs approximately 10 years later in women than in men, education about risk factors and healthy lifestyle modification are appropriate at any age.

Coronary Heart Disease Risk Factors

The physician should identify coronary heart disease risk factors (Table 1.1), clinically evaluate the patient for the presence of coronary heart disease, and recommend or refer the patient for appropriate intervention. The major risk factors for coronary heart disease are similar in women and men and include diabetes, hypertension, cigarette smoking, lipid profile, family history, and age. In addition, the hormonal fluctuations seen in postmenopausal women and in oral contraceptive users may affect the cardiac risk.

TABLE 1.1 Cardiac Risk Factors in Women

Risk Factors	Comments
Diabetes	Threefold increased risk of myocardial infarction and a fivefold increased risk of a fatal cardiovascular event, compared to nondiabetics
Hypertension	Two- to 10-fold increased risk of ischemic heart disease compared to normotensives
Tobacco smoking	No safe amount
Hyperlipidemia	Low HDL is an especially strong predictor of coronary heart disease in females
Family history	Increased risk if a family member had myocardial infarction at age 60 or younger
Oral contraceptives	In low doses has a small effect on lipids, but a prothombotic effect may increase the risk of vascular events
Obesity	Not an independent risk factor, but associated with other risk factors and an appropriate target for intervention

Diabetes is a potent risk factor for coronary atherosclerosis in women. Glucose intolerance accelerates the risk of myocardial infarction threefold compared to the risk in nondiabetic women of the same age. Moreover, there is a high prevalence of other risk factors, such as hyperlipidemia, obesity, and hypertension, among women with glucose intolerance.

Hypertension is also a strong risk factor for coronary heart disease. An elevated blood pressure is strongly associated with an increased risk of both recognized and unrecognized myocardial infarction. A systolic blood pressure greater than 160 mmHg or a diastolic pressure greater than 85 mmHg increases the risk of ischemic heart disease by 2- to 10-fold.[3]

There is a strong correlation between cigarette smoking and the risk of both fatal and nonfatal myocardial infarction. There appears to be no safe level of cigarette consumption. As few as 1–4 cigarettes per day may increase the risk of myocardial infarction by 2.5-fold, and more than 45 cigarettes per day increases the risk 11-fold.[4] Moreover, if the smoker is premenopausal, older than 35 years of age, and taking oral contraceptives, the risk of developing coronary heart disease is even greater.

Serum lipoprotein abnormalities are also a strong risk factor for coronary heart disease. In females, high density lipoprotein (HDL) cholesterol is especially important. For every increase in HDL of 10 mg/dl, there appears to be a 50% decrease in risk.[5] Estrogens increase HDL and decrease low density lipoprotein (LDL) cholesterol. Most progestins have the opposite effect. The ratio of LDL to HDL rises substantially after menopause. This may be one mechanism in the markedly increased risk of coronary atherosclerosis in postmenopausal women.

The coronary heart disease risk has a significant genetic component independent of other known risk factors. In females, the occurrence of myocardial infarction in a family member younger than 60 years of age indicates an increased coronary heart disease risk, whether the family member is a paternal, maternal, or other first-degree relative. Data also indicate familial clustering of atherosclerosis risk factors, especially hypertension, hyperlipidemia, and diabetes.

Oral contraceptives alter the cardiac risk primarily by affecting blood lipids. Alterations of the lipid profile are caused by the estrogen and progesterone content and are related to the adrenogenicity of the progestin. The current low-dose contraceptive formulations containing minimally androgenic progestins are probably not associated with a risk of coronary heart disease when used by healthy women.[6] However, adverse vascular events, including cardiac ischemia, may occur due to the prothrombotic effect of oral contraceptives. Current recommendations for oral contraceptive use[1] suggest prescribing preparations that lower LDL and raise HDL in women with risk factors for atherosclerosis. Oral contraceptives with levonorgestrel usually produce greater adverse effects on LDL and HDL than norethindrone-containing preparations.[1] Oral contraceptives with fixed levels of very-low-dose norethindrone (0.5 mg per dose or less) lower the LDL level and raise the HDL level.[1] Newer desogestrel- and norgestimate-containing contraceptives also favorably affect LDL and HDL cholesterol.[1] If appropriate alternative contraception can be utilized, it is preferable that oral contraceptives be avoided in women who smoke more than 10 cigarettes a day.

Obesity is probably not an independent risk factor for coronary heart disease, but it is a marker for the presence of other risk factors. Obesity is associated with hypertension, glucose intolerance, and hyperlipidemia. Weight gain itself produces an atherogenic risk profile with increased LDL, triglycerides, and total cholesterol, along with decreased HDL. The distribution of body fat is also a marker of risk. Increased abdominal fat, the typical male distribution pattern, is associated with an increased coronary heart disease risk. Increased fat on the hips and lower extremities, typical of obese females, is not as strong a coronary heart disease risk factor.

Clinical Presentation of Coronary Heart Disease

Chest pain is a common presentation of coronary heart disease, but there are many other causes of chest pain. The probability of coronary heart disease varies with the presenting symptoms. Chest pain may be typical of angina pectoris or may be atypical. Typical angina is substernal in location, often with radiation to the jaw, neck, and/or shoulders. It occurs with exertion and is relieved with rest or nitroglycerin. Angina-type pain may have an unusual distribution or may show a diminished response to the usual precipitating or ameliorating factors. Such pain is often labeled "probable angina." In contrast, atypical chest pain may occur at rest and may have an atypical location or an atypical response to exertion, rest, or nitroglycerin. In women, typical angina predicts the presence of coronary atherosclerosis in 60%, probable angina predicts it in 30%, and atypical pain predicts it in only 7%.[7]

Evaluation of Chest Pain

Treadmill electrocardiographic (ECG) testing is commonly used to evaluate the individual with chest pain. The exercise ECG test has a sensitivity and specificity for diagnosing coronary heart disease of 80% and 74% in men, and 76% and 64%, in women, respectively.[8] The lower accuracy in women is due, in part, to the low prevalence of coronary disease in premenopausal women and the consequent high rate of false-positive results. However, a negative test in a woman has a high predictive value for the absence of disease. Therefore, if the exercise test is negative with an adequate maximal heart rate and exercise level, then no additional testing is needed. A positive exercise ECG should be confirmed with a more accurate test.

Other diagnostic modalities that may be helpful include exercise or pharmacologic radionuclide scintigraphy, exercise or pharmacologic stress echocardiography, and coronary artery fluoroscopy. The nuclear studies utilize a radionuclide injected intravenously with the patient at rest, followed by scanning with a nuclear camera placed over the heart. A second injection of radionuclide is made at the peak exercise level, followed by scanning immediately after exercise. Abnormalities of perfusion may be present both after exercise and at rest, indicating a scar, or may be present only immediately after exercise, indicating ischemia. The sensitivity and specificity for diagnosing coronary atherosclerosis is 82% and 91%, respectively, in both men and women.[7]

Echocardiography can provide valuable information about wall motion abnormalities of the left ventricle. Both exercise and dobutamine have been used to evaluate cardiac function and diagnose ischemia. The exercise echocardiogram is obtained as a two-dimensional image along varied axes after exercise and compared with resting images. A dobutamine infusion is an alternative to exercise. Ischemia is diagnosed when new wall motion abnormalities occur with exercise or dobutamine stimulation. These forms of stress echocardiography have a higher sensitivity, specificity, and diagnostic accuracy than the exercise ECG test.[9] The stress echocardiogram is especially useful for patients who have a nondiagnostic exercise ECG. Dobutamine echocardiography may be used to evaluate patients who are unable to exercise.

Cardiac fluoroscopy may visualize calcified atherosclerotic lesions within coronary arteries. This is done with an image intensifier using cesium-iodide. Calcification indicates the presence of coronary atherosclerosis with 79% sensitivity and 83% specificity.[7] Cardiac fluoroscopy may be used to enhance the diagnostic accuracy of the treadmill test. Absence of coronary artery calcification significantly increases the likelihood that a positive ECG treadmill test result is a false-positive finding.[10]

Another diagnostic modality for identifying coronary artery calcification is ultrafast computed tomography. The sensitivity of coronary calcifications in diagnosing coronary atherosclerosis by this technique is 50% in women less than 60 years of age and 97% in women older than 60 years.[11] In men, the sensitivity is 87% in those less than 60 years of age and 96% in those above 60.[11] Specificity is 76% in younger women compared to 20% in older women.[11] Coronary calcification also has higher specificity in men below 60 years of age (58%) compared to men above 60 (33%).[11] Therefore, ultrafast computed tomography may be useful in screening for coronary calcification, and ultimately coronary heart disease, but additional confirmatory studies are needed.

When these noninvasive tests suggest that ischemia is severe or involves a large area of the left ventricle, coronary artery anatomy may be evaluated by coronary angiography.

PREVENTION OF CORONARY HEART DISEASE

The primary care physician's role in reducing coronary heart disease begins with the initial assessment of risk factors and patient education. As our population ages, the prevalence of coronary heart disease increases. Screening for modifiable risk factors, such as hypertension, hypercholesterolemia, diabetes, and tobacco use, is a part of good medical care. Early management of these problems could profoundly alter a patient's future health. Lifestyle modification, such as a diet low in saturated fat, increased physical activity, and smoking cessation may markedly lower the risk of coronary atherosclerosis. Pharmacologic treatment of hypertension, lipid abnormalities, and diabetes may also be appropriate.

Menopause has an unfavorable effect on lipid metabolism, which may contribute to an increase in coronary disease risk. The Postmenopausal Estrogen/Progestin Intervention Trial (PEPI)[12] was designed to assess the effects of different hormone replacement regimens on cardiovascular risk factors in healthy postmenopausal women. Participants were randomized to receive conjugated equine estrogen (Premarin), 0.625 mg daily; or conjugated equine estrogen, 0.625 mg daily, plus cyclic medroxyprogesterone acetate (Provera), 10 mg daily, for 12 days per month; or conjugated equine estrogen, 0.625 mg daily, plus medroxyprogesterone acetate, 2.5 mg daily; or conjugated equine estrogen, 0.625 mg daily, plus micronized progesterone, 200 mg daily, for 12 days per months; or placebo. Findings of this trial indicate that estrogen alone, or in combination with progestin, improves the lipoprotein profile and lowers the fibrinogen level, without detectable effects on blood pressure or insulin level. Unopposed estrogen (0.625 mg/day of conjugated equine estrogen) has a more favorable effect on HDL cholesterol than estrogen given with cyclic or continuous progestin. However, when cyclic progestin is used, micronized progesterone is associated with a significantly higher HDL cholesterol level than estrogen given with medroxyprogesterone acetate. All hormone treatments were associated with a significantly greater increment in mean HDL cholesterol compared to the results obtained with placebo. This is particularly significant since HDL cholesterol is a strong independent predictor of heart disease in women.

LDL cholesterol levels also decreased within the first 6 to 12 months of hormone replacement therapy. Decreases in LDL cholesterol averaging 15.9 mg/dl were found in all the treatment regimens compared to placebo. Triglyceride levels increased comparably in all active treatments. Estrogen treatment appears to increase triglycerides by increasing production, not by decreasing clearance, and these changes may not be atherogenic. However, women with high baseline triglyceride levels were excluded from this trial. Estrogen replacement may increase the risk of coronary atherosclerosis in patients with a history of hypertriglyceridemia. Fibrinogen levels were stable in the hormone replacement groups, but rose in participants treated with placebo.

Data on the clinical effects of hormone replacement have been derived primarily from epidemiologic studies, not prospective randomized interventional trials. The Nurses Health Study showed a lower rate of coronary heart disease among postmenopausal hormone users compared to nonusers.[13] The risk of fatal and nonfatal coronary heart disease was 50% lower in users. However, hormone users differed from nonusers in other ways that may affect the coronary disease risk. Specifically, hormone users were more likely to be lean and had a lower prevalence of hypertension, diabetes, and hyperlipidemia.[13] This group also appeared to be more health conscious, with more frequent physician visits and increased physical activity compared with the nonusers.[13] Underway are large clinical trials to determine how much or whether hormonal replacement therapy will reduce the risk of heart disease in women.

Overall, estrogen appears to reduce the risk of coronary heart disease. Recommendations for using hormone replacement to lower this risk must be individualized by considering the risks and benefits to each patient. Unopposed estrogen, as shown in the PEPI Trial, increases the risk of adenomatous and atypical endometrial hyperplasia. The patient should be counseled regarding this risk, and follow-up should include annual endometrial evaluation when the patient with an intact uterus is taking unopposed estrogen. This adverse experience is greatly diminished when cyclic or continuous progestin is used in combination with estrogen therapy.

Estrogen replacement therapy may also increase the risk of breast cancer, but findings have been inconsistent. One meta-analysis showed a small but significantly increased risk.[14] The relative risk of breast cancer may be higher in those who experience a natural menopause and use estrogen. Some studies suggest that the effect is dose dependent and that a dose of 0.625 mg/day of a conjugated estrogen causes no appreciable increase in the risk of cancer. While these factors must be considered in each patient, it should be emphasized that heart disease poses a much greater threat than does breast cancer and that the potential reduction in the risk of coronary heart disease statistically far outweighs the increase in breast cancer risk. Recommendations for the use of estrogen, and subsequent screening for breast cancer, will be different for the patient with a strong family history of breast cancer.

Aspirin reduces the risk of myocardial infarction, stroke, and death in both men and women with clinically evident vascular disease. Aspirin also reduces the risk of complications and death in acute myocaradial infarction in both men and women. However, the effect of aspirin on the primary prevention of myocardial infarction in women is uncertain. Observational studies have yielded inconsistent results. No prospective randomized trials of aspirin for primary prevention of myocardial infarction in women have been reported, although this issue is part of the ongoing Women's Health Study.

ARRHYTHMIAS

Atrial Fibrillation

Atrial fibrillation is the most common sustained arrhythmia in adults. Among women in the Framingham Heart Study, the 22-year incidence of atrial fibrillation was 17.1 per 1000.[15] The rate is quite low among younger adults but rises progressively with increasing age. Atrial fibrillation may be asymptomatic, but it often causes palpitations. In patients with heart disease, atrial fibrillation may significantly decrease cardiac output. In addition, even in asymptomatic individuals, atrial fibrillation is associated with a markedly increased rate of stroke and of total mortality. Therefore, the goals of therapy are to relieve the symptoms and hemodynamic consequences of atrial fibrillation by establishing and maintaining normal sinus rhythm, or at least by controlling the ventricular rate, and to use antiplatelet agents or anticoagulants to reduce the risk of stroke.

The onset of atrial fibrillation may precipitate heart failure in patients with mitral stenosis, aortic stenosis, or severe left ventricular dysfunction. In patients with coronary artery disease, atrial fibrillation may cause ischemia. In these clinical settings, prompt cardioversion may be necessary. However, in most cases, cardioversion is desirable but not urgent. If atrial fibrillation has been present for more than 48 h or if the duration is unknown, then the patient should be anticoagulated with warfarin to achieve an INR of 2.0 to 3.0 for 3 to 4 weeks prior to cardioversion.[16]

Sinus rhythm may be restored by direct-current (DC) electrical cardioversion or by antiarrhythmic drugs. DC cardioversion is the more effective and more rapid method of restoring sinus rhythm. Electrical cardioversion may be performed as an outpatient procedure, but general anesthesia is required.

An alternative method to rapidly restore sinus rhythm is intravenous administration of procainamide. Though less effective than DC cardioversion, this method does not require anesthesia. Close monitoring of the blood pressure and for ventricular arrhythmias is necessary.

Antiarrhythmic drugs may be administered orally to convert atrial fibrillation to sinus rhythm. All antiarrhythmic drugs have some proarrhythmic potential. This risk is greatest in patients with ischemic heart disease or with left ventricular dysfunction. Such patients should be hospitalized when antiarrhythmic drug therapy is initiated. Drugs that are effective in converting atrial fibrillation to sinus rhythm, and in maintaining sinus rhythm, include quinidine, procainamide, disopyramide, flecainide, propafenone, sotalol, and amiodarone. Each has significant potential toxicity, so there is no clear drug of first choice.

In many patients, sinus rhythm cannot be restored or atrial fibrillation invariably recurs after cardioversion, despite antiarrhythmic drug use. If atrial fibrillation is poorly tolerated, surgery may restore and maintain sinus rhythm. The maze procedure involves multiple incisions in the atria, creating blind alleys that prevent atrial fibrillation while allowing atrial activation. This restores sinus control of the rhythm and maintains atrial mechanical function. Experience with this procedure is limited. The corridor procedure creates a strip of atrial tissue connecting the sinus node to the atrioventricular node. This allows sinus impulses to reach the ventricles. However, the atria continue to fibrillate and the embolic risk is unchanged.

If sinus rhythm cannot be maintained, then ventricular rate control, along with anticoagulation to reduce the risk of emboli, is appropriate. The ventricular rate should be controlled both at rest and during activity. This can be achieved with a beta-adrenergic blocker, or with verapamil or diltiazem. Digoxin is considerably less effective, especially during activity.

Atrial fibrillation, whether chronic or paroxysmal, is associated with the risk of stroke. This risk is highest among patients with rheumatic mitral valve disease. Other markers of high risk include a history of an embolic event, hypertension, clinical heart failure, or echocardiographically detected left ventricular dysfunction, diabetes, and women over the age of 75 years. In untreated patients over age 75 with any one of these risk factors, the rate of stroke is approximately 8% per year compared to 2.5% per year in elderly patients with none of these risk factors. Therefore, in the presence of any of these risk factors, warfarin should be used unless contraindicated. The dose should be adjusted to produce an international normalized ratio of 2.0 to 3.0. In patients 60 years of age and older with none of these risk factors, the risk of stroke is 1.5% to 2.5% per year. In these patients, aspirin, 325 mg daily, appears to be a very reasonable alternative to warfarin in reducing the risk of total stroke, including both embolic and hemorrhagic etiologies. In patients less than 60 years of age with none of these risk factors, a condition referred to as *lone atrial fibrillation,* the risk of embolism is comparable to that of the age-matched population without atrial fibrillation, so neither aspirin nor warfarin appears to be necessary.

Ventricular Arrhythmias

Ventricular ectopy may occur in healthy individuals. They are usually of little consequence, and no treatment is required. In contrast, sustained ventricular arrhythmias may cause presyncope or syncope and may be a harbinger of sudden death in patients with underlying heart disease. These patients usually need extensive evaluation and treatment guided by an arrhythmia specialist. The primary care physician is often the first to discover the arrhythmia and initiate the evaluation.

Asymptomatic, isolated ventricular ectopic beats are a common finding on routine physical exam or ECG. If the history, physical exam, and ECG reveal no evidence of heart disease and the risk factor profile indicates a low probability of atherosclerotic heart disease, then no further evaluation or treatment is necessary. If this low-risk individual experiences palpitations, reassurance that the symptom is benign is usually the most appropriate treatment. Palpitations that are disturbing to the patient frequently respond to a beta-adrenergic blocker.

The patient who has underlying heart disease, or who has experienced presyncope or syncope, is at increased risk of sudden death and requires more extensive evaluation. The evaluation should assess the presence, etiology, and severity of any heart disease and determine the relationship between the arrhythmia and the symptoms. Cardiac disease is initially evaluated by the history, physical exam, ECG, and noninvasive tests. The history should evaluate any family history of premature sudden death and symptoms of coronary artery disease or heart failure. The physical exam should carefully evaluate any signs of heart failure, valvular disease, or hypertrophic cardiomyopathy. The ECG should be reviewed for evidence of prior myocardial infarction, ischemia, or a prolonged Q-T interval. Additional tests include echocardiography to evaluate the size and function of the cardiac chambers, as well as the valve anatomy and function, and exercise testing to uncover ischemia and determine the effect of exercise on the arrhythmia. The results of these tests may suggest that cardiac catheterization should be performed.

The relationship between symptoms and arrhythmia is often uncertain. This relationship may be elucidated by long-term ambulatory ECG recording in patients with frequent symptoms or by the use of a patient-activated portable recording device when symptoms are infrequent. In many patients these techniques are unrevealing, and a provocative method of arrhythmia detection may be used. These methods include exercise testing and electrophysiologic testing.

The goals of treatment of ventricular arrhythmia are alleviation of symptoms and prevention of sudden death due to ventricular fibrillation. The optimal form of treatment is uncertain. Antiarrhythmic drugs may suppress arrhythmias, as assessed by ambulatory monitoring, thereby reducing symptoms, but they may be associated with no decrease or even an increase, in the risk of arrhythmic death.[17] The risk of provoking serious arrhythmias is greatest in patients with recent myocardial infarction or significant left ventricular dysfunction.[17] Electrophysiologic testing appears to be no more successful than ambulatory monitoring in selecting antiarrhythmic drugs to prevent arrhythmic death.[18] One alternative to drug therapy is ablation of the site of the arrhythmia within the ventricle by either catheterization or surgery. Another alternative is the use of an implantable device that can detect and analyze arrhythmias and use either pacing, electrical cardioversion, or defibrillation to terminate the arrhythmia. Clinical trials comparing these treatment modalities are in progress.

MITRAL VALVE PROLAPSE

Mitral valve prolapse is present when a portion of a mitral leaflet crosses the plane of the mitral annulus and enters the left atrium during systole. This finding is best documented by two-dimensional echocardiography. Mitral valve prolapse usually indicates a structural abnormality of the mitral leaflet. However, prolapse may also occur with an anatomically normal mitral valve in the setting of hypovolemia, tachycardia, or geometric distortion of the left ventricle. Mitral valve prolapse is often an incidental finding on echocardiography that is clinically insignificant. This finding should not be confused with the mitral valve prolapse syndrome.

The mitral valve prolapse syndrome is a disorder with variable symptomatology, characteristic auscultatory findings, and anatomic and functional abnormalities of the mitral valve on echocardiography. Mitral leaflet histology reveals an increase in the spongiosa component, a condition termed *myxomatous degeneration*. This is associated with leaflet thickening and redundancy, elongated chordae tendineae, and ventricular endocardial friction lesions.

The symptoms associated with the mitral prolapse syndrome are nonspecific. They frequently include fatigue, atypical chest pain, palpitations, and dyspnea. Other associated symptoms are dizziness and anxiety. The symptoms usually cannot be ascribed to cardiac dysfunction but may be related to autonomic dysfunction, which includes increased adrenergic activity, decreased intravascular volume, abnormal renin and aldosterone regulation, and abnormal parasympathetic activity.

On cardiac auscultation, the characteristic findings are a systolic click and a murmur. The click is a mid- to late systolic, high-pitched sound over the apex. Multiple clicks may be present. The clicks are probably caused by a sudden tensing of the mitral leaflet and chordae. A high-pitched, blowing systolic murmur at the apex typically follows the click. In some patients, an apical whoop or honk is audible. The click and the murmur occur earlier in systole with maneuvers that reduce venous return, such as upright posture, or during the strain phase of a Valsalva maneuver.

The appearance and motion of the mitral leaflets on two-dimensional echocardiography are the standard for making the diagnosis of mitral valve prolapse. The echocardiogram shows systolic displacement of a portion of one or both mitral leaflets into the left atrium. The leaflets may appear to be thickened, and there may be redundant tissue on one or both leaflets. Doppler echocardiography may demonstrate the presence and severity of mitral insufficiency.

The mitral prolapse syndrome is most often a chronic, stable condition. Serious complications, which are uncommon, include progressive mitral insufficiency and heart failure; abrupt occurrence of severe mitral insufficiency due to chordal rupture; infective endocarditis; systemic embolism; and, rarely, sudden death.

Patient education and reassurance as to the benign nature of the condition is important. If the nonspecific symptoms persist and are troublesome to the patient, beta blockers may be helpful. Endocarditis prophylaxis is appropriate if mitral insufficiency is present or if the mitral leaflets appear thickened on echocardiography.

PREVENTION OF BACTERIAL ENDOCARDITIS

Bacterial endocarditis is a serious disease with a mortality rate of approximately 25%. Infective endocarditis results from blood-borne bacteria that may lodge on damaged, abnormal heart valves as well as prosthetic valves, or, less commonly, normal native valves. Bacteremia is most often transient and is due to instrumentation of mucosal surfaces. The risk of endocarditis is a function of predisposing cardiac lesions, the intensity of bacteremia, the characteristics of the blood-borne organism, and the host risk factors. Patients who are at higher risk for developing endocarditis should be treated prophylactically with antibiotics for procedures likely to cause bacteremia.

Endocarditis prophylaxis is recommended for patients with the following conditions[19]:

1. Prosthetic cardiac valves, including bioprostheses and homografts.
2. Congenital abnormalities including patent ductus arteriosus, ventricular septal defect, and tetralogy of Fallot.
3. A previous history of endocarditis, even in the absence of heart disease.
4. Rheumatic heart disease and other acquired valvular dysfunctions.
5. Mitral valve prolapse with regurgitation.
6. Hypertrophic cardiomyopathy.

Endocarditis prophylaxis is not recommended for patients with the following conditions[19]:

1. Isolated secundum atrial septal defect.
2. Surgical repair without residua beyond 6 months of secundum atrial septal defect, ventricular septal defect, or patent ductus arteriosus.
3. Previous coronary artery bypass surgery.
4. Mitral valve prolapse without regurgitation.
5. Physiologic or functional (innocent) heart murmurs.
6. Previous rheumatic fever without valve dysfunction.
7. Cardiac pacemakers or automatic defibrillator devices.
8. Previous Kawasaki disease without valve dysfunction.

Transient bacteremia occurs during certain procedures. In patients who are at risk for endocarditis, as indicated above, prophylaxis is recommended for the following procedures:

1. Dental procedures known to induce gingival or mucosal bleeding, including professional cleanings.
2. Tonsillectomy and/or adenoidectomy.
3. Involvement of the respiratory or intestinal mucosa during surgery.
4. Bronchoscopy with a rigid bronchoscope.
5. Esophageal sclerotherapy or esophageal dilation.
6. Gallbladder surgery.

7. Cystoscopy.
8. Urethral dilatation.
9. Urethral catheterization if urinary tract infection is present.
10. Urinary tract surgery if urinary tract infection is present.
11. Prostate surgery.
12. Incision and drainage of infected tissue.
13. Vaginal hysterectomy.
14. Vaginal delivery in the presence of infection.

Endocarditis prophylaxis is not recommended for caesarean section; uncomplicated vaginal deliveries without episiotomy; dilatation and curettage; therapeutic abortion; sterilization procedures; insertion or removal of intrauterine devices; or urethral catheterization in the absence of infection. Other procedures that do not require antibiotic prophylaxis are flexible bronchoscopy, cardiac catheterization, intubation, and endoscopy.

The standard prophylactic antibiotic regimen for dental, oral, or upper respiratory procedures is amoxicillin, 3.0 g orally 1 h before the procedure and 1.5 g 6 h after the initial dose. If the patient is allergic to penicillin or amoxicillin, then alternatives are erythromycin ethylsuccinate, 800 mg, or erythromycin stearate 1.0 g, orally 2 h before the procedure and then half the dose 6 h after the initial dose; or clindamycin, 300 mg orally 1 h before and then 150 mg 6 h after the initial dose.

An alternative regimen for prophylactic antibiotics for those unable to take oral preparations is intravenous or intramuscular ampicillin, 2.0 g 30 min before the procedure and then 1.0 g 6 h afterwards. For penicillin- or ampicillin-sensitive patients, intravenous clindamycin, 300 mg 30 min before the procedure and 150 mg 6 h after the initial dose may be used. An alternative regimen for penicillin-allergic patients is vancomycin, 1.0 g over 1 h starting 1 h before the procedure. This dose need not be repeated.

The standard regimen for genitourinary or gastrointestinal procedures is intravenous or intramuscular ampicillin, 2.0 g, plus gentamicin, 1.5 mg/kg (not to exceed 80 mg), 30 min before the procedure, followed by amoxicillin, 1.5 g orally 6 h after the initial dose. An alternative to the amoxicillin is to repeat the initial parenteral regimen 8 h after the initial dose. An alternative for penicillin-allergic patients is intravenous vancomycin, 1.0 g over 1 h, plus intravenous or intramuscular gentamicin, 1.5 mg/kg (not to exceed 80 mg), 1 h before the procedure, repeated 8 h after the initial dose.

There have been no adequate controlled clinical trials of antibiotic regimens for the prevention of bacterial endocarditis in humans. The recommendations are based on in vitro studies. Therefore, the practitioner must exercise clinical judgment in selecting antibiotics for individual patients and procedures. In addition, the clinician must maintain a high level of suspicion of endocarditis in patients who present with unusual symptoms after a procedure even when prophylactic antibiotics were administered.

REFERENCES

1. Eacker ED, Chesebro JM, Sacks FM, et al: Cardiovascular disease in women. AHA medical/scientific statement. *Circulation* 88(no. 4, Pt. 1):1999–2009, 1993.
2. Castelli WP: Cardiovascular disease in women. *Am J Obstet Gynecol* 158:1553–1560, 1988.

3. The Working Group on Risk and High Blood Pressure: An epidemiological approach to describing risk associated with blood pressure levels. *Hypertension* 7:641–651, 1985.
4. Willett WC, Green A, Stampfer MJ, et al: Relative and absolute excess risks of coronary heart disease among women who smoke cigarettes. *N Engl J Med* 317:1303–1309, 1987.
5. Kannel WB: Metabolic risk factors for coronary heart disease in women: Perspective from the Framingham Study. *Am Heart J* 114:413–419, 1987.
6. Mishell DR: Use of oral contraceptives in women of older reproductive age. *Am J Obstet Gynecol* 158:1652–1657, 1988.
7. Hung J, Chaitman BR, Lam J, et al: Noninvasive diagnostic test choices for evaluation of CAD in women: A multivariate comparison of cardiac fluoroscopy, exercise electrocardiography and exercise thallium myocardial perfusion scintigraphy. *J Am Coll Cardiol* 4:8–16, 1984.
8. Weiner DA, Ryan TJ, McCabe CH, et al: Correlations among history of angina, ST segment response and prevalence of coronary artery disease in the Coronary Artery Surgery Study (CASS). *N Engl J Med* 301:230–235, 1979.
9. Sawada SG, Segar DS, Ryan T, et al: Echocardiographic detection of coronary artery disease during dobutamine infusion. *Circulation* 83:1605–1614, 1991.
10. Taylor P, Becker RC: Noninvasive diagnosis of coronary heart disease in women. *Cardiology* 77(Suppl.2):91–98, 1990.
11. Fusman B, Wolfkiel C, Rich S, et al: Influence of gender and age in detection of coronary artery disease by UFCT calcification compared to angiography. *Circulation* 88:I–15, 1993.
12. The Writing Group for the PEPI Trial: Effects of estrogen or estrogen/progestin regimens on heart disease risk factors in postmenopausal women. *JAMA* 273:199–208, 1995.
13. Stampfer MJ, Colditz GA, Willett WC, et al: Postmenopausal estrogen therapy and cardiovascular disease: Ten year follow-up from Nurses' Health Study. *N Engl J Med* 325:756–762, 1991.
14. Sillero-Arenas M, Delgado-Rodriquez M, Rodigues-Canteras R, et al: Menopausal hormone replacement therapy and breast cancer: A meta-analysis. *Obstet Gynecol* 79:286–294, 1992.
15. Kannel WB, Abbott RD, Savage DD, et al: Epidemiologic features of chronic atrial fibrillation: The Framingham study. *N Engl J Med* 306:1018–1022, 1982.
16. Laupacis A, Albers GW, Dalen JE, et al: Antithrombotic therapy in atrial fibrillation. *Chest* 108:3525–3595, 1995.
17. Echt DS, Liebson PR, Mitchell LB, et al: Mortality and morbidity in patients receiving encainide, flecainide, or placebo—the Cardiac Arrhythmia Suppression Trial. *N Engl J Med* 324:781–788, 1991.
18. Mason JW for the ESVEM Investigators: A comparison of electrophysiologic testing with Holter monitoring to predict antiarrhythmic-drug efficacy for ventricular tachyarrhythmias. *N Engl J Med* 329:445–451, 1993.
19. Dajani AS, Bisno AL, Chung KJ, et al: Prevention of bacterial endocarditis. Recommendations by the American Heart Association. *JAMA* 264:2919–2922, 1990.

Chapter 2

Selected Pulmonary Complications During Pregnancy

Diego A. Diaz
Abraham Sanders

Oxygen delivery from the mother via the placenta to the developing fetus is necessary for its well-being. Inadequate oxygenation is detrimental to cell survival, morphogenesis, and organogenesis. Normal physiologic changes take place during pregnancy which can make it difficult to diagnose pulmonary complications. Dyspnea is normally seen in 50% of pregnant females by week 19 and in 71% by week 31 of gestation.[1] Even in those with dyspnea, the blood oxygen content is constant throughout pregnancy. Changes in pulmonary function during pregnancy are secondary to changes in airway pressure, thoracic cage excursion, respiratory drive, and diaphragmatic location.

Minute ventilation increases continuously throughout pregnancy, starting in the first trimester, with the greatest increase during the third trimester. This change in minute ventilation occurs in response to both increased metabolic demand and increased carbon dioxide production.[2] Serum progesterone is increased and contributes to an increased respiratory drive, which is seen as increased tidal volume with no change in the respiratory rate. Uterine enlargement causes diaphragmatic elevation, which is greatest during the last trimester; however, normal function continues throughout the pregnancy.[3] Arterial blood gases are characterized by a respiratory alkalosis secondary to increased carbon dioxide production and increased renal excretion of bicarbonate. Oxygen consumption increases throughout pregnancy and is greatest during the third trimester; however, a normal blood oxygen level is maintained. As the pregnancy advances the oxygen reserve decreases, making the patient more susceptible to hypoventilation or apnea with significant exertion.[4]

ASTHMA

Asthma is a disease of expiratory airflow obstruction that is usually reversible. The prevalence of asthma in the United States is 9–12 million, with 7% of patients being women of childbearing age[5]; it is estimated that 4% of all pregnancies are complicated by asthma. Hypoxemia is the complication of an exacerbation during pregnancy which can have serious effects on fetal development. Exacerbations are characteristically associated with the onset of dyspnea, wheezing, coughing, chest tightness, and decreased flow rates on spirometry. During severe attacks, accessory muscle use, pupillary dilation, mental status changes, and coma can be seen. Other common presentations include nocturnal coughing and wheezing secondary to respiratory infections, cold air, or exercise. Symptoms are secondary to airway hyperactivity and resultant bronchconstriction. Inflammation of airway mucosa is the hallmark of asthma. The goal of therapy is to suppress this inflammation and therefore decrease airflow obstruction. Histologically, the chronic inflammation seen in asthma is associated with thickening of the bronchial walls secondary to edema, glandular and muscular proliferation, and increased muscularity and vascularity. Cells found in the epithelium, such as polymorphonuclear cells (PMNs), mast cells, eosinophils, and activated T lymphocytes, maintain this inflammation by releasing a variety of mediators which promote continued inflammation and direct cytotoxic effects.

Effects of Asthma on Pregnancy

Asthma exacerbations during pregnancy can threaten the mother and fetus, leading to fetal distress and preterm labor. However, studies have shown that when asthma is controlled, the outcome of the pregnancy is the same as in the general population. The use of inhaled corticosteroids, with or without prednisone, to relieve the inflammatory component is the main therapy for asthma. Their use reduces and possibly prevents the increase in mortality reported in earlier studies. When asthma is unresponsive to conventional therapy during pregnancy, there is an increased incidence of preterm deliveries and growth retardation without any effect on organogenesis.[6]

Effects of Pregnancy on Asthma

Airflow obstruction may occur with an upper respiratory tract infection and may manifest as coughing and or wheezing. During pregnancy, there is worsening of asthma symptoms in 35% of patients, no change in 32%, and improvement in 28%, with 10% developing symptoms at the time of delivery.[7] Three months after delivery, the incidence of asthma returns to the prepregnancy state in 73% of these women.[7] Bronchial hyperactivity may increase or decrease during pregnancy, making it difficult to predict which patient will develop worsening of asthma symptoms. Infections and increased gastroesophageal reflux during gestation can change the character and/or increase the frequency and severity of asthma.

Treatment

Signs, symptoms, and offending agents can be identified with a thorough history and physical exam. A history of childhood allergies, food allergies, or aeroallergens, when identified and removed from the environment, can significantly improve the patient's quality of life. A goal of treatment is to remove any agents which may cause the airway hyperactivity. Once substances such as dust mites, animal dander, fungal elements,

TABLE 2.1 Step-Care Approach to the Management of Asthma

Step	Clinical Presentation	Goal	Drug Treatment
I	Mild intermittent asthma, less than 2 attacks per week	Treatment of acute symptoms	Inhaled beta_2-adrenergic agonist, anticholinergic agent, and theophylline
II	Frequent asthma attacks that affect patient's lifestyle with bronchodilator tolerance	Management of underlying inflammation	Inhaled corticosteroids, cromolyn sodium
III	Symptoms unresponsive to step II measures, resulting in dyspnea	Control of severe asthma exacerbations	Oral corticosteroids

Source: Adapted from Ref. 9.

medications, and aeroallergens are identified and removed, improvement is usually seen within 2 months, with resultant reduction in the medication requirement. If the symptoms are allergically mediated, then IgE levels should return to normal. The National Institutes of Health's recommendations for the treatment of asthma provide a step care approach to management according to the clinical presentation and disease severity[8,9] (Table 2.1). The goal of the step care approach is to reduce bronchospasm and airway inflammation. With the recognition that asthma is a disease of inflammation, the emphasis is now on treating symptoms by arresting the inflammatory process.

Pharmacotherapy

There are sufficient data to support the use of most antiasthma medications during pregnancy. No teratogenic effects have clearly been associated with the drugs used in the management of asthma. However, because drug toxicity studies are difficult to conduct in pregnancy, most of the drugs are termed "appropriate" rather than "safe."[10] Specific asthma management should exclude drugs whose teratogenicity is well established, such as sulfonamides, streptomycin, quinolones, clindamycin, and tetracycline.

The current management of asthma with beta_2-adrenergic agonists and inhaled corticosteroids is appropriate in most pregnant asthmatics. Beclomethasone diproprionate, an inhaled corticosteroid, in doses as high as four inhalations four times a day, was not associated with teratogenic risks in two series.[11] The systemic effects of beclomethasone are minimal in the mother even when used in doses as high as 12–20 inhalations per day. The majority of studies have not demonstrated teratogenic effects from inhaled beclomethasone or systemic corticosteroids. Human experience with the use of beta_2-adrenergic agonists is extensive, and there is no evidence of fetal injury from their use either systemically or by inhalation.

Cromolyn sodium by inhalation can be used safely as a prophylactic treatment, as there are no published teratogenic risks during pregnancy. The use of theophylline in the treatment of chronic asthma remains controversial. However, the general consensus is that it is not teratogenic and does not alter the outcome of the pregnancy. Theophylline does cross the placenta, and fetal and maternal levels are equivalent. Signs of intoxication in neonates have been reported in mothers with levels in excess of 12 mg/L (8–12 mg/L). Ipratropium bromide is not considered first-line therapy, although it may be necessary in patients difficult to manage with standard beta-agonist therapy. To date, there are no available data to support or reject its use during pregnancy.

The administration of corticosteroids is appropriate, although attention needs to be paid to hyperglycemia and hypokalemia. The typical starting dose is 30 to 60 mg of prednisone per day for 5 to 7 days, followed by a tapering regimen. If symptoms return, then long-term therapy may be indicated. Inhaled corticosteroids can be started to reduce the use and risk of complications from oral corticosteroids.

Initiation or continuation of immunotherapy, using subcutaneous injections of antigen, is not contraindicated in pregnancy. The major complication is anaphylaxis, which is uncommon. Immunotherapy is effective for the treatment of asthma induced by pollen, dust mites, and aeroallergens. Its benefits are small in the treatment of allergies to cat and dog dander. Immunotherapy is effective only in IgE-mediated asthma, and is used to reduce symptoms and medication requirements.

Acute Therapy of Asthma

An acute episode of asthma should be reversed as quickly as possible. Supplemental oxygen should be given and subcutaneous or inhaled beta-adrenergic agonist therapy begun. These drugs produce comparable changes in the improvement of forced expiratory volume in 1 sec (FEV_1) and relief of symptoms. Inhaled or parenteral beta agonists (terbutaline, 0.25 mg subcutaneously) can be used three times over 60–90 min, since only small amounts of these drugs reach the fetus. If symptoms do not improve, intravenous corticosteroids should be given and the patient admitted to the hospital. The role of theophylline in the setting of status asthmaticus is controversial; no significant improvement in airflow is seen when theophylline is used in addition to $beta_2$-adrenergic agonists. The recommended dose in patients not taking this drug is a loading dose of 5 mg/kg and a maintenance dose of 0.3–0.6 mg/kg/h. The serum level should be checked 4 h later and maintained at 8–12 mg/L.

PNEUMONIA AND PREGNANCY

Pneumonia is an uncommon infection in the pregnant female, but it can be a serious complication to the mother and fetus. Both mother and fetus tolerate the infection poorly because of the loss of respiratory reserve that occurs during pregnancy, especially during the last few months. The prevalence of pneumonia varies from 0.4% to 1% during pregnancy and it the most common cause of nonobstetric infection leading to maternal death.[12] In the preantibiotic era, maternal mortality was nearly 20%; it is now 3%.[12] Broad-spectrum antibiotics have also decreased the incidence of preterm labor associated with pneumonia from 70% to less than 10%.[12]

Invasion of the lower respiratory tract by microorganisms is responsible for the development of pneumonia. Only particles less than 10 μm in diameter, when inhaled, reach the alveoli. Particles not cleared by mucociliary cells are deposited in the alveolus and phagocytized by the lung macrophages. If infection develops, there is infiltration with PMNs and exudation of fluid.

Three main radiographic patterns are identified: (1) air space pneumonia with consolidation of the lung parenchyma secondary to an alveolar exudate, sparing the bronchi and producing a lobar infiltrate and an air bronchogram on the chest radiograph; (2) interstitial pneumonia with inflammation of the alveolar septa and a reticular appearance; and (3) bronchopneumonia with consolidation around and including the bronchial wall without air bronchograms.

Optimal antibiotic therapy depends on the specific sensitivity of the pathogen involved. Treatment is almost always empiric, as the causative organism is usually never identified on routine cultures. *Streptococcus pneumoniae* is responsible for 30–50% of all community-acquired pulmonary infections. The symptoms are classically abrupt and include the onset of fever, chills, cough, rusty sputum, and pleuritic chest pains. Radiographically, there is consolidation with air bronchograms or bronchopneumonia. The white blood cell count is elevated, with prominence of immature PMNs. *Hemophilus influenzae* is the next most common pathogen in community-acquired pneumonias, causing 10% of all infections, with a predilection for the lower lobes.

Staphylococcus aureus is often seen as a superimposed pulmonary infection following a viral pneumonia, usually influenza. Characteristically, there is an abrupt onset of symptoms including pleuritic chest pain and purulent sputum production following a viral illness. Hematogenous spread of infection is also seen in patients with intravascular catheters, in patients with endocarditis, and intravenous drug users. *Klebsiella pneumoniae* produces a destructive pneumonia which commonly leads to abscess formation and has a higher incidence in chronic alcoholics.

Atypical pneumonia pathogens, such as *Mycoplasma pneumoniae, Legionella pneumophila,* and *Chlamydia pneumoniae* (TWAR agent) are common in women of childbearing age, but their exact incidence in pregnancy is unknown. Their overall incidence in community-acquired pneumonias is 30%, with the majority of cases seen in young adults. *L. pneumophila* pneumonia is commonly preceded by an influenza-like syndrome. The onset of symptom is gradual, developing over 3 to 4 days, with fever and sore throat. The organism causes necrosis of the intra-alveolar septa, which can lead to fibrosis after resolution of the infection. *Mycoplasma* is the most common organism of the atypical pneumonias, with a higher incidence in children and young adults. It has an insidious onset and presents with low-grade fever, a nonproductive cough, and a mildly elevated white blood cell count. Bullous myringitis, cervical lymphadenopathy, and skin rash are sometimes seen. The most common viral pneumonia is influenza, generally type A, which is seasonal. However varicella, measles, and adenovirus pneumonias can also be seen.

Evaluation and Treatment

Therapy begins empirically, before the final microbiologic result is available. Sputum for Gram stain and culture is important to obtain during the initial assessment. An adequate sputum specimen is one with fewer than 10 epithelial cells and more than 25 PMNs per high-power field. If a good sputum sample is not obtained even after sputum induction, transtracheal aspiration or bronchoscopy may be necessary. Blood cultures should routinely be obtained prior to the initiation of therapy. Serology is helpful in the diagnosis of atypical pneumonias such as cold agglutinins for *Mycoplasma* and acute and convalescent titers for *Legionella,* but these are rarely available at presentation.

The selection of the antibiotic for coverage should be based in part on whether the infection is community or hospital (nosocomial) acquired. If it is nosocomial, then the antibiotic resistance pattern of the hospital must be identified. In community-acquired pneumonia, the most common organisms are *Strep. pneumoniae,* atypical organisms, *H. influenzae, K. pneumoniae,* and, less frequently, *S aureus;* all need to be considered when choosing an antibiotic regimen. The clinical presentation may provide a clue to the appropriate antibiotic coverage. The classic presentation, which is associated with bacterial infections, includes a sudden onset of fever, chills, a productive cough, and lobar consolidation. Most of the time, the symptoms are preceded by an upper respiratory tract infection. The atypical pneumonias have a slower onset and are associated with myalgias, headache, a nonproductive cough, and low-grade fever.

Regardless of the type of pneumonia, management must include hydration, proper oxygenation, and close monitoring. The goal is to maintain the partial pressure of oxygen (P_{O_2} above 70 mmHg to ensure the well-being of the mother and the fetus. Inability to maintain a P_{O_2} above 60 mmHg with maximum oxygen supplementation may be an indication for mechanical ventilation. If the patient's cardiovascular and pulmonary status continue to deteriorate even when maximum support is given, delivery of the infant may be necessary to ensure maternal and fetal survival.

Ampicillin, 1 to 2 g intravenously every 4–6 h for community-acquired pneumonias, should be the drug of choice to ensure coverage for *S. pneumoniae* and *H. influenzae.* If ampicillin resistance in the area is high, then a second-generation cephalosporin such as cefazolin can be used. If *Mycoplasma* or *Legionella* is suspected, then erythromycin in doses of 500–1000 mg intravenously every 6 h should be given. In the treatment of out-patient pneumonias, the new macrolide antibiotics are promising given their broad spectrum; however, their safety during pregnancy is not yet established. In nosocomial pneumonias, gram-negative organisms, anaerobes, and *S. aureus* need to be considered. In these patients antibiotic coverage should include third-generation cephalosporins, with the addition of an aminoglycoside, for a total of 7–10 days, with therapeutic peak and trough levels, pending results of culture and the clinical response. Amantadine is effective against influenza type A but must be used cautiously in pregnancy.[13] Yearly influenza immunization is recommended in women with chronic heart, lung, or renal disease.

TUBERCULOSIS

The incidence of tuberculosis in the United States is increasing. The reasons for this increase are immigration from countries with a high prevalence and the high incidence of tuberculosis in patients infected with the human immunodeficiency virus (HIV). From 1985 to 1990 the number of pediatric cases of tuberculosis increased by 27% implying a sharp increase in maternal transmission.[14]

In the pregnant female, the clinical presentation is the same as that in the nonpregnant female. Whether the outcome of the pregnancy is altered by tuberculosis is a topic of debate. What is known is that once chemotherapy for tuberculosis is started, the outcome of the pregnancy is the same as in the noninfected patient.[15] Maternal infection with tuberculosis does not alter the type of delivery.[16]

Transmission of tuberculosis to the fetus can occur via inhalation from an actively infected mother. Lymphangitic spread can also be seen from tuberculous endometritis. Hematogenous spread or "true congenital tuberculosis" can also occur from an infected placenta via the umbilical vein.[17] The signs and symptoms of congenital tuberculosis usually develop within the second and third weeks of life, the most common manifestations being respiratory distress, fever, hepatosplenomegaly, poor feeding, and lethargy.

Management of Infection

Early identification is essential for the prevention of disease. The Mantoux skin test is effective in identifying persons infected with *Mycobacterium tuberculosis,* but it does not define the extent of the disease. Skin testing, previously thought to be affected by pregnancy, is not, nor is there any effect on fetal development. Ideally, all pregnant females at risk should be skin tested and those positive treated, since 10% of infected individuals will ultimately develop disease during their lifetime. The decision to treat during pregnancy is based on whether the mother has active disease.

Antituberculous agents have made tuberculosis treatable and preventable. Isoniazid (INH) is highly effective in preventing reactivation. There is no evidence of increased congenital defects in the children of mothers treated with this drug. Preventive therapy is generally delayed until after delivery except in females with recent infections. In these women, INH is begun when infection is documented but after the first trimester. If the skin test is positive at the beginning of the pregnancy, then therapy is given postpartum. Some data suggest an increased incidence of hepatic toxicity from INH during pregnancy; therefore, liver function enzymes such as alanine transferase, aspartate transferase, and lactate dehydrogenase need be checked periodically. The incidence of INH-induced hepatitis is higher in patients 35 years of age or older. It has been suggested that there is an increased incidence of tuberculosis in the postpartum period.

The Advisory Committee for the Elimination of Tuberculosis recommends the following therapy for pregnant females[19]: Patients less then 35 years of age with a skin test reaction above 15 mm but with no other factors increasing their risk of tuberculosis should have preventive therapy. Those below 35 years of age with low-grade risk factors and/or those from high-prevalence areas should have prophylaxis if the skin reaction is above 10 mm. Those who are recent contacts of potentially infected individuals, who are HIV infected, or who have roentegraphic evidence of old tuberculosis but are inactive and asymptomatic, with negative sputum cultures, should be treated at any age if the skin reaction is above 5 mm. Females older then 35 years with a reaction of 10 mm and without risk factors should not be treated with INH because of the high incidence of hepatitis.

Management of Tuberculosis in Infants Born to Tuberculous Mothers

The prognosis of infants born to tuberculous mothers who are not treated and develop disease is poor. Treatment improves their outcome. The use of bacille Calmette-Guerin

(BCG) vaccine remains controversial despite many years of use worldwide, with protective effects ranging from 0% to 80%.

General guidelines suggest that if the mother is asymptomatic and has completed a course of therapy in the past, there is a minimal risk of transmitting the infection to the newborn. However, if the mother has been treated for tuberculosis during the pregnancy, the newborn must be evaluated for signs of congenital tuberculosis. The infant must be treated for 3 months until the sputum of the mother is smear and culture negative and she is compliant with therapy.[20] These infants must be skin tested at birth and at 3-month intervals. If the skin test is negative at 3 months and the mother's sputum smear and culture are negative, then INH can be stopped. Children whose tuberculin reaction is above 5 mm should be investigated for evidence of pulmonary or extrapulmonary tuberculosis; if the chest radiograph is abnormal, the child must be treated for 6 months with three bactericidal drugs. Temporary separation from the mother is recommended only when the newborn is exposed to a noncompliant, highly infectious mother and until her sputum is negative and compliance is assured.

Management of Active Disease During Pregnancy

Once the diagnosis of active tuberculosis is made, therapy is essential. Antituberculous therapy is associated with a number of side effects in both the mother and the infant; however, the effects of the disease are more hazardous than those of therapy. Chest radiography can be performed after the 12th week of gestation with abdominal shielding to exclude active pulmonary disease.

The guidelines for therapy of the pregnant female are as follows: (1) Active disease should be treated promptly; initial therapy should include INH, rifampin, and ethambutol. A fourth agent should be used if there is concern about antibiotic resistance. Pyrazinamide and streptomycin should be avoided during pregnancy due to fetal toxicity. (2) Active disease discovered at the time of delivery must be treated promptly. In this case, the mother must be isolated until her sputum is smear and culture negative. (3) The newborn must be isolated until the mother is noncontagious. (4) Complete evaluation of the infant's household is required. (5) If drug-resistant disease is present or the mother cannot take first-line therapy, then various combinations need to be employed based on susceptibility studies.

THROMBOEMBOLIC COMPLICATIONS DURING PREGNANCY[21,22]

Thromboembolism is one of the most dreaded complications of pregnancy. Pregnant women have a fivefold greater incidence than nonpregnant women. The incidence of superficial and deep thrombophlebitis is about 1 in 70 in both the antepartum and postpartum periods.[23] The incidence of pulmonary embolism (PE) is much lower, with an estimated incidence of about 1 in 2500 patients.[19]

Several factors are associated with an increased risk of thromboembolic disease during pregnancy. The most significant risk is a history of thrombophlebitis prior to the pregnancy. Several changes during pregnancy are responsible for hypercoagulability, such as venous stasis, increased levels of clotting factor, and decreased fibrinolytic activity. There is also a decrease in venous tone and flow in the lower extremities, which contribute to venous stasis. In addition, there is outflow obstruction of the inferior vena cava and the left iliac vein by the gravid uterus.

The epidemiology of deep venous thrombosis (DVT) and PE during pregnancy and in the postpartum period is unknown. For DVT most studies report the incidence to be less than 1 in 1000, with a higher incidence in the postpartum period. The incidence is higher in the left lower extremity than in the right lower extremity secondary to compression of the left iliac vein by the right iliac artery.[22]

Diagnosis of DVT

The clinical signs of thromboembolism are well known: pain, tenderness, swelling, and warmth of the affected limb; however, they are found in less than 50% of affected patients. Homan's sign—pain in the affected calf when the foot is sharply dorsiflexed—is significant but nonspecific. A history of previous superficial or deep thrombophlebitis, PE, or other factors such as bed rest and travel are also important. The useful diagnostic tests for DVT are contrast venography, impedance plethysmography (IPG), duplex ultrasonography, and radioactive fibrinogen uptake.

Contrast venography is the gold standard for the diagnosis of DVT, and a negative study excludes the diagnosis. A limited study allows visualization of vessels below most of the femoral veins but not the iliac vein. The problem with this test during pregnancy is the amount of radiation to which the fetus is exposed. The use of an abdominal shield may reduce the amount of fetal exposure. IPG is sensitive and specific for clots within the popliteal system in nonpregnant females. During pregnancy, because of obstruction of the iliac vein by the gravid uterus, false-positive results can occur. In pregnant females, the tests should to be done after the patient lies in the left lateral recumbent position for 30 min. Because the test is insensitive in calf pathology, serial testing should be performed over a 7- to 14-day period.

Duplex ultrasonography (a combination of real-time B-mode and Doppler ultrasound) is a sensitive and specific test for proximal DVT in symptomatic patients; however, this test is insensitive for the diagnosis of iliac vein disease. Doppler ultrasound is sensitive and specific for symptomatic outpatients with proximal DVT. Radioactive fibrinogen uptake scanning is contraindicated in pregnancy because of the amount of radiation involved.

Our recommendation is as follows: If IPG or duplex ultrasound is available and DVT is strongly suspected, then one of these tests should be performed. If the test is abnormal during the first two trimesters of pregnancy, the diagnosis of DVT is likely. If the test is abnormal during the last trimester, extrinsic compression must be ruled out with a limited venogram and abdominal shielding.

Diagnosis of Pulmonary Embolus

The diagnosis of PE in the obstetric patient can be difficult. The symptoms—tachypnea, tachycardia, chest pain, shortness of breath, hemoptysis, collapse, and severe anxiety—also may be present in other conditions. The chest radiograph is more helpful in evaluating other conditions which may have the same symptoms than in diagnosing an embolism. The electrocardiogram (ECG) may show sign of right ventricular strain, sinus tachycardia, or arrhythmias. The chest radiograph and ECG are frequently normal following PE. The best study for the diagnosis of PE is a pulmonary angiogram, but it is invasive and exposes the patient to very high doses of radiation. The most useful noninvasive test is the nuclear medicine ventilation and perfusion lung scan.

The ventilation and perfusion lung scan is the initial step in the diagnosis of a PE. A normal lung scan with low clinical suspicion excludes a PE; a high-probability scan, defined as a large segmental or 75% subsegmental defect, indicates a PE in the majority of cases. Unfortunately, 40–70% of patients have indeterminate scans. In this group, the incidence of PE is 20–40%.[23] The management of these patients is difficult, since therapy will expose those without embolism to the risks of anticoagulation therapy, whereas withholding therapy can be disastrous in those with embolism.

The options in patients with nondiagnostic scans are a pulmonary angiogram or investigation of the legs with Doppler ultrasound, IPG, or a venogram. These tests are useful in patients in whom PE is strongly suspected clinically, since DVT occurs commonly in patients with PE. A positive study calls for anticoagulant therapy.

The approach is to test the arterial blood gas to rule out hypoxia and hypercarbia, as well as a chest radiograph to exclude conditions which may manifest in the same manner as an embolus. In addition, an ECG and complete blood count should be obtained. If all these tests are nondiagnostic, then a ventilation-perfusion lung scan should be performed. If the scan is normal and there is a low clinical suspicion, PE is excluded. If there is a high probability of PE, anticoagulation should be started. If the scan is nondiagnostic, then studies of the lower extremities should be performed. If they are positive for DVT, anticoagulation therapy should be started. If studies of the lower extremities are normal or nondiagnostic, then a pulmonary angiogram should be considered.

Treatment

The use of anticoagulation during pregnancy is problematic. Heparin is safe for the fetus, as it does not cross the placenta.[24] Side effects to the mother include bleeding, thrombocytopenia, and osteoporosis, which is rare and is seen during chronic therapy. Heparin is given parenterally, either intravenously or subcutaneously. Following a loading dose of 5000 to 10,000 units, the recommended total dose of heparin is 24,000 to 32,000 units in a 24-h period, maintaining a partial thromboplastin time (PTT) of 1.5–2.5 times the control value. After 4–5 days of intravenous therapy, subcutaneous heparin can be given every 12 h and the PTT checked 6 h after the injection. Warfarin is contraindicated between 6 and 12 weeks of fetal development and during the second half of the third trimester due to the high incidence of embryopathy and the increased risk of bleeding at the time of delivery. Central nervous system abnormalities, both hemorrhage and malformations, have been reported after warfarin exposure at any time during the pregnancy; we therefore consider this drug contraindicated.

If the patient is receiving heparin every 12 h subcutaneously, treatment can be discontinued at the onset of true labor or it can be stopped 24 h before induction. After delivery, heparin should be restarted as soon as hemostatis is obtained. Warfarin should be started at the same time. Therapy should be continued for at least 3 months and up to 6 months after PE or DVT.

Other therapeutic modalities include thrombolytic agents which are relatively contraindicated during pregnancy. They are used in the setting of massive PE in which the patient is hemodynamically unstable. Low molecular weight heparin has been used extensively in Europe. The two advantages are the drug's long half-life, which allows once-a-day injection, and the lower incidence of thrombocytopenia. Vena cava interruption with mechanical filters is indicated in patients with absolute contraindication to anticoagulation therapy, such as those with neurosurgery and gastrointestinal bleeding, and in patients with recurrent PE while receiving adequate anticoagulation therapy.

REFERENCES

1. Milne J, Howie A, Pack A: Dyspnea during normal pregnancy. *Br J Obstet Gynaecol* 85:260–263, 1978.
2. Zeldis SM: Dyspnea during pregnancy; distinguishing cardiac from pulmonary causes. *Clin Chest Med* 13:657–585, 1992.
3. Contreras G, Gutierrez M, Beroiza T, et al: Ventilatory drive and respiratory muscle function in pregnancy. *Am Rev Respir Dis* 144:837–844, 1991.
4. Artal R, Wisweil R, Romen Y, et al: Pulmonary responses to exercise in pregnancy. *Am J Obstet Gynecol* 154:378–383, 1986.
5. Apter AJ, Greenberger PA, Patterson R: Outcomes of pregnancy in adolescents with severe asthma. *Arch Intern Med* 149:2571–2575, 1989.
6. Bahna SI, Bjerkedal T: The course and outcome of pregnancy in women with asthma. *Acta Allerg* 27:397–406, 1972.
7. Schatz M, Harden K, Forsythe A: The course of asthma during pregnancy, post partum, and with successive pregnancies: A prospective analysis. *J Allergy Clin Immunol* 81:509–517, 1988.
8. Bone RC: A step care strategy for asthma management. *J Respir Dis* 9:104–117, 1988.
9. Bone RC: Asthma: New treatments will improve disease management. *Clin Pulm Med* 2:249–257, 1995.
10. Greenberger PA: Asthma in pregnancy. *Clin Chest Med* 13:597–605, 1992.
11. Greenberger PA, Patterson R: Beclomethasone dipropionate for severe asthma during pregnancy. *Ann Intern Med* 98:478–503, 1983.
12. Benedetti TJ, Valle R, Ledger WJ: Antepartum pneumonia in pregnancy. *Am J Obtet Gynecol* 144:413–417, 1982.
13. Chow AW, Jeweson PS: Pharmacokinetics and safety of antimicrobial agents during pregnancy. *Rev Infect Dis* 7:287–313, 1985.
14. Centers for Disease Control: Tuberculosis morbidity in the United States: Final data, 1990. *MMWR* 40(SS-3):23, 1992.
15. Wilson EA, Thelin TJ, Dilts PV: Tuberculosis complicated by pregnancy. *Am J Obstet Gynecol* 115:526–529, 1973.
16. Wilson EA, Thelin TJ, Dilts PV: Tuberculosis complicated by pregnancy. *Am J Obstet Gynecol* 115:526–529, 1973.
17. Greenvile-Mather R, Haris WC, Trenchard HJ: Tuberculous primary infection in pregnancy and its relation to congenital tuberculosis. *Tubercle* 41:181–187, 1960.

18. Hamadeh MA, Glassroth J: Tuberculosis and pregnancy. *Chest* 101:1114–1120, 1992.
19. Centers for Disease Control: Screening for tuberculosis and tuberculous infection in high risk populations and the use of preventive therapy for tuberculous infection in the United States. *MMWR* 39(Suppl):1–12, 1990.
20. American Thoracic Society: Treatment of tuberculosis and tuberculosis infection in adults and children. *Am Rev Respir Dis* 134:355–363, 1986.
21. Aaro LA, Juergens JL: Thrombophlebitis associated with pregnancy. *Am J Obstet Gynecol* 109:1129, 1971.
22. Cocked FB, Thomas ML: The iliac compression syndrome. *Br J Surg* 52:816–821, 1965.
23. Hull RD, Hirsh J, Carter CJ, et al: Diagnostic value of ventiliation-perfusion lung scanning in patients with suspected pulmonary embolism. *Chest* 88:819–828, 1985.
24. Ginsberg JS, Hirsh J, Turner DC, et al: Risks to the fetus of anticoagulant therapy during pregnancy. *Thromb Haemost* 61:197–203, 1989.

Chapter 3

Common Gastrointestinal Problems

*Paul E. Zachary, Jr.**

Symptoms referable to the gastrointestinal system are common complaints of patients presenting to their primary caregivers. Abdominal pain and alterations in bowel habits are among the most common complaints. As the obstetrician-gynecologist (ob/gyn) is often a woman's only primary care physician, it is not unusual for him or her to see patients with varying gastrointestinal complaints. The purpose of this chapter is to familiarize the ob/gyn with the presenting signs and symptoms, differential diagnosis, basic diagnostic workup, and treatment of three common gastrointestinal tract disorders: cholelithiasis, gastroenteritis, and irritable bowel syndrome.

CHOLELITHIASIS

Cholelithiasis (stones in the gallbladder) is a common problem affecting approximately 10–15% of the population. A number of risk factors for gallstones have been identified[1] (Table 3.1). The prevalence of gallstones is two times higher in women than in men, largely due to the effect of estrogen, which increases cholesterol excretion in bile, and the effect of progesterone, which decreases gallbladder motility.[2] Multiparity, pregnancy at an early age, use of birth control pills, and postmenopausal estrogen replacement therapy are added risks.

While the majority of patients with gallstones are asymptomatic, gallstones should be considered in the differential diagnosis of patients with upper abdominal pain. The pain typically is located in the right upper quadrant (RUQ) or epigastric region and radiates to the RUQ. Radiation to the midback or right shoulder associated with nausea and vomiting is a typical complaint. Although often called biliary *colic*, biliary pain is usually steady, lasting for several hours, rather than spasmodic. Once typical symptoms appear, they tend to recur. Patients with symptomatic gallstones are more likely to have complications.[3] Indigestion, gas, bloating, and fatty and spicy food intolerance are common but are probably not related to the presence of gallstones.[4] Persistent upper abdominal pain lasting more than a few days is unlikely to be secondary to gallstones.

*I am very grateful to Drs. Bruce Bacon and Elizabeth Zachary for their comments and review of the manuscript.

TABLE 3.1 Risk Factors for Cholelithiasis

Cholesterol Stones	Pigment Stones
Native American descent	Hemolysis
Female sex	Biliary infection
Obesity	Age
Rapid weight loss	Cirrhosis
Gallbladder stasis	
Hypertriglyceridemia	
Spinal cord injury	
Estrogens	
Lipid-lowering agents	

Source: Adapted from ref. 1.

Complications

A number of complications may be associated with gallstones.[5] Obstruction of the cystic duct by a gallstone may lead to *acute cholecystitis*. This usually presents as severe RUQ abdominal pain, fever, and leukocytosis with nausea and vomiting. Patients examined during an acute attack often have tenderness in the RUQ, with cessation of inspiration on palpation (positive Murphy's sign).

Passage of gallstones into the common bile duct (CBD) may lead to infection and *ascending cholangitis*, which classically manifests as RUQ pain, fever, and jaundice (Charcot's triad). Common bile duct stones or even sludge or microlithiasis may also cause *acute pancreatitis*. Rarely, fistulization between an inflamed gallbladder and the intestine leads to *gallstone ileus*, giving rise to the triad of small bowel obstruction, air in the biliary tree, and an ectopic calcified gallstone on a plain abdominal radiograph. Eighty percent of patients with *gallbladder cancer* have gallstones, although a definite cause has not been proven.

Differential Diagnosis

A number of other gastrointestinal diseases should be considered in the differential diagnosis of upper abdominal pain. *Gastroesophageal reflux disease (GERD)* is one of the more common diseases and is frequently encountered in the obstetric population. Usually, a careful history can readily differentiate GERD from cholelithiasis. The pain associated with GERD is typically epigastric and substernal and is described as a burning sensation. Regurgitation of sour or bitter contents into the mouth is frequently present. Symptoms are often worse following meals and with recumbency. *Peptic ulcer disease (PUD)* is usually caused by infection with *Helicobacter pylori* or use of nonsteroidal anti-inflammatory agents. These patients typically complain of a gnawing upper abdominal pain that may be worsened (gastric ulcer) or improved (duodenal ulcer) with meals. Pain may also awaken them from sleep, usually in the early morning hours. Antacids frequently relieve the symptoms of both GERD and PUD. *Acute pancreatitis* is usually distinguished readily from biliary pain by elevation in the levels of amylase and/or lipase.

Frequently, patients have gastrointestinal symptoms that cannot be explained by structural or biochemical abnormalities and are classified as having functional disorders.[6] Some patients who undergo cholecystectomy will have persistent symptoms following surgery, the *postcholecystectomy syndrome*. Patients with functional disorders make up the majority of these patients. *Functional dyspepsia*, often called *nonulcer dyspepsia*, is very common and may present as a variety of complaints, including upper abdominal discomfort, nausea, vomiting, bloating, and early satiety. These patients often respond poorly to a variety of treatments. Every effort should be made to distinguish these less specific symptoms that may accompany gallstones from the typical biliary pain due to gallstones.

Functional biliary tract disorders may mimic gallstone disease. These disorders include *gallbladder dysfunction* and *sphincter of Oddi dysfunction*. These patients may have pain typical of biliary pain in the absence of gallstones. Elevation of liver or pancreatic enzymes during attacks makes the diagnosis more likely.

Diagnosis

Ultrasound of the gallbladder is the gold standard for evaluating the patient with suspected gallstones. It has a high sensitivity for demonstrating stones and can also show biliary ductal dilation, suggesting common bile duct (CBD) stones or stricture, and gallbladder wall thickening, suggesting cholecystitis. For the patient with suspected acute cholecystitis, nuclear cholescintigraphy is particularly helpful. Nonvisualization of the gallbladder constitutes a positive test. For the patient with suspected CBD stones due to ultrasound findings or elevated liver function tests, endosconic retrograde cholangiopancreatography (ERCP) is indicated.[7] To evaluate patients with suspected functional biliary tract disorders, additional specialized tests may be helpful. In patients with an intact gallbladder, calculation of a gallbladder ejection fraction using cholecystokinin-stimulated cholescintigraphy may be helpful. An ejection fraction of less than 40% is considered abnormal. Many of these patients will benefit from cholecystectomy. If the result is normal or if the patient has already had cholecystectomy, ERCP with sphincter of Oddi (SO) manometry can be performed to determine if an elevated sphincter pressure is present. An aspirate for biliary sludge or microlithiasis can also be obtained at this time. Patients with elevated SO pressure often benefit from sphincterotomy.

Treatment

Recent reviews of treatment are available, and the American College of Physicians has established guidelines for the treatment of gallstones.[5,7–10] No therapy is indicated for patients with asymptomatic gallstones. The primary treatment for symptomatic cholelithiasis is cholecystectomy. Only patients with typical biliary pain should be referred for surgery. Patients with atypical pain or dyspeptic symptoms alone will likely continue to have these symptoms following surgery.

Cholecystectomy is one of the most common operations performed and is increasing with the advent of laparoscopy. Although patient discomfort and recovery time are greatly reduced with the laparoscopic approach, the rate of complications is approximately the same as with an open procedure, and bile duct injuries may be higher than with the open approach.[3] Therefore, the indications for surgery remain the same, and patients should not be referred more often because of this new technique. Patients with acute cholecystitis are often "cooled off" with antibiotics and scheduled for elective cholecystectomy at a later date. Patients who are not surgical candidates or who desire not to have surgery may be considered for gallstone dissolution therapy with ursodeoxycholic acid.

Special Considerations in Pregnancy

Due to the hormonal effects described above, there is an increased incidence of gallstones in pregnant women. Development of biliary sludge is very common, but is usually asymptomatic and resolves following delivery.[11] Complications of gallstones, such as acute cholecystitis, occur at a low rate. Cholecystectomy is generally deferred until after delivery, with conservative management indicated particularly in the first trimester. ERCP with sphincterotomy can be safely performed in patients with gallstone pancreatitis or ascending cholangitis.[12]

Indications for Admission or Referral

Patients with suspected acute cholecystitis should be admitted for intravenous antibiotics and analgesics. Patients with suspected ascending cholangitis should receive similar treatment, along with prompt consultation with a gastroenterologist, as ERCP is indicated. Patients with suspected gallstone pancreatitis may also benefit from early ERCP.

Referral to a surgeon for cholecystectomy is appropriate in patients with symptomatic gallstones. If laparoscopy is desired, it is important to refer the patient to an experienced laparoscopic surgeon. Referral to a gastroenterologist may be helpful for patients with dyspeptic symptoms, atypical pain, or an uncertain diagnosis.

GASTROENTERITIS

Gastroenteritis manifesting as nausea, vomiting, and diarrhea is a common problem. Worldwide, diarrhea is a common cause of death. In Western countries, it accounts for many days lost from work. Day-care centers are a common source of outbreaks of rotavirus, *Shigella, Campylobacter, Giardia,* and *Cryptosporidium.*[13] Ob/gyns seeing young women with children therefore are likely to encounter patients with gastroenteritis.

The majority of cases of gastroenteritis are self-limited and are not investigated. Viral agents account for approximately 30–40% of cases in the United States.[14] Bacterial causes are less common but usually more severe. Protozoa may also cause gastroenteritis.[15] The etiology of presumed infectious diarrhea is unknown in approximately 40% of the cases.

Norwalk and Norwalk-like viruses are the most common viral causes of gastroenteritis in adults and usually occur as an epidemic resulting from contaminated water or food. Rotavirus, enteric adenovirus, calcivirus, and astrovirus typically cause diarrhea in infants and young children. Viral diarrheas are almost always noninflammatory.

Some bacterial and protozoal infections cause a noninflammatory diarrhea. Cholera and enterotoxigenic *Escherichia coli* are examples of bacteria that produce an enterotoxin stimulating small bowel secretion and inhibiting absorption, leading to diarrhea. *Giardia* is an example of an infectious agent causing diarrhea by interfering with absorption of the upper small intestine. Other bacteria or protozoa such as *Shigella, Salmonella, Campylobacter,* and amebas cause an inflammatory dysentery due to an invasive process or cytotoxin.

Clinical symptoms of diarrhea, frequently with nausea and vomiting, occur in patients with gastroenteritis. Signs and symptoms of dysentery include fever, bloody diarrhea, lower abdominal cramping, and tenesmus. It is important to assess the patient for signs of dehydration including dry mucous membranes, orthostatic changes in blood pressure and pulse, delayed capillary refill, and decreased urine output.

Differential Diagnosis

Some bacteria cause *food poisoning syndromes* in which nausea and vomiting may be more prominent than diarrhea.[15] Preformed heat-stabile toxins produced by *Staphylococcus aureus* or *Bacillus cereus* usually produce symptoms within the first 6 h of ingestion. *Clostridium perfringens* usually presents later, 6 to 72 h after ingestion.

Antibiotic-associated diarrhea is often associated with *Clostridium difficile* infection. The main antibiotics associated with *C. difficile* infection are ampicillin, cephalosporins, and clindamycin. However, many patients taking antibiotics will develop diarrhea, with or without colitis, in the absence of *C. difficile* infection. This usually resolves promptly upon withdrawal of antibiotics.

Diagnosis

The majority of patients with gastroenteritis will not require any evaluation. Table 3.2 lists situations in which further evaluation is indicated.[16] Tests include stool specimens for fecal leukocytes, ova and parasite examination times three (O & P × 3), culture for enteric pathogens, analysis for *C. difficile* toxin, and possibly flexible sigmoidoscopy.

Treatment

Most cases of gastroenteritis are self-limited, and most patients never seek medical attention. The majority of patients seeking medical attention may be reassured, encouraged to take liquids, and given symptomatic treatment with antidiarrheals such as loperamide (Imodium) or diphenoxylate/atropine (Lomotil). For patients with dehydration, intravenous replacement of fluids may be indicated, although in milder cases oral rehydration is preferred. Presumptive antibiotic therapy with a quinolone antibiotic should be considered for patients with signs and symptoms of dysentery.

TABLE 3.2 Indications for Evaluation of Acute Diarrhea

Any patient with:
Fever >39°C
Systemic illness
Tenesmus
Bloody diarrhea
Course >2 weeks
Dehydration
Patients with:
Overseas travel
Immunocompromised state
Raw seafood ingestion
Antibiotic use

Source: Adapted from ref. 16.

Special Considerations in Pregnancy

In the pregnant patient with diarrhea, significant volume depletion may be less apparent due to physiologic increased intravascular volume in the gravid state. Fetal tachycardia and an abnormal nonstress test may be among the first signs of maternal-fetal hypovolemia.[17] For specific bacterial infections, ampicillin and erythromycin are generally safe. Metronidazole, commonly used to treat protozoal infections, is teratogenic in animals and is therefore contraindicated in pregnant patients. For patients with documented protozoal infections, the appropriate drug of choice should be evaluated for its safety in pregnancy. Opiate antidiarrheals such as loperamide or diphenoxylate are best avoided, but kaolin and pectin may be used.[18]

Indications for Admission or Referral

Hospital admission may be indicated for patients with moderate to severe dehydration or signs of systemic toxicity. Patients with bloody diarrhea may need referral for sigmoidoscopy if the condition lasts for more than 2 to 3 days or is accompanied by systemic symptoms suggesting severe infection or inflammatory bowel disease. Referral to a gastroenterologist is appropriate for diarrhea without obvious etiology persisting for more than 2 weeks.

IRRITABLE BOWEL SYNDROME

Irritable bowel syndrome (IBS) is one of the most common disorders encountered by primary care physicians and may account for approximately 30–50% of a gastroenterologist's practice. Ob/gyns are likely to encounter this disorder, which is commonly seen in young women. The term *irritable bowel syndrome* is preferred to the older terms *spastic colon, spastic colitis,* or *mucous colitis.* The terms with *colitis* are to be especially avoided, as there is no inflammation in this disorder. IBS is a functional disorder and likely involves a number of pathophysiologic mechanisms including abnormal motility, abnormal visceral perception, and psychological distress.[19] A number of recent reviews are available.[20–23]

Clinical Manifestations

Irritable bowel syndrome is characterized by varying degrees of abdominal pain and alterations in bowel habits, sometimes with a predominance of diarrhea or constipation but often with cycles of alternating diarrhea and constipation. Manning identified six factors associated more commonly with IBS than with organic disease, including abdominal bloating, increased frequency of stool with onset of pain, looser stools with onset of pain, relief of pain with defecation, a sensation of incomplete evacuation, and passage of mucus in stools.[24] The more of these symptoms present, the higher the likelihood of IBS. These criteria are more reliable for female patients. An international working group proposed diagnostic criteria for IBS, the "Rome" criteria[6] (Table 3.3). Approximately 75–80% of patients with IBS are women, and many note worsening of symptoms during menses. Patients exhibiting weight loss, pain, or diarrhea interrupting sleep, blood in the stool (other than hemorrhoidal), or onset of symptoms after age 50 may still have IBS, but an organic cause is more likely.

Epidemiologic studies have shown that symptoms of IBS may be present in up to 15–20% of the general population. The majority of these people never seek medical attention. A number of factors may influence the patient to seek medical evaluation, including the presence and degree of pain, psychosocial disturbance, high life stress, or poor social support.[21]

Differential Diagnosis

The differential diagnosis of chronic diarrhea (lasting for more than 4–6 weeks) is extensive, but the most common disorder is IBS. *Lactose intolerance* may produce symptoms identical to those of IBS, and many patients with IBS have this condition, which contributes to their symptoms.

Patients with inflammatory bowel disease, particularly mild forms of *Crohn's disease*, are often initially labeled as IBS patients. Crohn's disease often presents with abdominal pain and diarrhea. Systemic symptoms such as weight loss, fever, and laboratory abnormalities such as elevated sedimentation rate or platelet count, anemia, or hypoalbuminemia should steer one away from the diagnosis of IBS. *Ulcerative colitis* presents with frequent, small volume, and bloody mucoid stools with prominent tenesmus. Typical patients are usually readily distinguished by the history, but some patients with

TABLE 3.3 Diagnostic Criteria for IBS

At least 3 months of continuous or recurrent symptoms of:

- Abdominal pain or discomfort relieved by defecation or associated with a change in the frequency or consistency of stool *and* two or more of the following on at least one-fourth of the occasions or days:
- Altered stood frequency
- Altered stool form
- Altered stool passage
- Passage of mucus
- Bloating or abdominal distention

Source: Adapted from ref. 6.

milder symptoms and less bleeding may be difficult to distinguish from those with IBS. Flexible sigmoidoscopy showing proctocolitis excludes IBS. A particular type of inflammatory bowel disease that may be encountered by gynecologic oncologists is *radiation colitis*. Patients with a history of pelvic irradiation may develop diarrhea due to injury of the ileum, which interferes with bile salt absorption. These patients often have a dramatic response to cholestyramine, which binds the bile salts. Strictures leading to bacterial overgrowth is another common factor contributing to diarrhea in these patients; an empiric trial of metronidazole is warranted in patients who do not respond to cholestyramine. Radiation proctitis can be quite severe and difficult to manage. It is usually poorly responsive to topical steroids and other anti-inflammatory agents. For persistent rectal bleeding, endoscopic treatment of rectal telangiectasias with contact probes or laser therapy may be palliative.

Diverticular disease in the absence of diverticulitis is more often clinically silent. However, some patients do have painful diverticular disease, with alterations in bowel habits, in the absence of overt diverticulitis. Some investigators have proposed that diverticular disease may be part of a spectrum including IBS.

Colon cancer may present with a change in bowel habits. In patients over age 50, with iron deficiency anemia, rectal bleeding, or a positive fecal occult blood test, colon cancer must be excluded.

Female patients often present to gynecologists for *chronic pelvic pain*. If a careful history is taken, with attention to bowel habits, many of these patients will be found to have IBS. An excellent review by Longstreth was recently published.[25]

Diagnosis

IBS is primarily diagnosed by the history. A limited evaluation including complete blood count, chemistry profile, thyroid function tests, and erythrocyte sedimentation rate should be performed in most patients. Patients with diarrhea-predominant symptoms should also have stool cultures (O & P × 3, enteric pathogens and *C. difficile* toxin) and flexible sigmoidoscopy with biopsy. Patients over age 50 or with a family history of colon cancer should have a full colonic evaluation with colonoscopy or flexible sigmoidoscopy plus a barium enema. Any positive finding requires further diagnostic evaluation. If these screening tests are negative, then IBS may be diagnosed with confidence. This diagnosis should be discussed with the patient to allay fears of another, more serious diagnosis.

Treatment

Patient education and positive reassurance are of the utmost importance. No placebo-controlled trials have shown benefit from drug therapies.[26] However, clinical experience has shown the usefulness of a number of agents. Treatment should focus on the patient's predominant symptom.[19,21] A trial of a lactose-free diet should be instituted in patients with diarrhea or gas/bloat-predominant symptoms, as some patients' symptoms will be related solely to lactose intolerance and many symptoms improve with avoidance of milk products. Fiber supplementation helps regulate bowel movements and is particularly helpful for constipation-predominant IBS. It may also help reduce diarrhea by adding bulk to the stool. Stool softeners and osmotic laxatives, such as milk of magnesia for constipation or loperamide and diphenoxylate/atropine for diarrhea, may also be used. Antispasmodics with an anticholinergic effect may be helpful for pain. Patients with more severe or refractory pain may benefit from low doses of antidepressants, as well as from behavioral therapy or psychotherapy.[20,27] An ongoing relationship with a trusted primary care physician is also important.

Special Considerations in Pregnancy

Symptoms of IBS, particularly constipation, may worsen during pregnancy.[17,28] Antispasmodics and antidepressants are best avoided during pregnancy because of their potential teratogenicity. Fiber supplementation and avoidance of offending foods are the mainstays of therapy in pregnancy.

Indications for Admission or Referral

Patients almost never require admission for IBS symptoms alone. Patients with onset of symptoms after age 50 and/or with weight loss, rectal bleeding, or anemia should be referred for gastroenterologic evaluation to exclude inflammatory bowel disease or cancer by colonoscopy or flexible sigmoidoscopy plus barium enema. Patients with more severe symptoms that do not respond to reassurance and the therapies outlined above likely have IBS. Gastroenterologic consultation to confirm the diagnosis or to consider other diagnostic possibilities is appropriate in these difficult patients.

SUMMARY

It appears that the pendulum is swinging back toward recognizing the importance of the primary care physician over that of the specialist. As ob/gyns are the sole providers of health care to many women, the ob/gyns' role as primary care physician is becoming more prominent. Gastrointestinal problems are common and therefore will likely be encountered by ob/gyns. Gallstones are a frequent cause of upper abdominal pain, but a number of other causes should also be considered. An attempt to identify patients with characteristic symptoms, as outlined above, should be made to avoid patient disappointment postcholecystectomy. Patients with uncertain symptoms, suspected common bile duct stones, or functional biliary tract disease benefit from gastroenterologic consultation.

Most patients presenting with acute diarrhea do not need workup and may be treated supportively. IBS, characterized by abdominal pain and alterations in bowel habits, is one of the most frequent disorders encountered in medicine and is the most common cause of chronic diarrhea. A thorough history, with careful attention to the criteria outlined above, will provide the diagnosis. Some patients with mild symptoms, a normal physical examination, and normal laboratory test results may be simply reassured. However, most patients, especially those with diarrhea, should also have referral for endoscopic evaluation.

REFERENCES

1. Goldschmid S, Brady PG: Approaches to the management of cholelithiasis for the medical consultant. *Med Clin North Am* 77:413–426, 1993.
2. Everson GT: Gastrointestinal motility in pregnancy. *Gastroenerol Clin North Am* 21:751–776, 1992.
3. Anonymous: NIH consensus conference. Gallstones and laparoscopic cholecystectomy. *JAMA* 269:1018–1024, 1993.
4. Diehl AK: Symptoms of gallstone disease. *Bailliere's Clin Gastroenterol* 6:635–657, 1992.
5. Johnston DE, Kaplan MM: Pathogenesis and treatment of gallstones. *N Engl J Med* 328: 412–421, 1993.
6. Drossman DA: *The Functional Gastrointestinal Disorders.* Boston, Little, Brown, 1994.
7. Gholson CF, Sittig K, McDonald JC: Recent advances in the management of gallstones. *Am J Med Sci* 307:293–304, 1994.
8. Plaisier PW, van der Hul RL, Terpstra OT, et al: Current treatment modalities for symptomatic gallstones. *Am J Gastroenterol* 88:633–639, 1993.
9. Randsohoff DF, Gracie WA: Treatment of gallstones. *Ann Intern Med* 119:606–619, 1993.
10. Anonymous: Guidelines for the treatment of gallstones. *Ann Intern Med* 119:620–622, 1993.
11. Maringhini A, Ciambra M, Baccelliere P, et al: Biliary sludge and gallstones in pregnancy: Incidence, risk factors, and natural history. *Ann Intern Med* 119:116–120, 1993.
12. Scott LD: Gallstone disease and pancreatitis in pregnancy. *Gastroenterol Clin North Am* 21:803–815, 1992.
13. Northrup RS, Flanigan TP: Gastroenteritis. *Pediatr Rev* 15:461–472, 1994.
14. Blacklow NR, Greenberg HB: Viral gastroenteritis. *N Engl J Med* 325:252–264, 1991.
15. Guerrant RL, Bobak DA: Bacterial and protozoal gastroenteritis. *N Engl J Med* 325:327–340, 1991.
16. Gorbach SL: Bacterial diarrhoea and its treatment. *Lancet* 2:1378–1382, 1987.
17. West L, Warren J, Cutts T: Diagnosis and management of irritable bowel syndrome, constipation, and diarrhea in pregnancy. *Gastroenterol Clin North Am* 21:793–802, 1992.
18. Baron TH, Ramirez B, Richter JE: Gastrointestinal motility disorders during pregnancy. *Ann Intern Med* 118:366–375, 1993.
19. Camilleri M, Prather CM: The irritable bowel syndrome: Mechanisms and a practical approach to management. *Ann Intern Med* 116:1001–1008, 1992.
20. Drossman DA: Irritable bowel syndrome. *Gastroenterologist* 2:315–326, 1994.
21. Drossman DA, Thompson WG: The irritable bowel syndrome: Review and a graduated multicomponent treatment approach. *Ann Intern Med* 116:1009–1016, 1992.
22. Lynn RB, Friedman LS: Irritable bowel syndrome. *N Engl J Med* 329:1940–1945, 1993.
23. Lynn RB, Friedman LS: Irritable bowel syndrome: Managing the patient with abdominal pain and altered bowel habits. *Med Clin North Am* 79:373–390, 1995.
24. Manning AP, Thompson WG, Heaton KW, et al: Towards positive diagnosis of the irritable bowel. *BMJ* 2:653–654, 1978.
25. Longstreth GF: Irritable bowel syndrome and chronic pelvic pain. *Obstet Gynecol Surv* 49:505–507, 1994.
26. Pattee PL, Thompson WG: Drug treatment of the irritable bowel syndrome. *Drugs* 44: 200–206, 1992.
27. Creed F: Irritable bowel or irritable mind? Psychological treatment is essential for some. *BMJ* 309:1647–1648, 1994.
28. Singer AJ, Brandt LJ: Pathophysiology of the gastrointestinal tract during pregnancy. *Am J Gastroenterol* 86:1695–1712, 1991.

Chapter 4

Viral Hepatitis, Human Immunodeficiency Virus and Acquired Immune Deficiency Syndrome

Paul Becherer

INTRODUCTION

Viral hepatitis and acquired immune deficiency syndrome (AIDS) are leading causes of morbidity and mortality in the United States. These viruses are most commonly contracted by young adults. As the primary care providers of many young women, obstetricians and gynecologists should be familiar with the epidemiology, clinical manifestations, diagnosis, prevention, and treatment of viral hepatitis and human immunodeficiency virus (HIV) infection.

VIRAL HEPATITIS

Definition of Hepatitis

Hepatitis, or inflammation with hepatocellular damage, is clinically defined by elevated activity of the serum aminotransferases alanine (ALT) and aspartate (AST). Drugs, toxins, bacteria, viruses, parasites, and other noninfectious agents are among the diverse causes of hepatitis. Five distinct hepatotropic viruses cause hepatic inflammation generally, without other clinical manifestations: hepatitis A (HAV), hepatitis B (HBV), hepatitis C (HCV), hepatitis D (delta hepatitis or HDV), and hepatitis E (HEV) (Table 4.1). Neither the risk of infectious hepatitis nor its clinical course is altered by pregnancy (with the exception of HEV noted below). Nor does viral hepatitis significantly increase the rate of fetal mortality or premature delivery.

TABLE 4.1 Viral Etiologies of Hepatitis

Etiology	Type
Hepatitis A (HAV)	Infectious
Hepatitis B (HBV)	Serum
Hepatitis C (HCV)	Posttransfusion non-A, non-B hepatitis
	Sporadic non-A, non-B hepatitis
	Community-acquired non-A, non-B hepatitis
Hepatitis D (HDV)	Delta hepatitis
Hepatitis E (HEV)	Enteric non-A, non-B hepatitis
	Endemic
	Waterborne

Liver Function Tests

Although clinically elevated serum aminotransferases generally reflect hepatic injury, their portrayal as a "liver function test" in medical jargon is a misnomer. ALT, AST, bilirubin, alkaline phosphatase, and gamma-glutamyl transpeptidase (GGT) levels do not reflect the true functional capacity of the liver and must be interpreted in the context of the clinical presentation.

Alanine aminotransferase (ALT or SGPT) is relatively well localized to the liver, but aspartate aminotransferase (AST or SGOT) can also be found in skeletal and myocardial muscle. The circulating half-life of ALT is longer than that of AST, so the ALT:AST ratio is elevated during the resolution phase following acute liver injury. When the ALT:AST ratio is less than 2, alcoholic hepatitis and perhaps cirrhosis and chronic viral hepatitis should be considered. Table 4.2 delineates some of the causes of ALT and AST elevation.

Bilirubin is the product of red blood cell and liver cytochrome heme catabolism and is made water soluble by conjugation with glucuronic acid. The conjugated bilirubin is excreted into the bile, resulting in brown stool. A fraction of the bilirubin is reabsorbed from the intestine as the bacterial metabolite urobilinogen and subsequently excreted by the urine. Pregnancy-related causes include acute fatty liver of pregnancy, pre-eclampsia, eclampsia, hepatic rupture, and intrahepatic cholestasis. Clues to the etiology of jaundice can be obtained by measuring the fraction of bilirubin that has been conjugated, as well as the level of urobilinogen in the urine. The liver maintains its ability to conjugate bilirubin even when hepatic function is severely compromised. When more than 80% of the bilirubin is unconjugated, a drug effect (rifampin), a genetic defect of bilirubin conjugation (Gilbert syndrome), and especially hemolysis must be considered. In a jaundiced individual, urobilinogen should be detectable unless the common bile duct is completely occluded, preventing conjugated bilirubin from reaching the intestine. The bilirubin level may rise by 1 mg/dL/day with liver failure. Increases exceeding 1 mg/dL/day suggest hemolysis.

Alkaline phosphatase is localized in the bile canaliculi, as well as in bone and placenta. Biliary obstruction causes the release of the enzyme. The source of alkaline phosphatase can be determined by performing isoenzyme analysis or heat fractionation or by measuring other enzymes associated with biliary canaliculi, such as GGT.

TABLE 4.2 Causes of ALT and AST Elevations

Level	Cause
Normal (0–50 U/L)	Does not exclude Genetic hemochromatosis Alcoholic hepatitis Cirrhosis from any cause
Mild elevation (50–400 U/L)	Drug-induced liver injury Parental nutrition Fatty infiltration Acute fatty liver of pregnancy Chronic viral, autoimmune, or alcoholic liver disease Autoimmune hepatitis Intrahepatic or extrahepatic obstruction Passive congestive (cardiac, etc.)
Moderate elevation (400–2000 U/L)	Acute biliary obstruction Acute viral hepatitis Drug-induced liver injury Toxin exposure Ischemia
High elevation (2000–30,000 U/L)	Acute viral hepatitis Drugs (e.g., acetaminophen) Toxins (e.g., mushroom poisoning) Shock liver

Clinical Presentation of Hepatitis

In an individual patient, the differentiation between each type of viral hepatitis based on clinical or histologic features is difficult. Nevertheless, several generalizations are possible. These are summarized in Table 4.3

The incubation period of HAV is approximately 1 month. Children tend to be asymptomatic and anicteric, while >75% of adults develop fever, abdominal pain, diarrhea, and jaundice. Hepatitis A infection is associated with a very low mortality rate and never progresses to chronic hepatitis.

By contrast, with HBV, symptoms develop insidiously without fever about 12 weeks after contracting the virus. Infection causes jaundice in only about 50% of infected adults and therefore is often not recognized. Occasionally, acute HBV infection is associated with glomerulonephritis or arthritis. While only about 5% of adults develop chronic hepatitis, 50–90% of infected children become carriers at risk of chronic hepatitis, cirrhosis, or hepatocellular carcinoma.

Approximately 8 weeks after exposure to HCV, about 10–25% of infected individuals become icteric. Despite the fact that the majority of infected individuals are unaware of their infection, most (50–70%) develop chronic hepatitis, which ultimately places them at risk for cirrhosis and hepatocellular carcinoma. Hepatitis C infection has also been associated with essential mixed cryoglobulinemia, glomerulonephritis, and porphyria cutanea tarda.

TABLE 4.3 Clinical Presentation of Viral Hepatitis

Virus	Average Incubation Period (weeks)	% of Adults Jaundiced	% of Adults with Chronic Infection	Sequelae
HAV	4	80%	0%	
HBV	12	50%	5–10%	Arthritis Glomerulonephritis Cirrhosis Hepatocellular carcinoma
HCV	8	20%	50%	Glomerulonephritis Mixed cryoglobulinemia Porphyria cutanea tarda Cirrhosis Hepatocellular carcinoma

HDV is a "defective" virus requiring a helper function from HBV, which provides HDV with an envelope surface antigen coat. The incubation period of HDV is roughly 5 weeks. Infection may present as a coinfection with HBV resulting in fulminant hepatitis with a high mortality rate, and rarely as a chronic carrier state or as a superinfection of a chronic HBV carrier leading to rapidly progressive subacute or chronic hepatitis due to persistent infection with both HBV and HDV.

The clinical presentation of HEV or enterically transmitted non-A, non-B hepatitis is similar to that of hepatitis A. Mortality is less than 1% except among pregnant women in the third trimester, whose mortality rate with HEV infection may exceed 20%.

Epidemiology

HAV is shed in high titers in the stool for several weeks preceding and for about 1 week following the onset of symptoms, but it causes only a transient viremia. This pattern of shedding coupled with the relatively stable characteristics of the viral particle account for the fecal-oral route of transmission. The risk of hepatitis A transmission decreases with improved sanitation. While food-borne or water-borne outbreaks of hepatitis A attract a great deal of local health department and media attention, person-to-person transmission accounts for the majority of cases. Employment or attendance at a day-care center, intravenous drug use, ingestion of raw or undercooked shellfish, and international travel are also recognized risk factors. Over 40% of patients have no known source of exposure. Perinatal transmission from contact with infectious blood or feces is conceivable, but the number of clinical reports is small.

HBV is excreted in the blood, as well as in body fluids, by persons with acute or chronic infection. Routes of transmission include blood (25%), homosexual and heterosexual activity (33%), and mother to infant. Children, in particular, may transmit HBV to other children during play, presumably due to inapparent blood contact. Transmission of HBV from mother to infant takes place at the time of birth. Caesarean section does not prevent transmission. Again, approximately 40% of patients with acute HBV infection have no recognized risk factor for acquisition.

Parenteral transmission via intravenous drug use or transfusion accounts for roughly half of the reported cases of acute, symptomatic HCV infections. While the sero-prevalence of anti-HCV among homosexuals and persons with multiple heterosexual contacts appears to be elevated, the risk of sexual transmission appears to be dramatically lower than that of HBV or HIV. Sexual transmission may be facilitated by coinfection with HIV. The current recommendations are that persons who are not in a mutually monogamous relationship should be counseled about the risk of HCV transmission, as well as other sexually transmitted diseases. They should be instructed to reduce their number of sexual partners. Theoretically, the proper use of condoms may further reduce the risk of transmission. Apparently vertical transmission occurs in 1–10% of births involving an infected mother, but the timing of this transmission remains to be defined. The presence of virus in human secretions is low or undetectable, explaining the apparent lack of household or horizontal transmission. Approximately 40% of patients with hepatitis C have no identifiable risk factor for infection.

HDV achieves high titers in the blood of patients also infected with HBV. HDV, which is transmitted predominantly by blood products, is seen in parenteral drug users and hemophiliacs, who receive pooled clotting factor concentrate. Sexual, perinatal, and household transmission have occasionally been reported.

HEV infection is endemic in Southeast and Central Asia, Africa, and Mexico. Confirmed cases in the United States have been limited to travelers returning from endemic regions. Large outbreaks in developing countries have been traced to contaminated water and poor sanitation. Mother-to-infant transmission has not been reported.

Hepatitis Serologies

The diagnosis of acute hepatitis A is based on the detection of IgM antibody which persists for about 6 months. IgG antibody may also appear early, but it persists for life and is an indication of lifelong immunity. Likewise, IgM anti-hepatitis B core (IgM anti-HBc) indicates acute HBV infection and becomes undetectable in 6 months. Hepatitis B surface antigen (HBsAg) disappears with recovery from the disease, generally with the appearance of anti-HBs, a neutralizing, protective antibody response. Seroconversion to anti-HCV occurs late in the acute disease (up to 6 months after development of the disease). Unfortunately, conditions associated with increased levels of gamma globulin, such as pregnancy, may be associated with false-positive anti-HCV enzyme-linked immunosorbent assay (ELISA) results. A supplementary assay, recombinant immunoblot assay (RIBA), may provide additional information. Diagnosis of HDV infection, and the distinction between coinfection and superinfection, depend on proper application and interpretation of both HBV and HDV serologic assays, which is beyond the scope of this chapter. A commercially available test is not available for HEV.

Viral hepatitis serologies represent a confusing alphabetic quagmire of antigens and antibodies. Before ordering hepatitis serologies, the first step is to determine whether the patient has acute or chronic hepatitis clinically. Fatigue, nausea, right upper quadrant abdominal pain, significant ALT elevation, and perhaps jaundice are characteristic

TABLE 4.4 Hepatitis Panels

Acute Hepatitis Panel Interpretation

Anti-HAV IgM	Anti-HBc IgM	HBsAg	Anti-HCV	
+	−	−	−	Acute HAV
−	+	+	−	Acute HBV
−	+	−	−	Acute HBV
−	−	+	−	Chronic HBV Consider HDV superinfection
−	−	−	+	Consider Acute HCV
+	−	+	−	Acute HAV in HBV carrier

Chronic Hepatitis Panel Interpretation

HBsAg	Anti-HCV	
+	−	Chronic HBV
−	+	Chronic HCV

of acute hepatitis, while asymptomatic ALT elevations or signs of cirrhosis such as spider angiomats, encephalopathy, ascites, varices, gynecomastia, and palmar erythema are more consistent with chronic hepatitis. The patient's history, including risk assessment, physical examination, and routine laboratory evaluations, is rarely so strongly predictive of a specific infectious agent that selected screening is warranted.

An acute hepatitis panel (Table 4.4) consisting of antihepatitis A IgM antibody (IgM anti-HAV), hepatitis B surface antigen (HBsAg), antihepatitis B core IgM antibody (IgM anti-HBc), and antihepatitis C (anti-HCV) provides cost-effective screening. The anti-HCV enzyme immune assay has a window period between the development of disease and a serologic response. Therefore, repeating the anti-HCV serology should be considered in patients without an identified etiology for their hepatitis. In patients with recent travel to areas endemic for HEV, additional testing may be warranted.

Chronic hepatitis can be caused by HBV, with or without HDV and HCV. An appropriate screen for chronic hepatitis might include HBsAg and anti-HCV (Table 4.4). Other hepatitis serologies (Table 4.5) are available but clinically are not particularly relevant.

Prevention

Pooled serum globulin which contains HAV antibodies has proven protective against disease when given before exposure or early in the incubation period. Effective inactivated whole-virus vaccines have been licensed in Europe since 1991 and in the United States in 1996.

Hepatitis B immune globulin (HBIg) is effective if administered prior to exposure or early in the incubation period. The availability of recombinant HBV vaccines which induce neutralizing HBsAg antibodies in over 95% of immunocompetent adults, infants, and neonates has unfortunately failed to significantly reduce the incidence of hepatitis B infection. Because about 40% of infected patients have no identified risk factors, and because many of the high-risk groups such as injecting drug users are difficult to identify, educate, and target for prevention programs, the failure of prevention

TABLE 4.5 Additional Hepatitis Serologies

Test	Interpretation of a Positive Result
Hepatitis A total antibody (total anti-HAV)	Does not distinguish between current and past HAV infection
Hepatitis B e antigen (HBeAg)	Acute or chronic hepatitis B with active viral replication
Anti-hepatitis B e (anti-HBe)	Suppression of hepatitis B replication: does not exclude infectivity
Hepatitis B core total antibody (total anti-HBc)	Does not distinguish between current and past HBV infection

strategies involving immunization of high-risk groups is understandable. Thus, the U.S. Public Health Service recommends universal immunization of infants and adolescents, leading to immunity before these individuals participate in risk-taking behavior.

Passive-active neonatal immunization reduces the risk of perinatal HBV transmission by nearly 95%. The Centers for Disease Control (CDC) recommends that all pregnant women be screened for HBsAg during a prenatal visit. For infants of HBsAg-positive mothers, HBIg should be administered within 48 h, and the vaccine should be given during the first 7 days and repeated at 1, 6, and 12 to 15 months. If HBsAg results are not available within 48 h of delivery, HBIg should probably be administered to infants of high-risk mothers such as intravenous drug users, as well as mothers from Asia, Haiti, sub-Saharan Africa, and the Alaskan Eskimo population.

The effectiveness of pooled immune globulin in preventing HCV infection has never been clearly demonstrated. Recently, in fact, anti-HCV-positive donors have been excluded from the donor pools for such products. Challenge experiments in chimpanzees indicate that antibody immune responses are probably not protective, making hepatitis C vaccine development problematic.

Effective HBV prevention also protects against HDV infection. The role of immune globulin in preventing HEV infection remains to be defined.

HIV AND AIDS

AIDS Surveillance Definition

In 1993, the CDC expanded the surveillance definition of AIDS among adolescents and adults in the United States to reflect more accurately the number of persons with severe HIV-related immune suppression. Many of these patients could not be defined by the previous AIDS-defining diagnostic criteria despite evidence of advanced disease. The major change was the inclusion of persons with a CD4+ count of fewer than 200 cells/mm^3 or a CD4+ percentage of less than 14. Thus, immune monitoring plays an increasing role in staging the disease progression as well as in therapeutic interventions, as will be discussed below. Pulmonary tuberculosis and recurrent pneumonia (two or more episodes with 12 months) in an HIV-infected individual were added to

TABLE 4.6 Conditions Included in the 1993 AIDS Surveillance Case Definition

Candidiasis of bronchi, trachea, or lungs
Candidiasis, esophageal
Cervical cancer, invasive
Coccidioidomycosis, disseminated or extrapulmonary
Cryptococcosis, extrapulmonary
Cryptosporidiosis, chronic intestinal (>1 month's duration)
Cytomegalovirus disease (other than that of the liver, spleen, or nodes)
Cytomegalovirus retinitis (with loss of vision)
Encephalopathy, HIV-related
Herpes simplex: chronic ulcer(s) (>1 month's duration) or bronchitis, pneumonitis, or esophagitis
Histoplasmosis, disseminated or extrapulmonary
Isosporiasis, chronic intestinal (>1 month's duration)
Kaposi's sarcoma
Lymphoma, Burkitt's (or equivalent term)
Lymphoma, immunoblastic (or equivalent term)
Lymphoma, primary, of brain
Mycobacterium avium complex or *M. kansasii,* disseminated or extrapulmonary
Mycobacterium tuberculosis, any site (pulmonary or extrapulmonary)
Mycobacterium, other species or unidentified species, disseminated or extrapulmonary
Pneumocystis carinii pneumonia
Pneumonia, recurrent (two episodes in 12 months)
Progressive multifocal leukoencephalopathy (PML)
Salmonella septicemia, recurrent
Toxoplasmosis of the brain
Wasting syndrome due to HIV

Source: Adapted from CDC. *MMWR* 41(No. RR-17), 1992.

the other 23 clinical conditions listed in the previous definition (Table 4.6). Finally, invasive cervical cancer was added as a criterion. Several studies had indicated an increased risk of cervical dysplasia associated with increasing immunosuppression. This expanded definition, as expected, transiently increased the number of cases reported to the CDC by 50–75%.

HIV infection causes a gradual deterioration in immune status. While the surveillance definition provides important information, there is no clinical or laboratory difference between a CD4+ count of 190/mm^3 and 210/mm^3. Therefore, in an individual patient, the focus should not be on diagnostic criteria for AIDS but on the person's own clinical status in conjunction with a crude marker of immune dysfunction, with an understanding of the variability of CD4+ determinations.

Current Trends in HIV/AIDS Epidemiology

As the number of reported AIDS cases has increased each year, the relative number of patients reporting homosexual contact or intravenous drug use has plateaued. Heterosexual HIV transmission is the most rapidly increasing mode of HIV exposure. Cases attributed to heterosexual contact are increasing throughout the United States, rising at alarming rates in the South, including rural areas. The impact among minority populations is escalating, with rates among Hispanics and African Americans being approximately three and four times, respectively, the rate among whites.

During the past decade, the toll of AIDS on women has increased dramatically. HIV infection is now the fourth leading cause of death among women 25–44 years of age. As might be expected, the incidence of HIV infection among children—virtually all infected through perinatal transmission—has likewise mushroomed; HIV is now the seventh leading cause of death among children 1–4 years of age. African American and Hispanic women have been disproportionately affected; HIV infection is now the leading cause of death among African American women 25–44 years of age and the third leading cause among Hispanic women in this age group. These same populations have a high incidence of sexually transmitted disease and tuberculosis, including multidrug-resistant tuberculosis.

Nearly half of AIDS cases among women have been attributed to intravenous drug use compared to 20% from sex with an IV drug user and 20% from other heterosexual encounters. In younger women (13–25 years old) heterosexual transmission is even more critical. A growing proportion of perinatally acquired AIDS cases have been reported among children born to mothers who acquired HIV infection through heterosexual contact, often without knowledge of their partner's infection status or risk behaviors. By the end of 1995, maternal AIDs-related deaths had orphaned approximately 25,000 children and 21,000 adolescents in the United States.

Heterosexual Transmission

Anal intercourse, lack of condom use, genital ulcerative disease and other sexually transmitted disease, intrauterine contraceptive devices, advanced HIV disease, and cervical ectopy increase the risk of HIV transmission. Sexual intercourse during menses may increase the risk of female-to-male transmission but apparently not male-to-female transmission. While nonoxynol-9 spermicide has antiviral activity, it may cause vaginal irritation, particularly when used frequently, thus theoretically increasing the risk.

Perinatal Transmission of HIV

The rate of perinatal transmission has been estimated to be 13–40%. Although HIV transmission from an infected woman to her fetus can occur early during pregnancy, studies suggest that most infections occur late in pregnancy or during the birth process. Breast-feeding may also transmit HIV. Several risk factors have been suggested to be associated with an increased rate of transmission, including premature rupture of membranes, premature delivery, placental membrane inflammation, and increased exposure of the fetus to maternal blood, as well as markers of advanced disease in the woman including the presence of p24 antigen in the serum, a high viral titer, a low CD4+ lymphocyte count, and an AIDS diagnosis. Cesarean section delivery and therapy with zidovudine may decrease the risk of HIV transmission.

Counseling and HIV Testing

Because of the physical and psychosocial implications of HIV seropositivity, testing should be performed after providing counseling, obtaining informed consent, and ensuring confidentiality. Counseling should be culture, education, language, and age appropriate in order to obtain truly informed consent. Pretest counseling involves assessing the person's relative risk of infection, as well as reviewing the perceived and actual purpose for, meaning of, and impact of test results. Information should include the routes of HIV infection and options for reducing the risk of transmission. The psychosocial implications of testing HIV positive, such as discrimination, abandonment, and domestic violence reported in 4–13% of women, should also be discussed. Partner notification, legal, social, and psychological services as well as sexually transmitted disease, substance abuse, and HIV treatment services should be offered if warranted. Most studies have suggested a high acceptance of HIV testing when the health care provider has given appropriate counseling and encouragement to be tested for HIV infection.

Screening is initiated with an HIV enzyme immunoassay (EIA or ELISA) which is highly sensitive (>99%) and specific (>99%). Serum which is repeatedly reactive by EIA is then submitted for confirmatory testing using a Western blot or immunofluorescence assay (IFA). Both tests detect HIV-specific antibodies. Persons who test negative by EIA or have repeatedly positive EIA but negative confirmatory tests should be considered uninfected. An indeterminate Western blot test result can be due to the nonspecific reactions seen more often in pregnant women (<1 in every 4000 EIA-positive specimens) or to an incomplete immune response caused by recent infection, end-stage HIV disease, or perinatally exposed infants who are losing maternal antibodies. The IFA is less likely to provide an indeterminate result and thus may helpful in patients with indeterminate Western blot findings. Alternatively, tests such as viral culture, polymerase chain reaction, and p24 antigen may help diagnose or exclude HIV infection. Posttest counseling should be provided to all women. A negative HIV screen should not be perceived to legitimize high-risk behavior since continued exposure carries a cumulative risk.

Counseling and Voluntary Testing of Pregnant Women

For many young women, their only interaction with the health care system is with gynecologic, prenatal, or obstetric clinics. Since most individuals do not seek HIV screening until they become ill, often within months of their AIDS diagnosis, most HIV-infected women are not aware of their infection status. Strategies which offer testing only to women who report high-risk behavior fail to recognize 50–75% of infected women. Generally, these women are not aware of previous sexual contact with an HIV-infected person or are reluctant to admit to engaging in high-risk behavior. Therefore, the U.S. Public Health Service recommends a more sweeping, universal, voluntary screening approach.

Besides the counseling considerations discussed above, reproductive options and the availability of therapy to reduce the risk of perinatal transmission should be discussed. Screening should be performed as early in the pregnancy as possible so that informed therapeutic and reproductive choices can be made. Women who test positive for HIV or who refuse to be screened should not be discriminated against by denying health care or reporting them to child protective service agencies. HIV-negative women who continue to participate in high-risk behaviors should be retested during the third trimester. HIV infection is more common among women who have not received prenatal care. Therefore, counseling and screening should be performed promptly. If infection is not identified until the time of labor and delivery, intrapartum and neonatal zidovudine use could still be considered.

Every attempt should be made to resolve any uncertainty regarding the patient's HIV serostatus given the implications of a positive test for the woman, the fetus, and the decisions regarding zidovudine therapy, pregnancy termination, or other interventions.

Acute Primary HIV Infection

Primary infection with HIV may be asymptomatic, but more often it is probably not recognized by the patient or the clinician. The symptoms of acute infection are nonspecific and include fever (97%), pharyngitis (73%), lymphadenopathy (77%), arthralgias/myalgias (58%), malaise, and anorexia—a mononucleosis-like syndrome that typically develops 2 to 4 weeks after exposure. Other systems may include an erythematous maculopapular rash (70%), diarrhea (33%), nausea (20%), headache (30%), mucocutaneous ulcers (35%), and thrush.

Laboratory abnormalities are also nonspecific and suggestive of an acute viral illness. Leukopenia, thrombocytopenia, and transaminase elevations may be noted. The screening HIV EIA may be negative during the first several weeks of symptoms. Serum p24 HIV antigen, viral isolation from blood, and detection of viral sequence by the polymerase chain reaction are more sensitive but not widely available. If there is clinical suspicion of acute HIV infection, antibody testing should be repeated in 4–8 weeks. After resolution of the acute illness, most patients become asymptomatic for many months to years, but progressive immune dysfunction occurs at extremely variable rates. The treatment of acute HIV is supportive, and the role of anti-retroviral therapy remains to be defined.

HIV-Related Disease Presentation Among Women

Although studies of disease progression in women are limited, most investigations that match for socioeconomic status, risk group, and access to care demonstrate no significant difference in disease course. *Pneumocystis* pneumonia remains the leading AIDS-defining diagnosis in women, perhaps reflecting a decreased awareness of risk and lack of access to medical care. Otherwise, the risk of opportunistic infections does not seem to differ significantly between men and women. Kaposi's sarcoma, which is seen relatively frequently in homosexual men, is rarely reported in HIV-infected women.

Some authors have suggested that menstrual disorders occur more frequently in HIV-infected women. Severe ulcerative genital herpes occurs in both men and women with HIV. The clinical presentation and therapeutic response of pelvic inflammatory disease do not appear to be altered by HIV infection. Vaginal candidiasis may be particularly problematic. In fact, frequent infection in the absence of diabetes or concomitant antibiotic therapy or refractory *Candida* infection should prompt HIV screening.

Cervical neoplasia and cervical intraepithelial neoplasia (CIN) are more frequent in HIV-positive women with severe immunosuppression. In recognition of this association, the CDC included cervical neoplasia as a AIDS-defining diagnosis for surveillance purposes. Currently, the CDC recommends annual Pap smears for HIV-infected women. If inflammation is present, treatment should be initiated and the Pap smear repeated in 3 months. If it is then normal, the Pap smear should be repeated at 6-month intervals. If two Pap smears 6 months apart are normal, the examination may be repeated annually. If a squamous interstitial lesion is found, colposcopy should be considered.

Initial Evaluation of HIV-Infected Patients

During the first encounter with an HIV-infected individual, the clinician should provide counseling, discuss the natural history of HIV infection, stage the disease, initiate preventive care measures, and consider antiretroviral therapy and opportunistic infection prophylaxis. Many questions remain, particularly regarding the timing of antiretroviral therapy and the cost benefit, efficacy, and timing of some preventive interventions.

Rather than conceptualizing HIV infection as progressing in distinct stages, the infection should be viewed as a dynamic but progressive deterioration of immune function. Approximately 50% of patients progress to AIDS in 10 years, but the rate of progression in an individual patient is difficult to predict. A complete baseline medical history and physical examination may provide important clues regarding the stage of infection. Several clinical manifestations are indicators of HIV disease progression, including persistent fever, thrush, unexplained diarrhea, oral hairy leukoplakia, herpes zoster, and involuntary weight loss.

Once HIV infection is documented, the CD4+ count should be measured. This parameter correlates with HIV-related immune dysfunction and disease progression, guides medical management, and is one of the criteria for the CDC surveillance case definition of AIDS. CD4+ lymphocyte count determinations are marked by significant laboratory variability and influenced by concomitant illnesses. Therefore, any determination must be interpreted in the context of the clinical findings and repeated if the validity of the test is questioned.

Routine chemistry studies and blood cell counts serve as baseline values or as indicators of disease. Many patients have an elevated polyclonal gamma globulin level and an increased erythrocyte sedimentation rate. Testing the glucose-6-phosphate dehydrogenase level may be helpful since dapsone and certain sulfas, useful for the treatment and prophylaxis of *Pneumocystis carinii* pneumonia (PCP), is contraindicated in patients with low levels. (Table 4.7).

Additional evaluation should include the detection of other disease processes that occur in the patient's particular HIV risk group, as well as other infections that might recur with advancing immune dysfunction. These may include syphilis (rapid plasma reagin test or VDRL), or HBV, and HCV serology. A (5-TU) purified protein derivative (PPD) skin test with controls should be performed, along with a chest radiograph. A patient with a reactive PPD skin test (defined by induration greater than 5 mm in an

TABLE 4.7 Evaluation At the Time of Diagnosis

Medical history and examination
Complete blood count with differential
CD4 cell count
Routine chemistries (LFT, Cr), urinalysis
PPD ± controls
Syphilis serology (RPR or VDRL)
Hepatitis serology
Anti HCV
Anti HBcore—if positive HBsAg and anti-HBs
Toxoplasma IgG antibody
Glucose-6-phosphate dehydrogenase
Chest x-ray
Update vaccination, pneumovax, hepatitis B, *Haemophilus B*

HIV-positive individual) without evidence of active disease should receive 1 year of prophylaxis with isoniazid. *Toxoplasma* (IgG) serology identifies patients at risk of developing toxoplasmosis as their immune status deteriorates.

Besides updating any childhood immunizations, pneumococcal vaccine, hepatitis vaccine, and *Haemophilus* B vaccines should be considered.

Approach for Evaluation and Prevention of Opportunistic Infections Based on Stage of Infection

Once again, the CD4+ count in conjunction with the history and physical examination guides decisions regarding initiation of anti-retrovirals and prophylactic therapies, as outlined in Table 4.8. Individuals with a normal examination and a CD4+ count above 500/mm^3 warrant evaluation every 4–6 months. As symptoms develop or the CD4+ count drops into the 200–500/mm^3 range, more frequent evaluation may be warranted.

Since the introduction of prophylactic therapy for PCP, the incidence of PCP among patients with advanced HIV disease has dropped dramatically. Adults, including pregnant women, with a CD4 count below 200/mm^3 should receive chemoprophylaxis. Trimethoprim-sulfamethoxazole (TMP-SMZ), which provides protection against PCP and toxoplasmosis, as well as many bacterial infections, is the drug of choice. Multiple alternative agents are also available for PCP prophylaxis, as noted in Table 4.8. HIV-infected persons who have IgG antibodies to *Toxoplasma* and a CD4+ count below 100/mm^3 should receive prophylaxis. Again, TMP-SMZ is recommended, but alternatives are available if the patient cannot tolerate this regimen. Pyrimethamine-containing regimens should be avoided during pregnancy, however. Infants born to HIV-infected women with serologic evidence of toxoplasmosis should be evaluated for congenital toxoplasmosis.

Exposure to the ubiquitous *Mycobacterium avium* complex (MAC) organisms is difficult to avoid, and MAC infection is extremely common among HIV-infected individuals with CD4+ counts below 50/mm^3. Unfortunately, rifabutin, related to rifampin, provides only partial protection. Expense, potential drug interactions, and concerns related to the development of resistance are considerations.

Patients infected with HIV can take an active role in avoiding exposure to opportunistic pathogens (Table 4.9). Certainly, safe-sex precautions should be discussed, and

TABLE 4.8 Preventive Medicine in HIV-Infected Patients

Timing	Agent	Drug of First choice	Drug of Second choice
Diagnosis	*Strep. pneumoniae* *Haemophilus B* Hepatitis B Influenza Update childhood vaccinations	Vaccine Vaccine Vaccine Vaccine	
CD4+ 200–500	Consider antiretroviral therapy		
CD4+ <200	PCP	TMP-SMZ	Dapsone* aerosolized pentamidine
CD4+ <100	*Toxoplasma*†	TMP-SMZ	Dapsone plus pyrimethamine and leucovorin
CD4+ <50	MAC	Rifabutin	Clarithromycin Azithromycin

*Dapsone—patient should have normal glucose-6-phosphate dehydergenase.
†If patient is *Toxoplasma* seropositive.

continuously reviewed and assessed, to reduce the risk of further transmission of HIV and lessen exposure to other sexually transmitted (HBV, herpes simplex, human papilloma virus), as well as orally-anally transmitted agents (hepatitis A, giardia, cryptosporidium). In addition, the patient should be informed about the potential environmental and food-associated exposures listed in Table 4.9.

Reptiles, young farm animals, and young (<6 months of age) cats and dogs, particularly those with diarrhea, should be avoided to decreased exposure to *Cryptosporidium, Salmonella,* and *Campylobacter. Toxoplasma, Cryptosporidium,* and *Bartonella* (cat scratch–like organisms) remain potential risks for cat owners. Transmission may be reduced by changing the litter box daily, preferably by a nonpregnant, non-HIV-infected individual, or at least by good hand washing. Preferably, the cat should be kept indoors, not be fed raw or undercooked meat, not scratch or bite, not be flea infected, and not be allowed to lick any skin wounds on the patient. Gloves should be worn when cleaning aquariums, pools, or saunas to decrease the risk of *Mycobacterium marinum,* and hands should be washed following contact with soil. Chicken coops, bird roosts, caves, and excavation sites should be avoided to protect against exposure to *Cryptococcus,* as well as endemic fungal infections *(Histoplasma, Coccidiomyces).* Water obtained directly from lakes and rivers may harbor *Cryptosporidium* and *Giardia.* Even municipal water supplies may be contaminated with *Cryptosporidium.*

The relative risk of occupational exposures must be weighed in conjunction with financial, psychological, and social considerations. Health care workers, as well as workers in homeless shelters and correctional institutions, are at risk of exposure to tuberculosis. Good hygienic practices should be emphasized to child-care providers, who might be at increased risk for giardiasis, hepatitis A, and cryptosporidiosis. Animal contact poses a risk of bacterial, fungal, and parasitic infection.

TABLE 4.9 Potential Exposures to Opportunistic Pathogens

Exposure	Agent
Reptiles	*Salmonella*
Young animals	*Salmonella* *Cryptosporidium* *Campylobacter*
Cats	*Cryptosporidium* *Bartonella* *Salmonella* *Campylobacter* *Sporotrichosis* *Toxoplasma*
Hot dogs, cold cuts	*Listeria*
Raw eggs; unpasteurized milk; undercooked poultry, meat, seafood	*Salmonella*
Uncooked bivalve molluscs	HAV *Vibrio* *Salmonella*
Aquariums	*Mycobacterium marinum*
River, lake water	Cryptosporidium *Giardia*
Municipal water	*Cryptosporidium*
Undercooked meat; fruits, vegetables not rinsed	*Toxoplasma*

Antiretroviral Therapy

In the United States, early intervention with zidovudine in asymptomatic individuals has been widely, if not universally, advocated. This recommendation, however, has been questioned by the results of some recent studies. Decisions regarding the initiation of antiretroviral therapy and the acceptability of side effects as they may develop requires a partnership between the patient and the health care provider, and should be based on a frank, informative discussion.

Multiple drugs are now available, including reverse transcriptase inhibitors, zidovudine (Retrovir, AZT), didanosine (Videx, ddI), zalcitabine (Hivid, ddC), lamivudine (Epivir, 3TC), and stavudine (d4T), as well as a protease inhibitor (Inviraise). Due to the tremendous burden of HIV virus in infected individuals and the high mutation rate of HIV, resistance develops rapidly when single agents are used. Therefore, just as in certain antimicrobial therapies and cancer chemotherapy, the concept of combination or sequential therapy, which might provide synergy, is gaining acceptance.

Recommendations for HIV-Infected Pregnant Women

HIV infection does not greatly influence the birth weight, gestational age at delivery, incidence of hypertension, or complications such as abruption. Pregnancy does induce a relative state of immune compromise, with declines in CD4+ cell counts. Pregnancy may therefore accelerate the progression of HIV infection.

Several reports have suggested that cesarean section may reduce the risk of HIV infection of the neonate, presumably by decreasing exposure to infected blood and secretions. Surgery in an immune-compromised individual, however, may have inherent risks; thus, further studies are warranted.

A multicenter placebo-controlled trial demonstrated that zidovudine administered during pregnancy, labor, delivery, and then to the newborn decreased the risk of perinatal HIV transmission by approximately two-thirds. This therapy was well tolerated, causing only mild anemia in some infants, which resolved without intervention. The U.S. Food and Drug Administration and the U.S. Public Health Service subsequently approved and recommended zidovudine therapy. Women should be informed, however, that the long-term safety of this regimen remains to be defined.

Recommendations for Follow-Up of Infected Women and Perinatally Exposed Children

Children perinatally infected with HIV may develop rapidly progressive disease and AIDS by 24 months of age. As in adults, PCP is the most common opportunistic infection in HIV-infected infants and often strikes during the first 6 months of life. Since infants born to HIV-infected mothers acquire maternal antibody and will test antibody positive for up to 18 months of age, guidelines now suggest prophylaxis against PCP in all children born to HIV-infected mothers beginning at 4–6 weeks of age. Regular follow-up and prompt evaluation for other HIV-related illnesses, such as severe bacterial infections and tuberculosis, can decrease the need for hospitalization.

Ultimately, uninfected infants will lose maternal antibodies, while infected infants will remain seropositive. The presence of at least two positive assays, such as polymerase chain reaction, viral culture, and p24 antigen, may also help to identify HIV infection during infancy.

Conclusion

Viral hepatitis and HIV, which are most often contracted by young adults, affect the health of patients and their children. As professionals providing perinatal as well as primary care to many young women, obstetricians and gynecologists have an obligation to provide compassionate, effective counseling, testing, and treatment that has significant measurable impact.

BIBLIOGRAPHY

Hepatitis

Alter M, Mast E: The epidemiology of viral hepatitis in the United States. *Gastroenterol Clin North Am* 23:437–455, 1994.

Centers for Disease Control: Prevention of perinatal transmission of hepatitis B virus: Prenatal screening of all pregnant women for hepatitis B surface antigen. *MMWR* 37:341–351, 1988.

Centers for Disease Control: Hepatitis B control: A comprehensive strategy for eliminating transmission in the United States through universal childhood vaccination. *MMWR* 40:1–25, 1991.

Iwarson S, Norkrans G, Wesjstal R: Hepatitis C: Natural history of a unique infection. *Clin Infect Dis* 20:1361–1370, 1995.

Mishra L, Seeff L: Viral hepatitis, A through E, complicating pregnancy. *Gastroenterol Clin North Am* 21:873–887, 1992.

Neuschwander-Tetri BA: Common blood tests for liver disease: Which ones are useful. *Postgrad Med* 98:49–63, 1995.

Scott GR: The sexual transmission of hepatitis C virus. *Int J STD AIDS* 6:1–3, 1995.

Simms J, Duff P: Viral hepatitis in pregnancy. *Semin Perinatol* 17:384–393, 1993.

HIV and AIDS

Centers for Disease Control (CDC): 1993 revised classification system for HIV infection and expanded surveillance definition for AIDS among adolescents and adults. *MMWR* 41(No. RR-17), 1992.

CDC: Recommendations for HIV testing services for inpatients and outpatients in acute care hospital settings and technical guidance for HIV counseling. *MMWR* 42(No. RR-2), 1993.

CDC: Recommendations of the ACIP: Use of vaccines and immune globulins in persons with altered immunocompetence. *MMWR* 42(No. RR-4), 1993.

CDC: Recommendations of the USPHS Task Force on the use of zidovudine to reduce perinatal transmission of HIV. *MMWR* 43(No. RR-11), 1994.

CDC: 1994 revised classification system for human immunodeficiency virus infection in children less than 13 years of age. *MMWR* 42(No. RR-12), 1994.

CDC: USPHS recommendations for human immunodeficiency virus counseling and voluntary testing for pregnant women. *MMWR* 44(No. RR-7), 1995.

CDC: Update: AIDS among women—United States, 1994. *MMWR* 44:81–84, 1995.

CDC: USPHS/IDSA guidelines for the prevention of opportunistic infections in persons infected with human immunodeficiency virus: A summary. *MMWR* 44(No. RR-8), 1995.

CDC: Revised guidelines for prophylaxis against *Pneumocystis carinii* pneumonia for children infected with or perinatally exposed to human immunodeficiency virus. *MMWR* 44(No. RR-4), 1995.

Newell, et al: Caesarean section and risk of vertical transmission of HIV-1 infection. *Lancet* 343:1464–1467, 1994.

Ruff AJ: Breast milk, breast-feeding, and transmission of viruses to the neonate. *Semin Perinatol* 18:510–516, 1994.

Sande MA, Carpenter CCJ, Cobbs CG, et al: Antiretroviral therapy for adult HIV-infected patients: Recommendations from a state of the art conference. *JAMA* 270:2583–2589, 1993.

Ugen KE, et al: Diagnosis and prediction of pediatric HIV-1 infection and AIDS: Current status. *J Clin Lab Anal* 8:309–314, 1994.

Chapter 5

Primary Care Nutrition for Women

Maureen A. Murtaugh

Primary care obstetricians and gynecologists are in a unique position to improve the health of women. The most important nutrition objectives for primary care obstetricians and gynecologists are primary prevention of disease and identification of patients with nutrition-related problems. This chapter will discuss the importance of providing consistent health messages, nutrition in primary prevention, and methods for identification of nutrition-related problems among women.

EFFECTIVE NUTRITION MESSAGES

Communicating effective nutrition messages to patients has become more difficult given the current level of consumer interest in nutrition. Consumers receive nutrition messages from the government, the food industry, professional health-related volunteer organizations such as the American Heart Association and the American Diabetes Association, and special interest consumer groups. The credibility of nutrition messages is compromised not only by the competing interests of these groups but also by the evolution of messages as scientific knowledge advances.[1] The results include consumer confusion, skepticism, and the perception that the scientific community cannot make up its mind.

Effective health care messages, including nutrition messages, are translated into changes in behavior. Health communicators have learned that short, straightforward, positive statements focusing on one behavior are effective and that additional qualifiers should be resisted.[2] Therefore, for primary care providers and educators, the basis of nutrition messages must be consistent with that of the U.S. Department of Agriculture's food guide pyramid.[3] More specific messages can be related to the framework of the food guide pyramid to achieve consistency. For example, patients can be advised to reduce fat intake by choosing low-fat dairy and meat servings, as suggested by the food guide pyramid.[3]

DIETARY EFFECTS ON THE MENSTRUAL CYCLE

Nutrition for women deserves special consideration due to the effect of diet on sex hormone levels and the menstrual cycle. A recent detailed review[4] of this topic highlights our poor understanding of the mechanisms whereby diet affects the key hormones and thus regulation of the menstrual cycle. For instance, energy intake varies across the menstrual cycle, but we have little information about which specific macro- and micronutrient intakes are changed. Extreme alterations in body weight (overweight and underweight) reduce fertility, but the mediating mechanisms are unclear. Reduced dietary fat intake compared to higher fat intake in omnivores[5,6] and in meatless[7] or vegetarian diets[8] seem to increase the cycle length, particularly in the duration of menstruation and the follicular phases of the cycle. Clinical recommendations at this time are to investigate the dietary patterns of patients with irregular menstrual patterns and to refer patients for nutrition counseling to correct severe alterations in body weight or dietary patterns inconsistent with adequate nutrition. As scientists come to understand more clearly the relationship between dietary intake and hormonal status, our understanding of the role of sex hormones in chronic diseases in women may improve.

COMMON NUTRITION-RELATED PROBLEMS

Obesity

One of the most common and most problematic nutrition problems among women is overnutrition in the form of obesity. Obesity, an increase in body fat, differs from overweight, which is merely a body weight which exceeds an arbitrary standard. Accurate determination of body composition necessary to distinguish the two requires expensive and often time-consuming methods such as measurement of body density, use of bioelectric impedance, radioactive isotopes, or neutron activation analysis.[9]

Clinical Classification of Obesity For clinical purposes, several weight/height ratios are available for classification of body weight compared to ideal or reference standards. Body mass index (BMI) or Quetelet's index, which expresses weight relative to height (kg/m^2), is preferred, since it correlates well with body fat and is the least biased by height.[10] Using this tool (Fig. 5.1), the National Center for Health Statistics and the National Health and Nutrition Examination Survey III define desirable weight for women aged 20–65 as a BMI between 19.1 and 27.3 kg/m^2. A BMI greater than 27.3 kg/m^2 is considered overweight.[11] Some, however, suggest that this range of BMI is too high.

While BMI is useful in classifying obesity, it does not reflect the distribution of subcutaneous and intra-abdominal fat, whereas the waist-hip ratio does.[12] The waist and hip circumferences are measured midway between the lowest rib margin and the iliac crest and the point yielding the maximum circumference around the hips, respectively[13,14] and are expressed as a ratio. Ratios greater than 0.8 in women are associated with an increased risk of cardiovascular complications and death,[15] as well as an increase in the risk of diabetes, hypertension, and hyperlipidemia.[16]

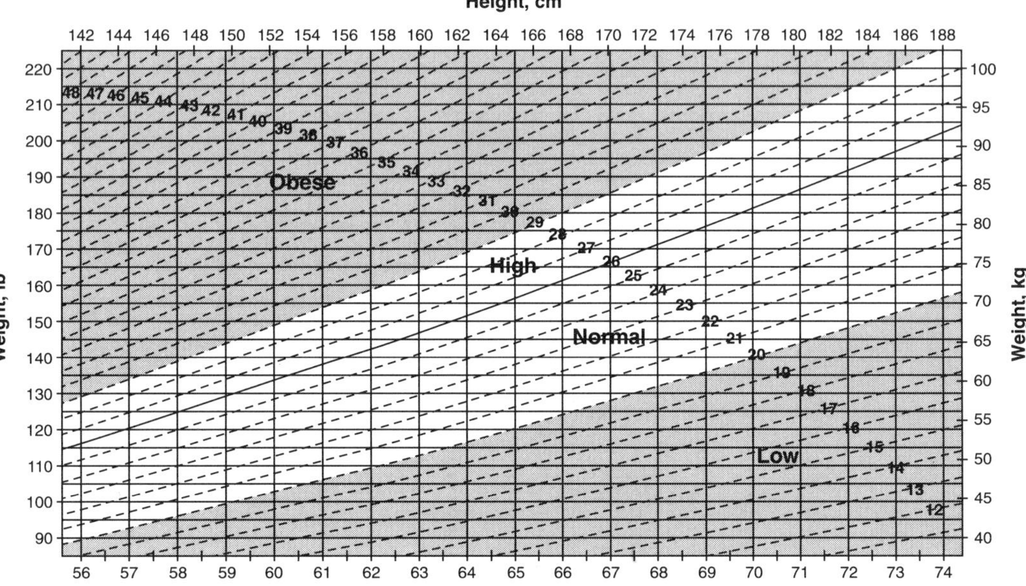

Figure 5.1 Chart for estimating body mass index (BMI) category and BMI. (Reprinted with permission from *Nutrition During Pregnancy and Lactation: An Implementation Guide*, National Academy Press, 1992.)

Directions

To find BMI category (e.g., obese), find the point where the woman's height and weight intersect. To estimate BMI, read the bold number on the dashed line that is closest to this point.

Incidence of Obesity Among Women in the United States The incidence of women who exceed the population's 85th percentile for BMI is rising.[17] Obesity among all women rose 8% (from 27% to 35%) between 1987 and 1992. Obesity rose from 15% to 21% in adolescents 12 to 19 years old despite the Healthy People 2000 goal to maintain the incidence of adolescent obesity at 15%.[17] In minority women aged 20 to 74, obesity has continued to rise to an estimated incidence of 48% in black women and 47% in Mexican American women. These rises occur despite the fact that 31–40% of women claim to be dieting on a given day of questioning.[18,19]

Health Risks of Obesity/Benefit of Weight Loss The rising incidence of obesity among women highlights the failure of the health care community in general in the primary prevention of obesity. This failure has led to the reevaluation of obesity and weight loss with respect to their health risks and benefits, respectively. The Nurses Health Study found that increasing body weight was directly and positively associated with an increase in all-cause mortality even after correction for smoking.[20] When BMI reached 27.0 kg/m^2, the risk of death due to coronary heart disease, other cardiovascular diseases, and cancer was increased. This study also suggested that young women with a BMI of 22.0 kg/m^2 or more at the age of 18 have the greatest increase in risk for cardiovascular disease. Similarly, a 10-kg weight gain from the age of 18 was associated with an increased risk of all-cause mortality. While these data from the Nurses Health Study may not be generalizable to all groups of women, they demonstrate that weight management is an integral component of primary prevention.

Health benefits can be realized through a weight loss equal to or greater than 10% of body weight.[21] Significant improvements have been identified in patients (both male and female) with non-insulin-dependent diabetes mellitus, hypertension, hypercholesterolemia, and cardiovascular disease with 10% weight losses.[21] Any weight loss which results in health improvement should be positively reinforced.

Treatment for Obesity

The high recidivism rate following weight loss programs is discouraging. The options range from diet, exercise, and pharmacologic agents to jaw wiring, behavior modification, and surgery. The most effective methods for weight loss appear to be long-term multidisciplinary intensive treatment programs including behavior modification and exercise coupled with diet.[22] Commercial programs are widely available, but their safety, efficacy, and long-term success are not well established. In 1992, the cost of weight loss ranged from none to $25.50/kg in the Boston area.[23] In general, one should encourage patients to seek counseling from qualified professionals who view weight loss as a lifelong issue which is best addressed through lifestyle modifications, such as diet and exercise. Individual energy needs are calculated to achieve a weight loss of 0.5 to 1.0 kg per week while meeting vitamin and mineral requirements and providing fewer than 30% of calories from fat.[24]

Heart Disease Among Women

Heart disease accounts for the death of 500,000 women per year, with half of those deaths due to coronary artery disease.[25] Additional dietary recommendations to reduce the risk of heart disease include reducing salt intake to 7.5 g/day (3 g Na), consuming fewer than two alcoholic drinks per day, and increasing the intake of complex carbohydrates from legumes and peas, grains, and fruits and vegetables.[26] Modification of dietary fat (less than 30% of total calories, less than 10% saturated fat) and cholesterol (less than 300 mg/day) is important in modifying the risk of heart disease, cancer, and diabetes.

Dietary Fat Intake The World Health Organization and Food and Agriculture Organization Joint Consultation on Fats and Oils in Human Nutrition have provided guidelines for fat intake which are appropriate for primary prevention of obesity, cardiovascular disease, and cancer.[27] In order to preserve fertility and optimize the fetal outcome, women of reproductive age should consume at least 20% of their calories as fat. For all women, fewer than 10% of total calories should come from saturated fat and 30% or less of their total energy from fat, particularly if a large proportion is derived from animal sources.

Osteoporosis

Women over the age of 45 are the segment of the population most commonly affected by osteoporosis. A diet providing adequate calcium and other nutrients is essential in preventing osteoporosis[28] and fractures due to osteoporosis.[29] Generally, women should consume sufficient calcium (RDA for females aged 11–24 years, 800 mg; for those over 24 years, 1200 mg; for pregnant women, 1200 mg[30]) by making high-calcium choices from the food guide pyramid. Dairy products are excellent and bioavailable sources of calcium, especially low-fat or skim milk and/or yogurt. Higher-fat dairy products are similar to lower-fat dairy products in calcium content (1 cup of skim milk has 296 mg calcium versus 288 mg calcium in 1 cup of whole milk), but lower-fat dairy products are superior choices due to the reduced saturated fat content. Other foods such as spinach, beet greens, and kidney beans are relatively rich in calcium but are also high in oxalates, phytates, or soluble fiber, which decrease the absorption of calcium.[31]

Women who cannot consume adequate calcium in their diet can take supplemental calcium with meals to enhance calcium absorption. Calcium as carbonate contains 40% calcium and is better absorbed than tricalcium phosphate, calcium citrate, or calcium gluconate; therefore, calcium carbonate is an appropriate choice for calcium supplementation of healthy women.[31] Supplement dietary calcium intake with amounts to increase the total intake to the RDA levels, up to 1 g daily. More details regarding calcium supplements, their safety, their availability, and medical conditions which influence the choice of calcium supplement are available in a recent review.[31]

Iron Deficiency Anemia in Women of Childbearing Age

The prevalence of iron deficiency anemia in women of childbearing age persists at 4–10%.[32] In an effort to prevent anemia, all women should be screened once between the ages of 15 and 25 years.[33] Screening at 2- to 3-year intervals is appropriate for individuals with risk factors for anemia such a high menstrual blood loss, high parity, or

TABLE 5.1 Cutoff Values for Identifying Anemia in Women

Nonpregnant Women	Hemoglobin (g/dL)*		Hematocrit (%)*
	White	Black	All Races
Nonsmokers	12.0	11.2	36
10–20 cigarettes/day	12.3	11.5	37
20–40 cigarettes/day	12.5	11.7	37.5

*Add 0.5 g/dL to hemoglobin and 1.5% to hematocrit for elevations above 5000 ft. (Reprinted with permission from *Iron Deficiency Anemia*. Copyright 1993 by the National Academy of Sciences. Courtesy of the National Academy Press.)

frequent blood donations. Screening laboratory results must be considered according to stage of menstruation, as indices of iron status are influenced by the phase of the menstrual cycle.[34] Hemoglobin (3 g/L) and ferritin (5 μg/L) levels drop from late luteal phase to menses.

Mild anemia, or hemoglobin and hematocrit or ferritin screening laboratory levels below recommended levels (Table 5.1) by no more than 2 g/dL should be treated with a therapeutic dose of 60 mg elemental iron twice daily, along with nutrition education.[33] Promote a varied diet (following the food pyramid guidelines) and recommend that patients avoid coffee and tea with meals to enhance iron absorption. Include meat and fruit juice or fruit, which are high in ascorbic acid, in meals.[33] An increase in hemoglobin (1 g/dL) and hematocrit (3%) should be evident in 4 to 6 weeks. Continue iron therapy until the hemoglobin reaches 12.0 g/dL. Then reduce the supplement to 30 mg daily for 6 months and check the ferritin level prior to terminating supplementation to document repleted stores.

If no hematologic response to iron supplementation occurs within 1 to 1.5 months despite compliance with the iron supplement regimen, check the ferritin level and consider other causes. It is important to recognize that severe anemia (more than 2 g/dL below recommended levels [Table 5.1] may not be due to iron deficiency. Physical, nutritional, and biochemical data should be considered to determine the cause of anemia. Serum ferritin levels are altered by inflammation and chronic disease. Therefore, results can be interpreted as follows: less than 15 μg confirms iron deficiency and 100 μg or more rules out iron deficiency; results between these levels mandate further workup.[35]

Iron Status and Supplementation in Postmenopausal Women Iron status and supplementation must be considered differently for women after menopause. After the childbearing years, the frequency of iron deficiency decreases and the possibility of iron overload increases.[36] For this reason, no iron supplements should be prescribed to postmenopausal women without checking their iron status.

Neural Tube Defects in Offspring

Women with inadequate folate stores are at greater risk of having children with congenital anomalies such as neural tube defects. The primary goal of prevention is to ensure adequate folate intake during embryonic neural tube closure, which may occur before pregnancy is confirmed (6 weeks after conception). Therefore, the U.S. Public

Health Service recommends that all women of childbearing age consume at least 0.4 mg/day of folate.[37] Researchers, however, indicate that the average American woman consumes only about 0.2 mg folate daily from food.[38] To ensure adequate dietary folate intake, encourage women to eat 3 to 5 servings of vegetables and 2 to 4 servings of fruit daily, with 6 to 11 servings of grains daily. Women's choices should include folate-rich foods such as raw green leafy vegetables (spinach, turnips, and mustard greens), citrus fruits (oranges), and fortified cereals and whole grains. It is important to note that raw leafy greens are high in folate but that heat destroys folate; losses can be as high as 50–90% during cooking.

Women of childbearing age who are unable to consume adequate dietary folate from foods should choose a multivitamin containing 0.4 mg folate. Higher levels are not recommended, as an upper limit of safety for total folate intake is 1.0 mg daily.[37] While hypersensitivity to folic acid is rare, susceptible individuals[39] may have fever, urticaria, erythema, and respiratory distress from oral doses ranging from 1 to 10 mg.[40] The secondary prevention strategy for women who have had a prior neural tube defect that affected pregnancy is a pharmacologic dose of 4.0 mg supplemental folate daily. In this setting, the risk of neural tube defect outweighs the concern about folic acid given in excess of 1 mg daily.[41]

IDENTIFYING PATIENTS AT RISK FOR MALNUTRITION

In healthy persons of ideal body weight, daily variations in weight are generally less than 0.5 kg.[14] However, in illness, negative nitrogen or energy balance often occurs with a loss of body weight. The cause for unintentional weight loss must be investigated and identified, but assessing the degree of unintentional weight loss is important. Death occurs at approximately 70% of usual body weight in total starvation and at approximately 50–60% of usual weight with chronic undernourishment. Criteria exist to distinguish significant and severe weight loss (Table 5.2). These criteria are useful for the identification of patients who might benefit from the use of oral, enteral, or parenteral nutrition. Patients identified as having significant weight loss in any care setting should be referred to a registered dietitian for medical nutrition therapy.

EATING DISORDERS

Eating disorders are gross disturbances in eating and include anorexia nervosa (anorexia), bulimia nervosa (bulimia), and eating disorders not otherwise specified (EDNOS).[42] Binge eating disorder, pica, and rumination disorder of infancy fall under the EDNOS category. Pica and rumination disorder of infancy are found primarily in children and are considered unrelated to anorexia and bulimia. Pica is occasionally identified in pregnant women who eat baking soda, baking powder, matches, ice, starch, or other nonnutritive substances. While some suggest that pica results from iron or some other micronutrient deficiency, objective evidence is not available to support this theory. The major focus in dealing with patients with pica is to rule out nutritional

TABLE 5.2 Criteria for Evaluating Clinically Significant Unintentional Weight Loss

Time	Significant Weight Loss (%)	Severe Weight Loss (%)
1 week	1–2	>2
1 month	5	>5
3 months	7.5	>7.5
6 months	10	>10

Source: Adapted with permission from Blackburn GL, Bistrain BR, Maini BS, et al: Nutritional and metabolic assessment of the hospitalized patient. *J Parent Ent Nutr* 1:11–22, 1977.

problems such as iron deficiency anemia and change the eating behavior. Anorexia and bulimia commonly present during adolescence or adulthood and predominate in middle- and upper-class women. This section will discuss how a primary care gynecologist can identify eating disorders.

Anorexia Nervosa

To date, the most plausible etiologic explanation for anorexia is that the clinical manifestations of several different illnesses are set off by the stress of the desire for autonomy and individualization or the development of sexuality.[43] Anorexia nervosa occurs in two forms. The first form is restricting-type behaviors, in which no binge eating or purging occurs. The second form is accompanied by regular binging, purging, or misuse of diuretics, laxatives, or enemas.[42] Patients with anorexia often refuse to disclose any problems related to being underweight, are preoccupied with food, and have an intense fear of becoming fat. The diagnostic criteria for anorexia (Table 5.3) include refusal to maintain body weight, disturbed perception of body weight, and obsessive-compulsive behavior. The disturbance in body shape perception can be either an unnatural influence of body weight or shape on self-evaluation or denial of the seriousness of underweight. Ask direct questions about fear of fat or body perception or use the Eating Attitudes Test, a psychological questionnaire, to help identify high-risk eating attitudes in patients.[44]

Although there are no specific tests for the diagnosis of anorexia, there are many physical symptoms, in addition to weight loss, which may accompany the disordered eating behaviors. A medical history of three consecutive missed menstrual periods in females past menarch is the fourth criterion for diagnosis. Patients complain about fullness, constipation, abdominal pain, insomnia, or feeling cold even on hot days.[45] Physical symptoms related to severe weight loss include dry skin and hair, cold hands and feet, generalized weakness, and nausea. A history of fractures may be caused by calcium depletion and/or low estrogen levels.

While biochemical tests are not included in the diagnostic criteria, laboratory testing identifies decreases in baseline thyroid-stimulating hormone, growth hormone, and prolactin. In addition, other hormonal abnormalities are sometimes found in patients with anorexia.[46] For instance, a drug screen for laxatives, diuretics, and drugs of abuse is helpful in identifying patients who have the binge/purge form of anorexia.

TABLE 5.3 DSM-IV Diagnostic Criteria for Anorexia Nervosa and Bulimia Nervosa

Anorexia Nervosa	Bulimia Nervosa
A. Refusal to maintain body weight at or above a minimally normal weight for age and height (e.g., weight loss leading to maintenance of body weight less than 85% of that expected, or failure to make expected weight gain during growth, leading to body weight less than 85% of that expected). B. Intense fear of gaining weight or becoming fat, even though underweight. C. Disturbance in the way in which one's body weight or shape is experienced, undue influence of body weight or shape on self-evaluation, or denial of the seriousness of the current low body weight. D. In postmenarchal females, amenorrhea, i.e., the absence of at least three consecutive menstrual cycles. (A woman is considered to have amenorrhea if her periods occur only following hormone, e.g., estrogen, administration.) *Specify* Type: **Restricting Type:** during the current episode of Anorexia Nervosa, the person has not regularly engaged in binge-eating or purging behavior (i.e., self-induced vomiting or the misuse of laxatives, diuretics, or enemas) **Binge-Eating/Purging Type:** during the current episode of Anorexia Nervosa, the person has regularly engaged in binge-eating or purging behavior (i.e., self-induced vomiting or the misuse of laxatives, diuretics, or enemas.	A. Recurrent episodes of binge eating. An episode of binge eating is characterized by both of the following: (1) eating, in a discrete period of time (e.g., within any 2-hour period), an amount of food that is definitely larger than most people would eat during a similar period of time and under similar circumstances (2) a sense of lack of control over eating during the episode (e.g., a feeling that one cannot stop eating or control what or how much one is eating) B. Recurrent inappropriate compensatory behavior in order to prevent weight gain, such as self-induced vomiting: misuse of laxatives, diuretics, enemas, or other medications; fasting or excessive exercise. C. The binge eating and inappropriate compensatory behaviors both occur, on average, at least twice a week for 3 months. D. Self-evaluation is influenced by body shape and weight. E. The disturbance does not occur exclusively during episodes of Anorexia Nervosa. *Specify* Type: **Purging Type:** during the current episode of Bulimia Nervosa, the person has regularly engaged in self-induced vomiting or the misuse of laxatives, diuretics, or enemas. **Nonpurging Type:** during the current episode of Bulimia Nervosa, the person has used other inappropriate compensatory behaviors, such as fasting or excessive exercise, but has not regularly engaged in self-induced vomiting or the misuse of laxatives, diuretics or enemas.

Bulimia Nervosa

Bulimia is similar to anorexia in onset, occurring in adolescence or early adulthood, with fear of overweight, preoccupation with dieting, restrictive eating or purging behavior, and distorted body image.[45] Bulimics may have low self-esteem, high anxiety levels, and communication problems; they characteristically lack self-control and discipline. Diagnostic criteria[42] differ from those for anorexia in recurrent episodes of eating large amounts of food in a 2-h period (amounts larger than most people could eat under similar circumstances) or a sense of lack of control during the eating episode.[47] The bulimic repeats inappropriate behaviors to prevent weight gain, such as self-induced vomiting, laxative and diuretic abuse, and enema use, for an average of twice a week for 3 months. Nonpurging bulimics use fasting or excessive exercise during the present episode of bulimia rather than the other compensatory behaviors.

The physical and medical profiles of bulimics differ from those of anorexics. Weight fluctuations of up to 9 kg per week may be observed.[48] The medical history may reveal depression; coexisting personality disorder; overweight in the past; excessive exercise, diuretic, or laxative use; or drug or alcohol abuse.[42] Useful tests to support the diagnosis include the Eating Attitude Test,[44] electrolyte levels, urine dipstick for ketones, protein and specific gravity, as well as a complete blood count. Advanced cases of bulimia are characterized by electrolyte abnormalities, elevated cholesterol levels, anemia, positive urine ketones and protein, and elevated urine specific gravity. Physical manifestations include lower esophageal tears, dental erosion, difficulty swallowing, and swollen salivary or parotid glands.

Eating Disorders Not Otherwise Specified

Eating behaviors of clinical significance but not meeting the specific criteria for anorexia or bulimia fall into the EDNOS category. For instance, women who meet the weight criteria for anorexia and the psychological profile, but who have not had three consecutive missed menstrual periods, fall into this category. Others who do not meet the criteria for the frequency or severity of bulimia also are considered to have EDNOS.

Binge Eating Disorder Binge eating disorder differs slightly from bulimia and is listed as a proposed diagnostic criteria in the appendix of DSM-IV.[42] *Binge eating disorder* is used by researchers to describe individuals who have regular binges, as defined by DSM-IV[42] under bulimia disorder (Table 5.3), but without the purging and other extreme behaviors designed to control body shape and weight.[49,50] These episodes are regular, occur over a period of at least 6 months, and appear as part of a more general tendency to overeat, compared to bulimia, in which strict attempts to diet occur.[51] The relationship between bulimia and binge eating disorder is not yet defined.

Referral for Eating Disorders

Denial by patients and their families often complicates the initiation of treatment for anorexia or bulimia. Discussion of the signs, symptoms, and laboratory findings may create an awareness of the disorder and acceptance of treatment.[52] Referral to a multidisciplinary team specializing in eating disorders is necessary for treatment. Centers for treatment can be located by contacting the American Anorexia/Bulimia Association in New York City or by obtaining the National Institutes of Health information on binge eating disorder.[52]

CONCLUSION

Primary care obstetricians and gynecologists have a great potential to influence women's health through nutrition and preventive care. A tremendous impact can be achieved by gathering and providing appropriate nutrition educational resources. Provide consistent messages along with written information. When issues extend beyond the normal nutrition guidelines, refer patients to licensed or registered dietitians. Qualified nutrition professionals can be located in your area by contacting your state's or city's dietetic association.

REFERENCES

1. Goldberg JP: Nutrition and health communication: The message and the media over half a century. *Nutr Rev* 50:71–77, 1992.
2. Neilson JL, Larson-Brown LB: College students' perception of nutrition messages: How motivating are they? *J Nutr Educ* 22:30–34, 1990.
3. U.S. Department of Agriculture Human Nutrition Information Service: *The Food Guide Pyramid.* Hyattsville, MD, U.S. Government Printing Office. 1992.
4. Tangney CC: Diet, the menstrual cycle, and sex steroid hormones. In Krummel D (ed): *Nutrition in Womens' Health.* Gaithersburg, MD, Aspen, 1995, p 141.
5. Jones DY, Judd JT, Taylor PR, et al: Influence of dietary fat on menstrual cycle and menses length. *Hum Nutr Clin Nutr* 47:341–345, 1987.
6. Reichmann ME, Judd JT, Taylor PR, et al: Effect of dietary fat on length of the follicular phase of the menstrual cycle in a controlled diet setting. *J Clin Endocrinol Metab* 74: 1171–1175, 1992.
7. Hill PB, Garbaczewski L, Haley N, et al: Diet and follicular development. *Am J Clin Nutr* 39:771–777, 1984.
8. Hill PB, Garbaczewski L, Daynes G, et al: Gonadotrophin release and meat consumption in vegetarian women. *Am J Clin Nutr* 43:37–41, 1986.
9. Heymsfield SB, Waki M: Body composition in humans: Advances in the development of multicompartment chemical models. *Nutr Rev* 49:97–108, 1991.
10. Garrow JS, Webster J: Quetelet's index (Wt/H^2) as a measure of fatness. *Int J Obes* 9: 147–153, 1985.
11. Kuzmarski RJ, Flegal KM, Campbell SM, et al: Increasing prevalence of overweight among U.S. adults. The National Health and Nutrition Examination Surveys, 1960 to 1991. *JAMA* 272:205–211, 1994.
12. Larsson B, Svardsudd K, Welin L, et al: Abdominal adipose tissue distribution, obesity and risk of cardiovascular disease and death: 13-year follow-up of participants in the study of men born in 1913. *Br Med J* 288:1401–1404, 1984.
13. Lohman TG, Roche AF, Martorell R: *Anthropometric Standardization Reference Manual.* Champaign, IL, Human Kinetics Books, 1988.
14. Gibson RS: *Nutritional Assessment. A Laboratory Manual.* New York, Oxford University Press, 1993.
15. Björntorp P: Regional patterns of fat distribution: *Ann Intern Med* 103:994–995, 1985.
16. Bray GA: Pathophysiology of obesity. *Am J Clin Nutr* 55:488S–494S, 1992.
17. U.S. Department of Health and Human Services: *Healthy People 2000 Review 1994.* Hyattsville, MD, Public Health Service. 1995, p 13.
18. Berg F: Who is dieting in the United States? *Obesity Health* 5:48–49, 1992.

19. Blackburn GL, Wilson GT, Kanders BS, et al: Weight cycling: The experience of human dieters. *Am J Clin Nutr* 49:1105–1109, 1989.

20. Manson JE, Willet WC, Stampfer MJ, et al: Body weight and mortality among women. *N Engl J Med* 333:677–685, 1995.

21. Goldstein D: Beneficial health effects of modest weight loss. *Int J Obes* 16:397–415, 1992.

22. Wing R: Obesity and weight gain during adulthood: A health program for United States women. *Women's Health Issues* 2:114–122, 1992.

23. Spielman AB, Kanders B, Kienholz BA, et al: The cost of losing: An analysis of commercial weight-loss programs in a metropolitan area. *J Am Coll Nutr* 11:36–41, 1992.

24. Zeman FJ: Disorders of energy balance and body weight. In Zeman FJ (ed): *Clinical Nutrition and Dietetics,* ed 2. New York, Macmillan, 1991, pp 470–516.

25. Legato MJ: Cardiovascular disease in women: What's different? What's new? What's unresolved? *Ann NY Acad Sci* 736:147–157, 1994.

26. Chait A, Brunzell JD, Denke MA, et al: Rationale of the diet-heart statement of the American Heart Association. Report of the nutrition committee. *Circulation* 88:3008–3029, 1993.

27. WHO and FAO joint consultation: Fats and oils in human nutrition. *Nutr Rev* 53:202–205, 1995.

28. Dawson-Hughes B, Dallal GE, Krall EA, et al: A controlled trial of the effect of calcium supplementation on bone density in postmenopausal women. *N Engl J Med* 323:878–883, 1990.

29. Chapuy MC, Arlot ME, Duboeuf F, et al: Vitamin D_3 and calcium to prevent hip fractures in elderly women. *N Engl J Med* 327:1637–1642, 1992.

30. Food and Nutrition Board: *Recommended Dietary Allowances,* ed 10. Washington, DC, National Academy of Sciences, 1989.

31. Levenson DI, Bockman RS: A review of calcium preparations. *Nutr Rev* 52:221–232, 1994.

32. Institute of Medicine: *Iron Deficiency Anemia. Recommended Guidelines for the Prevention, Detection, and Management Among U.S. Children and Women of Childbearing Age.* Washington, DC, National Academy Press, 1993.

33. Institute of Medicine. *Nutrition During Pregnancy. Report of the Committee on Nutrition during Pregnancy and Lactation, Food and Nutrition Board.* Washington, DC, National Academy Press, 1990, p 293.

34. Kim I, Yetley EA, Calvo MS: Variations in iron-status measures during the menstrual cycle. *Am J Clin Nutr* 58:705–709, 1993.

35. Guyatt GH, Oxman AD, Ali M, et al: Laboratory diagnosis of iron-deficiency anemia: An overview. *J Gen Intern Med* 7:145–153, 1992.

36. Edwards CQ, Griffen LM, Kushner JP: Disorders of excess iron. *Hosp Pract* 26(Suppl 3):30–36, 1991.

37. Centers for Disease Control: Use of folate for prevention of spina bifida and other neural tube defects 1983–1991. *MMWR* 40:513–516, 1991.

38. U.S. Department of Agriculture, Human Nutrition Information Service: *Nationwide Food Consumption Survey, Continuing Survey of Food Intakes by Individuals, Women 19–50, and Their Children 1–5 Years, 4 Days.* Washington, DC, 1988.

39. Zimmerman MB, Shane B: Supplemental folic acid. *Am J Clin Nutr* 58:127–128, 1993.

40. Sesin GP, Kirschenbaum H: Folic acid hypersensitivity and fever: A case report. *Am J Hosp Pharm* 36:1565–1567, 1979.

41. MRC Vitamin Study Research Group: Prevention of neural tube defects: Results of the Medical Research Council Vitamin Study. *Lancet* 338:132–137, 1991.

42. American Psychiatric Association: *Diagnostic and Statistical Manual of Mental Disorders,* Fourth Edition. Washington, DC, American Psychiatric Association. 1994, pp 544–550.

43. Slaby AE, Dwenger R: History of anorexia nervosa. In Giannini AJ, Slaby AE (eds): *The Eating Disorders.* New York, Springer Verlag, 1993, pp 1–17.

44. Button EJ, Whitehouse A: Subclinical anorexia nervosa. *Psychosomatic Med* 11:509–516, 1981.

45. de Pheils PB: Eating disorders: In Star W, Lommel LL, Shannon MT (eds): *Women's Primary Health Care: Protocols for Practice.* Washington, DC, American Nurses Publishing, 1995, pp 14.31–14.39.

46. Martin DM, Turner CE, Long BK: Clinical laboratory aspects of eating. In Giannini AJ, Slaby AE (eds): *The Eating Disorders.* New York, Springer Verlag, 1993, pp 76–92.

47. American Psychiatric Association: *Diagnostic and Statistical Manual of Mental Disorders,* Fourth Edition. Washington, DC, American Psychiatric Association, 1994, pp 549–550.

48. Yates AJ, Sambrailo F: Bulimia nervosa: A description and therapeutic study. *Behav Res Ther* 22:503–577, 1984.

49. Spitzer RL, Devlin MJ, Walsh BT, et al: Binge eating disorder: To be or not to be in DSM-IV? *Int J Eat Disord* 10:627–629, 1991.

50. Spitzer RL, Devline M, Walsh BT, et al: Binge eating disorder: A multisite field trial of the diagnostic criteria. *Int J Eat Disord* 11:191–203, 1992.

51. Fairburn CG, Walsh BT: Atypical eating disorders. In Brownell KD, Fairburn CG (eds): *Eating Disorders and Obesity. A Comprehensive Handbook.* New York, Guilford Press, 1995, pp 135–140.

52. Powers P: Anorexia nervosa: Evaluation and treatment. *Neuropsych Comp Ther* 16:24–34, 1994.

Chapter 6

Rheumatic and Autoimmune Disorders

Elise Belilos
Steven E. Carsons

ARTHRITIS

Rheumatoid Arthritis

Rheumatoid arthritis (RA) is the most common chronic inflammatory joint disease affecting young and middle-aged women.[1] Although its most prominent feature is joint deformity, RA is also a systemic disease and may be accompanied by fever, weight loss, adenopathy, and extra-articular manifestations. The onset of RA usually occurs between the ages of 35 and 55; however, it may also occur in elderly persons and children. RA affects women approximately three times more often than men. The first symptoms of RA usually are pain and stiffness affecting the small joints of the hands, wrists, and feet. The knees, ankles, and elbows frequently are involved as well. The pattern of joint involvement is classically symmetrical, but exceptions, especially in early disease, are common. The onset is most often insidious, with pain, stiffness, and the number of involved joints increasing over weeks to months. Occasionally, however, RA presents as an explosive polyarthritis with disabling consequences. Early morning stiffness is characteristic of RA, as is the return of stiffness following sitting for a prolonged period of time. The long-term course of RA is punctuated with disease flares and partial remissions overlying a chronic course. On occasion, the disease may remit spontaneously or show a nearly complete response to antirheumatic therapy. In many cases, pregnancy has an ameliorative effect on RA. Approximately one-third of RA patients experience a significant reduction in their disease during gestation due to a combination of immunogenetic, hormonal, and anti-inflammatory mechanisms.[2]

RA may be complicated by a spectrum of extra-articular manifestations including ocular involvement (scleritis, sicca syndrome), cardiopulmonary involvement (nodules, pleuritis, pericarditis), neuropathy, vasculitis, and subcutaneous nodules. Subluxation of the atlantoaxial joint in the cervical spine may lead to cord compression and severe neurologic impairment including paraplegia. RA patients scheduled for surgery with general anesthesia should undergo radiologic evaluation for atlantoaxial subluxation.

Differential Diagnosis The differential diagnosis of RA includes other causes of chronic inflammatory polyarthritis. These conditions will now be discussed.

Spondyloarthropathies: The spondyloarthropathies are a group of disorders linked by a common genetic predisposition (HLA-B27) and spinal involvement (sacroiliitis and spinal ankylosis).[3] Spondyloarthropathies include ankylosing spondylitis, reactive arthritis (Reiter's syndrome), psoriatic arthritis, and the arthritis of inflammatory bowel disease. In addition to the predilection for spinal involvement, the spondyloarthropathies are generally more asymmetrical and involve the lower extremities to a greater extent than does RA.

Polymyalgia Rheumatica: Polymyalgia rheumatica (PMR) is a disorder of older individuals involving progressive stiffness of the cervical spine, shoulder and hip girdles.[4] Patients are generally 55 years of age or older and are most often older than 65. The erythrocyte sedimentation rate is almost always elevated and may reach levels as high as 75–100 mm/hr. Mild synovitis of the shoulders and wrists may be seen. Approximately 20% of patients with PMR develop temporal arteritis (TA), manifested by headache, scalp tenderness, and difficulty chewing solid food (jaw claudication). Sudden visual loss may occur due to occlusion of the ophthalmic branch. Elderly patients with chronic headache should be evaluated for possible TA. PMR and TA are treated with corticosteroids; however, the doses are significantly different. PMR generally responds dramatically to low doses (10–15 mg of prednisone per day), whereas TA requires higher doses (40–80 mg) for 1 month prior to tapering.

Crystalline Arthritis: Occasionally, patients with long-standing crystalline-induced arthritis have joint disease that may resemble RA. Acute crystalline arthritis (gout and calcium pyrophosphate disease [CPPD]) usually begins with a monoarthritis. In cases of long-standing disease, however, many joints may become involved, including the wrists, hands, and knees. In some instances, the involvement may be quite symmetrical and may resemble RA. Gout is more common in older men, especially those who are obese, hypertensive and have abused ethanol.[5] CPPD (pseudogout) is more common in older women with preexisting osteoarthritis.[6] The finding of crystals in a synovial fluid aspirate is diagnostic.

Septic Arthritis: Septic arthritis most commonly presents as a monoarthritis.[7] The most common organisms in adults are gram-positive cocci. The affected joint is usually acutely painful, erythematous, and warm. Often the patient is febrile. The knee, hip, elbow, and wrist are most often involved. Bursae adjacent to the knee (prepatellar) and the elbow (olecranon) also may become infected due to cutaneous abrasions at pressure points. In some cases, the presentation of septic arthritis may be atypical. Elderly and immunosuppressed patients (patients with malignancy, diabetes, human immunodeficiency virus, renal insufficiency, or taking immunosuppressive medications including corticosteroids) may not display a typical inflammatory response. Fever, leukocytosis, and local inflammation may be diminished or absent. Patients with preexisting rheumatic diseases such as RA and patients with joint prostheses are at increased risk of developing a septic joint or may develop an infection with an unusual organism. Therefore, patients with chronic polyarthritis who develop apparent monoarticular flares should be evaluated for a possible septic joint. Arthrocentesis with synovial fluid white blood cell count and differential, Gram stain, and culture and sensitivity should be performed. Patients with disseminated gonococcal infection (DGI) are usually younger and sexually active. The arthritis of DGI may be polyarticular, often involving the wrists and knees. On careful inspection, wrist involvement is often found to be secondary to a tenosynovitis. Other features include cutaneous pustule, fever, and symptomatic genital infection. Women have a higher risk of developing DGI while pregnant or during menses. Treatment of septic arthritis consists of a course of intravenous antibiotics and joint drainage. The latter can be accomplished by repetitive needle drainage or may require arthroscopic or open debridement.

Lyme Disease: Lyme disease is associated with characteristic musculoskeletal symptoms.[8] In early Lyme disease, myalgias and arthralgias (often resembling flue-like symptoms) occur together with the rash of erythema chronicum migrans (ECM). At this time, fever, chills, anorexia, and headache are also common. In late disease, a variety of musculoskeletal manifestations can be seen. Approximately 50% of untreated patients develop a transient and migratory pain syndrome involving the axial and appendicular skeleton. Peripheral manifestations include pain in joints, bursae, tendons, entheses, and muscles. The affected area is painful on motion, but there is little objective evidence of joint swelling. In 60% of untreated patients with ECM, this syndrome progresses to a transient arthritis within several months. This arthritis is monoarticular or oligoarticular and commonly involves the knee, shoulder, ankle, elbow, temporomandibular joint, wrist, and hip. Episodes commonly last for a few months and intervals between episodes become shorter as time goes on. Ten percent of patients with untreated ECM develop chronic arthritis within 4 years. The mean time of onset is approximately 1 year from the development of ECM.

Treatment The treatment of RA begins with aspirin and nonsteroidal anti-inflammatory agent therapy (see the section on osteoarthritis). Usually, this results in symptomatic relief, but generally it does not alter the course of the illness. In most instances, patients require disease-modifying antirheumatic drugs (DMARDs) to significantly control disease activity. DMARDs are generally derived from two main pharmacologic categories: antimicrobials and antineoplastics. Gold, the first drug used as a long-term disease-modifying agent, was initially developed as an antimycobacterial drug. It is available in an injectable form, given weekly at first and then as a monthly maintenance injection, and in oral form administered daily. Other DMARDs in common use which also have antimicrobial properties are hydroxychloroquine (Plaquenil), sulfasalazine (Azulfidine), and minocycline (Minocin). Among the antineoplastic agents used to treat RA, methotrexate has achieved the widest use and currently is the most commonly prescribed DMARD. Methotrexate is given orally once a week, starting at 7.5 mg, with doses increasing to 25 mg/week if necessary. Patients are monitored for the development of macrocytic anemia, thrombocytopenia, leukopenia, and transaminase elevations. Other antineoplastics that have been used to treat refractory RA are azathioprine

(Imuran), chlorambucil (Leukeran), and cyclophosphamide (Cytoxan). The immunosuppressive agent cyclosporine A has also been used to treat refractory RA.

Osteoarthritis and Soft Tissue Rheumatic Disorders

Osteoarthritis (OA) is generally regarded as the most prevalent rheumatic disease affecting the geriatric population; however, adults of all ages may be affected. It is useful to think of OA as not just one disease but as having three major subgroups based on the type of joint involved. OA commonly involves the small joint of the hands, the weight-bearing joints of the lower extremity (hips and knees), and the spine. The distribution of OA of the hands is characteristic, with proximal and distal interphalangeal involvement resulting in the formation of Bouchard's and Heberden's nodes, respectively. The carpometacarpal joint at the base of the thumb also is commonly involved, especially in individuals who work with their hands. Hand OA appears to be familial and affects several generations, usually with a female predominance. In such families, symptoms may first appear at an early age (late 20s or early 30s). Occasionally, these joints can become quite inflamed, resulting in an erythematous appearance. This condition is often referred to as *erosive osteoarthritis.* OA of the weight-bearing joints usually occurs later in life unless there is an underlying congenital or posttraumatic abnormality of the hips or knees. Obesity is an important risk factor for the development of hip and knee OA. Spinal OA usually involves the lower segments of the cervical (C5-C8) and lumbar (L4-S1) spine. The term *spinal osteoarthritis,* as usually used clinically, encompasses degenerative disease of the intervertebral disc space and the facet joints. Either can be a cause of chronic low back pain. In younger individuals, management of low back pain should include weight loss, posture training, and exercise. Physical therapy, along with judicious use of muscle relaxant and anti-inflammatory medication, may be warranted.[9] In older individuals, other organic diseases such as osteoporosis, with resultant fracture, tumor, infection, and referred visceral pain, must be excluded as potential causes of back pain. Plain films of the spine and basic laboratory studies including a complete blood count, erythrocyte sedimentation rate, urinalysis, and chemistries including calcium, total protein, and alkaline phosphatase, constitute a cost effective screening workup.

Fibromyalgia and Soft Tissue Rheumatism

Soft tissue rheumatic disorders constitute a heterogeneous group of syndromes resulting in musculoskeletal pain in the absence of true joint inflammation. Bursitis and tendinitis are common following overuse secondary to occupational, recreational, or chronic pressure. Local injection of corticosteroids is often the most effective means of treating these disorders. Table 6.1 lists the most common forms of bursitis/tendinitis and the usual approach for local steroid therapy. An extremely common cause of nonarticular musculoskeletal pain is fibromyalgia (FM) (fibrositis).[10] This condition usually affects young and middle-aged women and presents as a diffuse pain syndrome accompanied by fatigue. Sleep is usually poor or disturbed, and the onset of FM may follow an illness such as a severe viral syndrome or emotional trauma. FM may coexist with the irritable bowel syndrome, migraine headaches, and Raynaud's-like symptoms. Diagnosis depends on the exclusion of other systemic rheumatic disorders and

TABLE 6.1 Common Forms of Bursitis and Tendinitis

Region	Disorder	Approach for Injection Therapy
Shoulder	Subacromial bursitis/supraspinatus tendinitis	Subdeltoid bursa
Shoulder	Bicipital tendinitis	Biceps tendon sheath
Elbow	Epicondylitis (tennis and golfer elbow)	Lateral or medial epicondylar soft tissue
Wrist	DeQuervain's tendinitis	Radial styloid tendon sheath
Hip	Trochanteric bursitis	Greater trochanter of the femur
	Ischial bursitis	Sacroiliac area
Knee	Pes anserinus bursitis	Medial condylar soft tissue
Foot	Plantar fasciitis	Calcaneal soft tissue

the demonstration on exam of characteristic soft tissue trigger points at the cervical, trapezial, scapular, epicondylar, gluteal, trochanteric, and anserine regions. The treatment of FM relies on the administration of low doses of tricyclic antidepressants or muscle relaxants, usually in the evening. Exercise is also very useful in motivated patients.

Nonsteroidal Anti-Inflammatory Drug Therapy

Nonsteroidal anti-inflammatory agents (NSAIDs) are the mainstay of treatment for OA and related soft tissue inflammatory conditions. Nearly two dozen NSAIDs are available for routine clinical use; the basic principles of prescribing anti-inflammatory therapy apply to all of these agents. To achieve sustained anti-inflammatory action, medications should be given on a consistent basis for multiple half-lives (usually several days). To minimize gastrointestinal (GI) toxicity, NSAIDs should always be given with food. For patients at higher risk for GI complications (prior ulcer or GI bleed; frail elderly patients; or those with multiple medical problems), prophylaxis with misoprostol (Cytotec) should be considered. NSAIDs may blunt the antihypertensive response to blood pressure–lowering drugs and may cause fluid and potassium retention. NSAIDs may also exacerbate bronchospasm in susceptible patients. Aspirin and other NSAIDs should be discontinued approximately 1 week prior to surgery to avoid bleeding problems. For the patient in whom chronic NSAID therapy may be hazardous, simple analgesics (acetaminophen, proproxyphene, codeine, tramadol) or the use of NSAID on a prn basis alone provides alternative treatment strategies.

AUTOIMMUNE CONNECTIVE TISSUE DISEASES

Systemic Lupus Erythematosus

Systemic lupus erythematosus (SLE) is an autoimmune disorder which can affect many different organ systems and is associated with the presence of multiple autoantibodies. SLE most commonly occurs in young and middle-aged women, with a female:male ratio between 8:1 and 15:1.[11] SLE more commonly affects African-Americans and

TABLE 6.2 Important Clinical and Laboratory Features of SLE

Cutaneous involvement
Photosensitivity
Malar rash
Discoid lesions
Oral ulcers
Serositis
Pleurisy
Pericarditis
Abdominal serositis
Arthritis
Hematologic involvement
Leukopenia
Thrombocytopenia
Hemolytic anemia
Renal disease
Proteinuria
CNS disease
Seizures, psychosis, other conditions
Serologic abnormalities
ANA
Anti-DS-DNA antibodies
Anti-Smith antibodies
Hypocomplementemia (↓ C3, C4)
Biologic false-positive test for syphilis

Asians than Caucasians or Hispanics.[11] The presentation of SLE can be quite variable, and diagnosis can sometimes be difficult. The diagnosis of SLE should be based on a combination of clinical signs and symptoms, as well as laboratory findings (see Table 6.2).

Cutaneous manifestations are common and include photosensitivity, malar (butterfly) rash, discoid lupus (DLE), and subacute cutaneous lupus (SCLE). Malar erythema occurs on the cheeks and over the bridge of the nose, characteristically sparing the nasolabial folds. DLE lesions tend to scar and typically occur on the face, scalp, and extremities; they are characterized by scaling, central atrophy, and follicular plugging. Vasculitic lesions and digital ulcerations may also occur, especially in patients who are systemically ill. In addition to vasculitis, severe Raynaud's phenomenon and the antiphospholipid syndrome can contribute to nonhealing digital ulcers. Livedo reticularis is also often associated with the antiphospholipid syndrome and appears as a lacy, mottled rash generally seen on the extremities.

Serositis and mucosal lesions are common in SLE. Patients should be carefully examined for the presence of oral and nasal ulcerations, as these lesions tend to be painless and may be overlooked by the patient. Pleurisy and pericarditis are common in SLE, but pericardial tamponade is rare. Abdominal serositis may mimic an acute abdomen and should always be considered in a patient with SLE and abdominal or pelvic pain.

The arthritis of SLE may mimic that of RA. It is a symmetrical polyarthritis which occurs in a distribution similar to that of RA, including the small joints of the hands (especially the metacarpophalangeal and proximal interphalangeal joints) and wrists. Like RA, it is generally characterized by prominent morning stiffness and gelling, as well as swelling, warmth, and erythema of the joints. In contrast to the fixed deformities seen in RA, the deformities seen in SLE (such as Jaccoud's arthropathy) are generally reducible. Another important distinguishing feature is that the arthritis of SLE is generally non-erosive.

Patients with SLE often have systemic features such as fever, weight loss, fatigue, lymphadenopathy, and hepatosplenomegaly. Raynaud's phenomenon (triphasic color change in response to cold) and alopecia are not specific but occur in many patients with SLE.

More serious manifestations of SLE include hematologic involvement, manifested as leukopenia (especially lymphopenia), thrombocytopenia, or hemolytic anemia. It is important to rule out medication-induced hematologic abnormalities in SLE patients before attributing these conditions to the patient's underlying disease, since many of the agents used to treat SLE can cause bone marrow suppression.

Lupus Nephritis Nephritis is a major cause of morbidity and mortality in patients with SLE. Patients may present with hypertension, peripheral edema, proteinuria, and urinary sediment abnormalities (casts, red and white blood cells). Patients may develop renal insufficiency later in their disease course. Hypocomplementemia and high-titer anti-dsDNA antibodies have been associated with the development of significant renal disease and may correlate with disease activity in individual patients. A variety of renal lesions can occur in SLE; renal biopsy findings can be categorized by the World Health Organization classification system as class I through V. The most worrisome renal lesion is class IV lupus nephritis (diffuse proliferative glomerulonephritis); aggressive therapy with cyclophosphamide and high-dose corticosteroids is indicated for this lesion.[12]

Central Nervous System Lupus Classically, seizures and psychosis have been described as the major central nervous system (CNS) manifestations of SLE. However, it is becoming increasingly clear that a variety of neurologic abnormalities occur in patients with SLE, including headache, depression, and aseptic meningitis. Stroke and transverse myelitis are CNS manifestations that are strongly associated with the antiphospholipid syndrome (see below). In patients with diffuse cerebral disease or meningeal signs, it is extremely important to rule out infection, especially since many patients with SLE are taking potent immunosuppressive medications. Side effects of the medications used should also be considered as cause of CNS dysfunction, for example, steroid psychosis. In SLE patients, aseptic meningitis (manifested by headaches and stiff neck) may be precipitated by NSAID use.

Lab Testing for SLE Serologic testing should be used to confirm the clinical suspicion of SLE. The antinuclear antibody (ANA) is a useful screening test, since more than 95% of patients with SLE will have a positive ANA. The major limitation of the ANA is its lack of specificity. A positive ANA may be seen in many other connective tissue diseases, organ-specific autoimmunity (e.g., thyroiditis, pulmonary fibrosis, chronic hepatitis), chronic infections (e.g., subacute bacterial endocarditis [SBE], Epstein-Barr virus [EBV], human immunodeficiency virus [HIV]), aging, malignancy, and with the use of certain medications (see below). Antibodies such as anti-dsDNA and anti-Smith antibodies are specific for the diagnosis of SLE but are present in only 50% and 30–40% of cases, respectively.[11] A biologic false-positive test for syphilis can also be seen in SLE and should prompt an investigation for an associated antiphospholipid syndrome (see below).

Differential Diagnosis of SLE When arthritis is the major manifestation of SLE, confusion with RA can occur. In addition, some patients with RA may have a positive ANA. As mentioned above, several features of SLE arthritis can help distinguish it from RA. In addition, a careful review of systems will often reveal other manifestations suggestive of SLE and should lead the examiner to obtain further serologic tests. Anti-dsDNA and anti-Smith antibodies, if present, can be very helpful in establishing the diagnosis, since they are highly specific for SLE.

Fibromyalgia may be confused with SLE, especially in patients with a variety of nonspecific complaints who are incidentally found to have a low positive ANA. FM is a soft tissue pain syndrome (see above) which is extremely common in young and middle-aged women. Thus, it occurs with an age and sex distribution similar to that of SLE.

Because of their multisystem involvement and their tendency to have false-positive serologies (i.e., ANA), several *infections* (most notably SBE, EBV, and occasionally HIV) can mimic SLE.

Certain *medications* can induce a syndrome which is indistinguishable from SLE. The drugs most commonly implicated are procainamide, hydralazine, methyldopa, chlorpromazine, isoniazid, and anticonvulsants. Drug-induced lupus is generally characterized by fever, arthritis, and serositis; renal and CNS diseases are distinctly absent. Anti-histone antibodies are seen in the majority of patients with drug-induced lupus (>90%), but they may also be seen in some patients with native SLE.

Treatment of SLE The treatment of SLE should begin with patient education. Reassurance that a wide spectrum of clinical disease occurs, and that not everyone with SLE has life-threatening disease, helps the patient adjust to the diagnosis. Patients should be instructed to avoid excessive sun exposure, wear a potent suncreen, and wear wide-brimmed hats when necessary. Medical management of SLE depends on the specific manifestations and should be individualized for each patient.[13] Arthritis, serositis, and constitutional symptoms can be treated with NSAIDs or antimalarials (hydroxychloroquine). Many of the cutaneous manifestations of SLE also respond well to treatment with hydroxychloroquine. Topical corticosteroid preparations are a useful adjunct in treating skin disease. Systemic corticosteroids are used in two ways in SLE.[14] First, low-dose steroids (prednisone, <10 mg/day) are used to treat arthritis, serositis, and constitutional symptoms that are unresponsive to treatment with NSAIDs or hydroxychloroquine. Second, high-dose steroids (prednisone, 1–2 mg/kg/day) are used to treat major organ involvement or life-threatening diseases including nephritis, cerebritis, and systemic vasculitis. The use of steroids is associated with many potential side effects, including hypertension, hyperglycemia, weight gain, osteoporosis, infection, and avascular necrosis. Patients with major organ involvement generally require additional immunosuppressive therapy; azathioprine (Imuran) and intravenous pulse cyclophosphamide (Cytoxan) have been used extensively to treat SLE. As mentioned above, intravenous pulse cyclophosphamide in combination with high-dose steroids is the treatment of choice for diffuse proliferative glomerulonephritis.[12] Azathioprine and cyclophosphamide are potent immunosuppressive therapies and should be given only by physicians experienced in their use. Both agents may be associated with significant bone marrow suppression and the risk of serious infection and may lead to an increased risk of subsequent malignancy. Cyclophosphamide is also associated with a significant risk of ovarian failure, an issue of obvious concern, since SLE is a disease which most commonly occurs in women of childbearing age.

SLE and Pregnancy SLE may flare during pregnancy and in the postpartum period. In addition, patients with SLE have a higher risk of miscarriage and of premature delivery.[15] Despite these problems, many women with SLE have successful pregnancies and, in general, lupus patients who desire pregnancy should not be discouraged. However, several important issues need to be considered before pregnancy is planned. Patients with SLE should be counseled that the timing of their pregnancy is critical. The optimal time for pregnancy is when their disease is completely quiescent; the absence of active renal disease is particularly important. Women with SLE who desire pregnancy should be screened for the presence of anti-SSA and SSB antibodies, which have been associated with the neonatal lupus syndrome including congenital heart block. However, even the presence of these autoantibodies does not preclude pregnancy, since less than 10% of mothers who are SSA/SSB positive will have infants who develop congenital heart block.[16] Patients should also be screened for an associated antiphospholipid syndrome (see below) because of the increased risk of spontaneous abortion.

The Antiphospholipid Syndrome (Anticardiolipin Syndrome; Lupus Anticoagulant Syndrome)

The antiphospholipid (APL) syndrome can occur in association with SLE or other autoimmune diseases (secondary APL). However, it should be emphasized that the APL syndrome also occurs commonly in the absence of any other systemic disease (primary APL). The APL syndrome is characterized by the presence of an antibody that inhibits coagulation in vitro (circulating anticoagulant) and thus prolongs phospholipid-dependent tests of coagulation (such as the partial thromboplastin time [PTT]). Paradoxically, this is associated with thrombotic events in vivo such as recurrent venous and/or arterial thromboses (including stroke and myocardial infarction in young individuals). In addition to thromboses, the APL syndrome is characterized by recurrent spontaneous miscarriages (especially in the second and third trimesters), thrombocytopenia, migraine headaches, and livedo reticularis. In addition, Libman-Sacks endocarditis and chorea may occur, but less commonly. Patients with the APL syndrome may have a variably positive ANA (usually in low titer). In this syndrome, a positive ANA alone (in the absence of signs or symptoms of lupus) does not necessarily indicate that the patient has underlying SLE.

Several laboratory tests are available to evaluate patients for suspected APL syndrome. Since only one or any combination of tests may be positive in an individual patient, those suspected of having this syndrome should be screened using multiple tests. An adequate laboratory evaluation for this syndrome includes a PTT, a lupus anticoagulant (or dilute Russel viper venom time, dRVVT), a (VDRL), and anticardiolipin antibodies. A numerical platelet count should also be measured in all patients. A biologic false-positive test for syphilis can be seen in the APL syndrome, i.e., a positive VDRL or rapid plasma reagin test with a negative fluorescent treponemal antibody. In patients with the lupus anticoagulant, the addition of normal plasma does not correct the PTT.

Treatment of the APL syndrome depends on the specific manifestations in individual patients. For example, patients who are incidentally found to have a circulating lupus anticoagulant or anticardiolipin antibodies in the absence of recurrent thromboses or spontaneous abortions need not be treated. By contrast, patients who have had recurrent thrombotic events associated with high-titer anticardiolipin antibodies or a lupus anticoagulant are candidates for lifelong anticoagulation, generally with coumadin. During pregnancy, the management of the APL syndrome is complex and depends on the individual patient's medical and obstetric history.[17] In general, patients who are incidentally found to have anticardiolipin antibodies or a lupus anticoagulant, and who have not had previous thrombotic events or pregnancy loss, may be either observed or treated with a baby aspirin per day. Patients with a history of prior miscarriage (especially second- and third-trimester miscarriages) are generally treated with a combination of low-dose aspirin and subcutaneous heparin. A combination of prednisone and low-dose aspirin has also been used, but this may be associated with increased maternal morbidity. In general, the use of steroids in this syndrome is reserved for significant thrombocytopenia or associated SLE activity.

Other Autoimmune/Connective Tissue Diseases

Sjögren's Syndrome Sjögren's syndrome is an autoimmune disease which occurs more commonly in women and is characterized by lymphocytic infiltration into glandular tissue and the production of autoantibodies. It may occur as a primary syndrome or in association with another autoimmune disease, most commonly RA. Infiltration of the salivary glands leads to parotid swelling and symptoms of xerostomia (dry mouth). Patients may also report a sudden increase in dental caries or a history of oral candidiasis including angular cheilits. Xerostomia may be assessed more objectively by measuring salivary flow rates or by salivary scintigraphy or magnetic resonance imaging. However, a simple bedside assessment can be made by asking the patient to raise her tongue and noting any decrease in salivary pooling. Infiltration of the lacrimal glands leads to symptoms of xerophthalmia (dry eyes). This can also be measured objectively utilizing a simple bedside test, the Schirmer's test. This test is performed by inserting a sterile strip of filter paper under each of the lower eyelids and measuring the amount of tear production in 5 min. (Less than 8–10 mm in 5 min is considered abnormal). In patients who are found to have dry eyes by the Schirmer's test, ophthalmologic evaluation with rose bengal staining should be performed to assess for corneal abrasion secondary to dryness. It is important to realize that extraglandular features may also occur, including pulmonary involvement, renal tubular acidosis, neuropathies, cutaneous involvement (hypergammaglobulinemic purpura), cryoglobulinemia, autoimmune thyroiditis, and primary biliary cirrhosis. Patients with Sjögren's syndrome may also develop pseudolymphoma and have a 44-fold greater risk of developing lymphoma. Serum protein electrophoresis and immunoelectrophoresis should be performed to look for a monoclonal protein, and patients should be followed clinically for the development of lymphadenopathy.

Laboratory testing can be helpful in diagnosing Sjögren's syndrome. Approximately 70% of patients will have SSA (anti-Ro) antibodies and 40% will have SSB (anti-La) antibodies.[18] Patients with Sjögren's syndrome also frequently have high-titer rheumatoid factors and positive ANAs. In addition to the serologic tests, a minor salivary gland biopsy (lip biopsy) can be helpful in confirming the diagnosis of Sjögren's syndrome.

The differential diagnosis of Sjögren's syndrome includes other causes of keratoconjunctivitis sicca and parotid gland swelling, including sarcoidosis, tumor (often unilateral), preexisting lymphoma, and HIV infection. These diagnoses should be carefully considered, especially in patients who are seronegative (negative SSA and SSB).

Treatment of Sjögren's syndrome is generally symptomatic, with artificial tear replacement, home humidifiers, and a program of intensive oral hygiene. In general, systemic corticosteroids are not used to treat Sjögren's syndrome, with the exception of life-threatening manifestations such as vasculitis, hemolytic anemia, and pleuropericarditis resistant to treatment with NSAIDs.[19]

Progressive Systemic Sclerosis (Scleroderma) Progressive systemic sclerosis is a systemic disorder of unknown etiology characterized by widespread fibrosis of the skin and internal organs. It is three to four times more common in women and commonly presents between the ages of 30 and 60.[20] Limited scleroderma, formerly termed the *CREST variant* (calcinosis, Raynaud's phenomenon, esophageal dysmotility, sclerodactyly, telangiectasias), generally follows a more indolent course, with less internal organ involvement and a better prognosis. One notable exception is that patients with limited scleroderma more frequently develop pulmonary hypertension. In the early stages of the disease the skin may appear edematous, but it eventually becomes thickened or "hidebound." In the diffuse form of scleroderma, thickening of the skin extends proximal to the forearms and often involves the trunk, as well as the extremities and face. Raynaud's phenomenon is extremely common in patients with scleroderma. Chronic vascular insufficiency can lead to acrolysis with resorption of the distal tufts of the digits. Involvement of the GI tract leads to esophageal, small bowel, and large bowel dysmotility. Pulmonary fibrosis can be a major cause of morbidity and mortality. Scleroderma renal crisis presents as accelerated hypertension (often with headache, blurred vision, or encephalopathy) and renal abnormalities (rapid rise in serum creatinine, proteinuria, microscopic hematuria). The treatment of choice for scleroderma renal crisis is ACE inhibitors.

The majority of patients with scleroderma will have a positive ANA. Scl-70 (antibody to topoisomerase I) is seen more commonly in the diffuse form of scleroderma but is present in only approximately 20% of cases. Anti-centromere antibodies are seen in approximately 80% of patients with limited scleroderma and are useful prognostically, since they are rarely seen in the diffuse form.

Unfortunately, overall treatment of scleroderma has been disappointing, and there is no drug or combination of drugs of proven value in treating these patients.[21] D-Penicillamine has been reported to be successful in some patients, especially those with early diffuse disease or interstitial lung disease.[21] In general, systemic corticosteroids are of little benefit and, in fact, have been associated with renal failure and other vaso-occlusive complications of the disease.[21] Treatment of specific manifestations, such as esophageal symptoms or Raynaud's phenomenon, can offer symptomatic relief for patients with scleroderma.

Polymyositis and Dermatomyositis Polymyositis and dermatomyositis are inflammatory myopathies characterized by symmetric proximal weakness. Patients often complain of difficulty raising their arms to comb their hair or difficulty arising from a chair. It is important to distinguish polymyositis from polymyalgia rheumatica, in which patients may have difficulty with similar activities but on the basis of pain and stiffness rather than weakness. It is also important to rule out a drug-induced myopathy in evaluating patients with proximal weakness. Drugs which can cause a myopathy include many of the antihyperlipidemics (nicotinic acid, gemfibrozil, lovastatin), zidovudine (AZT), cocaine, corticosteroids, colchicine, and hydroxychloroquine.

Polymyositis and dermatomyositis are systemic diseases which can affect internal organs, most commonly involving the heart, lung, and GI tract. In addition, an increased risk of malignancy has been reported. All patients should have a comprehensive history and physical exam, as well as routine screening procedures.[22]

A variety of cutaneous manifestations can be seen in dermatomyositis, including the classic heliotrope rash (purplish discoloration over the eyelids) and an erythematous or dusky discoloration of the face and upper chest in a "shawl" distribution. Gottron's papules are violaceous, flat papules seen over the dorsal surface of the interphalangeal joints of the fingers and are said to be pathognomonic for dermatomyositis.

Laboratory data usually reveal elevated creatine phosphokinase and aldolase in patients with polymyositis and dermatomyositis. A subset of patients have antibodies to Jo-1 (antihistidyl tRNA synthetase), which has been associated with an increased incidence of interstitial lung disease. Electromyograms show characteristic findings in patients with myositis and can be helpful in establishing the diagnosis. However, the most definitive diagnostic test in these disorders is the muscle biopsy; biopsy should be performed in almost all patients before long-term and potentially toxic therapy is begun. The biopsy specimen should be taken from a muscle that is moderately weak and is on the contralateral side to where the electromyogram was performed.

Polymyositis and dermatomyositis are generally treated with high-dose corticosteroids (prednisone, 1–2 mg/kg/day) and physical therapy. This dose of steroid is generally continued until muscle enzymes normalize and/or clinical strength improves; it is then tapered to the lowest possible dose which controls the disease. In patients who fail to respond or who have unacceptable side effects of the steroid, the addition of another immunosuppressive agent may be necessary.

Mixed Connective Tissue Disease Mixed connective tissue disease (MCTD) is an overlap syndrome characterized by puffy hands, polyarthritis, Raynaud's phenomenon, and myositis. Pulmonary involvement, including pulmonary hypertension, occurs frequently. Patients with MCTD often have features of other rheumatic disorders, especially SLE or scleroderma (see above), and may eventually develop one of these disorders. A positive ANA with a speckled pattern is generally found in patients with MCTD. In addition, this syndrome is characterized by high titers of antibody to the extractable nuclear antigen ribonuleoprotein (anti-RNP) in the absence of other autoantibodies.

Undifferentiated Connective Tissue Disease Not uncommonly, patients may present with positive serologies (i.e., ANA, RF) who do not meet the criteria for the diagnosis of a specific rheumatic disorder at the time of initial evaluation. For example, a young woman may present with Raynaud's phenomenon, mild joint aches, and a low positive ANA. Such patients are often classified as having early or undifferentiated connective tissue disease. These patients should be followed over time since some of these patients may develop classic rheumatic syndromes, especially SLE, scleroderma, or RA.

REFERENCES

1. Harris, ED Jr: Clinical features of rheumatoid arthritis. In Kelly WN, Harris ED Jr, Ruddy S, et al (eds): *Textbook of Rheumatology,* ed 4. Philadelphia, WB Saunders, 1993, pp 874–911.
2. Klippel GL, Cecere FA: Rheumatoid arthritis and pregnancy. *Rheum Dis Clin North Am* 15(No. 2):213–239.
3. Calin A: Ankylosing spondylitis and the spondyloarthropathies. In Schumacher HR Jr (ed): *Primer on the Rheumatic Diseases,* ed 9. Atlanta, Arthritis Foundation, 1988, pp 142–147.
4. Hunder GG: Polymyalgia rheumatica and temporal (giant cell) arteritis. In Schumacher HR Jr (ed): *Primer on the Rheumatic Diseases,* ed 9. Atlanta, Arthritis Foundation, 1988, pp 134.
5. Tate G, Schumacher HR Jr: Gout: Clinical features. In Schumacher HR Jr (ed): *Primer on the Rheumatic Diseases,* ed 9. Atlanta, Arthritis Foundation, 1988, pp 198–202.
6. Moskowitz RW: Diseases associated with the deposition of calcium pyrophosphate or hydroxyapatite. In Kelly WN, Harris ED, Jr, Ruddy S, et al (eds): *Textbook of Rheumatology,* ed 4. Philadelphia, WB Saunders, 1993, pp 1337–54.
7. Carsons S, Malone B: Septic arthritis. *Infect Dis Pract* 15:1–14, 1991.
8. Steere AC: Lyme disease. In Schumacher HR, Jr (ed): *Primer on the Rheumatic Diseases,* ed 9. Atlanta, Arthritis Foundation, 1988, pp 188–190.
9. Lipson SJ: Low back pain. In Kelly WN, Harris ED Jr, Ruddy S, et al (eds): *Textbook of Rheumatology,* ed 4. Philadelphia, WB Saunders, 1993, pp 441–458.
10. Yunus MB, Masi AT: Fibromyalgia, restless legs syndrome, periodic limb movement disorder, and psychogenic pain. In McCarty DJ, Koopman WJ (eds.): *Arthritis and Allied Conditions,* ed 12. Philadelphia, Lea & Febiger, 1993, pp 1383–1405.
11. Schur PH: Clinical features of SLE. In Kelly WN, Harris ED Jr, Ruddy S, et al (eds): *Textbook of Rheumatology,* ed 4. Philadelphia, WB Saunders, 1993, pp 1017–1042.
12. Wallace DJ: Cytotoxic drugs. In Wallace DJ, Hahn BH (eds.): *Dubois' Lupus Erythematosus,* ed 4. Philadelphia, Lea & Febiger, 1993, pp 588–599.
13. Hahn BH: Management of systemic lupus erythematosus. In Kelly WN, Harris ED Jr, Ruddy S, et al (eds): *Textbook of Rheumatology,* ed 4. Philadelphia, WB Saunders, 1993, pp 1043–1056.
14. Quismorio FP Jr: Systemic corticosteroid therapy in systemic lupus erythematosus. In Wallace DJ, Hahn BH (eds): *Dubois' Lupus Erythematosus,* ed 4. Philadelphia, Lea & Febiger, 1993, pp 574–587.
15. Mintz G, Rodriguez-Alvarez E: Systemic lupus erythematosus. *Rheum Dis Clin North Am* 15(2):255–274.
16. Mintz G, Kitridou RC: The neonatal lupus syndrome. In Wallace DJ, Hahn BH (eds): *Dubois' Lupus Erythematosus,* ed 4. Philadelphia, Lea & Febiger, 1993, pp 516–522.
17. Lockshin M: Antiphospholipid antibody syndrome. *Rheum Dis Clin North Am* 20(1):45–59.
18. Carsons SE: The medical workup of Sjögren's syndrome. In Harris EK, Carsons SE, Scuibba JJ, et al (eds): *The Sjögren's Syndrome Handbook.* New York, Sjögren's Syndrome Foundation, 1989, pp 19–25.

19. Fox RI, Kang HI: Sjogren's syndrome. In Kelly WN, Harris ED Jr, Ruddy S, et al (eds): *Textbook of Rheumatology*, ed 4. Philadelphia, WB Saunders, 1993, pp 931–942.

20. Medsger TA Jr: Systemic sclerosis (scleroderma), localized forms of scleroderma, and calcinosis. In McCarty DJ, Koopman WJ (eds): *Arthritis and Allied Conditions*, ed 12. Philadelphia, Lea & Febiger, 1993, pp 1253–1292.

21. Seibold JR: Scleroderma. In Kelly WN, Harris ED Jr, Ruddy S, et al (eds): *Textbook of Rheumatology*, ed 4. Philadelphia, WB Saunders, 1993, pp 1113–1143.

22. Cronin ME, Miller FW, Plotz PH: Polymyositis and dermatomyositis. In Schumacher HR, Jr (ed): *Primer on the Rheumatic Diseases*, ed 9. Atlanta, Arthritis Foundation, 1988, pp 120–123.

Chapter 7

Resuscitation in the Office

Kathleen M. Kelly

There's nothing like the adrenaline generated when a patient or staff member collapses in the office. This chapter is designed to explain simple techniques of resuscitation that will enable you to maintain the ABCs—airway, breathing, circulation—while help is summoned. The equipment and skills needed are familiar to you—basic life support (BLS) with intravenous fluids. Being able to intubate, perform and interpret electrocardiograms (ECGs), or administer advanced cardiac life support is rarely essential. Understanding what caused your patient's or colleague's collapse is also usually secondary to the immediate problems of securing an airway, ensuring good air exchange, and maintaining heart rate and systemic blood pressure. Anaphylaxis, however, must be recognized and treated early, since standard ABC maneuvers will not be effective due to upper airway edema and circulatory collapse. Epinephrine, benadryl, and/or steroids must be given (see the section on anaphylaxis).

AIRWAY

Supplemental Oxygen

Your office should be able to deliver supplemental oxygen via nasal cannula or venti-mask and bag-valve mask. To do this, you need an oxygen tank, a regulator, tubing, and the delivery devices. Good portable pulse oximetry will tell you whether your resuscitative efforts are maintaining good oxygen saturation.

If the patient is breathing easily, at an acceptable rate, with no airway obstruction, place a nasal cannula at 4 L/min or a 100% nonrebreather mask. Monitor oxygen saturation via pulse oximetry. Keep oxygen saturation on pulse oximetry greater than or equal to 92% (S_P0_2 >, 92%). The pulse oximetry heart rate should agree with the palpated heart rate. If not, the $Sp0_2$ may not be accurate.

Airway Obstruction

If the patient shows signs of airway obstruction—stridor, snoring, noisy airflow, contractions of accessory respiratory muscles (struggling to breathe), vomitus, or food particles in the back of the mouth—you must clear the airway. Here is the sequence to follow:

1. Suction the oropharynx with a Yankauer suction catheter. This maneuver presupposes that you have a suction apparatus with tubing and a catheter. It also assumes that the patient's oropharynx is accessible. Remember, you may need to remove large food pieces manually.
2. Perform a head-tilt with chin lift or jaw thrust to pull the tongue and epiglottis away from the airway (Figure 7.1). Do not tilt the head if neck injury is possible (falls).
3. If steps 1 and 2 do not open the airway, insert an oropharyngeal or nasopharyngeal airway (Figure 7.2A and 7.2B). The nasopharyngeal airways are much easier to place properly. Use surgilube. To choose an oral or nasal airway of the proper size, select a length that equals the distance from the corner of the mouth to the top of the ear.
4. Reassess the patient's condition. If the patient is breathing easily and independently after opening the airway, start supplemental oxygen and measure the oxygen saturation by pulse oximetry (S_pO_2). S_pO_2 should be 92% or higher.

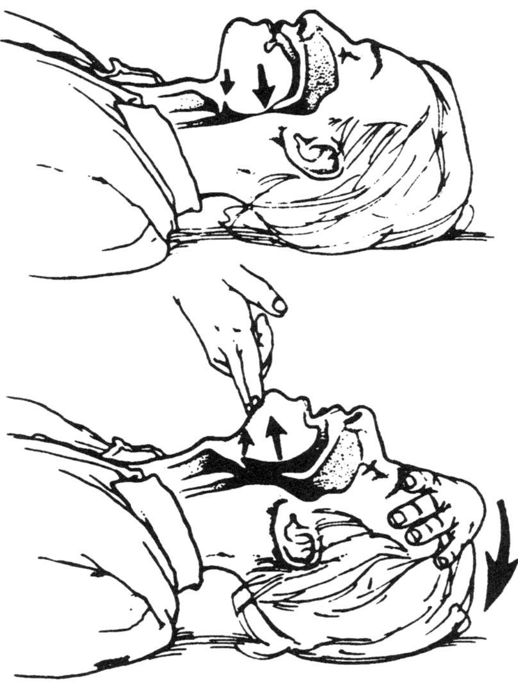

Figure 7.1 Opening the airway. *Top:* Airway obstruction produced by tongue and epiglottis. *Bottom:* Relief by head tilt/chin lift. Reproduced with permission from: *Textbook of Advanced Cardiac Life Support,* American Heart Association, 1987, p 27.

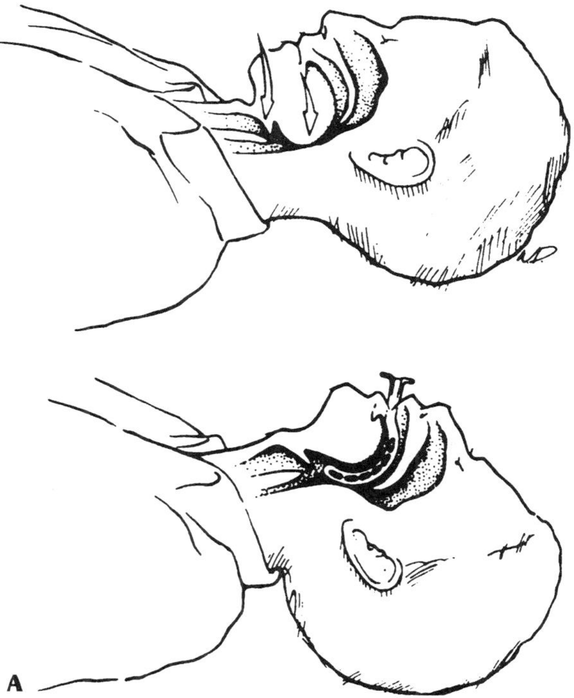

Figure 7.2A Placement of correctly inserted oropharyngeal airway. *Top:* Before insertion, incorrect head position. *Bottom:* After insertion, showing head tilted and oropharyngeal airway in place.

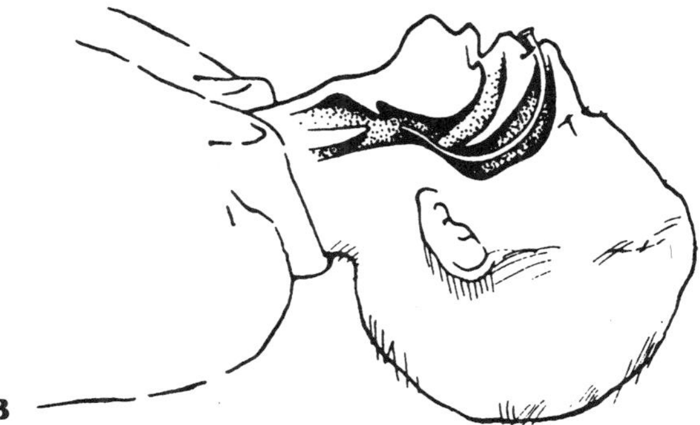

Figure 7.2B Nasopharyngeal airway in place. Note head tilted back for proper insertion. Reproduced with permission from: *Textbook of Advanced Cardiac Life Support,* American Heart Association, 1987, p. 28.

5. If you cannot maintain a pulse oximetry oxygen saturation greater than 92%, begin positive-pressure ventilation. If the patient is not breathing well, or is cyanotic despite an unobstructed airway and supplemental oxygen, begin positive–pressure ventilation.

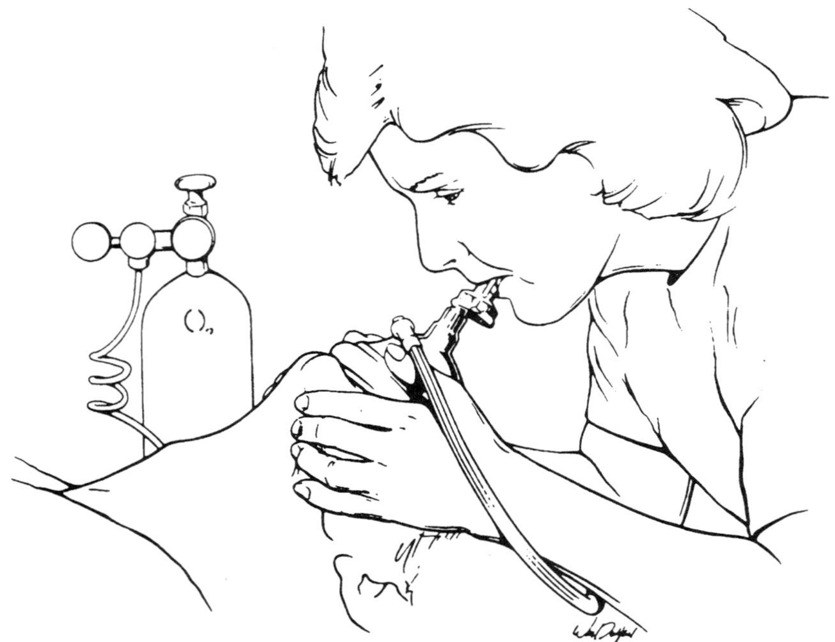

Figure 7.3 Mouth-to-mask ventilation with a one-way valve. Reproduced with permission from: *Textbook of Advanced Cardiac Life Support,* American Heart Association, 1987, p. 36.

Positive-Pressure Ventilation

Positive-pressure ventilation pushes air into the lungs and allows passive exhalation. One of the easiest techniques for delivery of positive-pressure ventilation is mouth-to-mask ventilation with a one-way valve. You can administer supplemental oxygen, avoid direct contact with the patient's mouth/nose, and obtain good head tilt, chin lift, and mask seal (Figure 7.3).

The one-way valve is connected to the mask, and supplemental oxygen is added by connecting your oxygen source to the O_2 inlet on the mask (10 L/min flow provides approximately 80% oxygen). The operator stands at the patient's head and tilts the head towards himself/herself. (Remember, don't tilt head, use jaw thrust only if there is a possibility of cervical spine injury.) As shown in Figure 7.3, using both hands, press the mask with your thumbs to the face and pull the mandible up with the fingers. Then blow in through the one-way valve, with pauses between breaths to allow exhalation. You may need an oropharyngeal or nasopharyngeal airway to ensure an open passage, since the mouth may close or the nares occlude with efforts to obtain a good skin-to-mask seal. If possible, an assistant should apply cricoid pressure (Sellick maneuver) by placing the thumb and index finger over the cricoid cartilage and pressing toward the spine. Since the cricoid cartilage is the only tracheal ring which is complete, this maneuver occludes the esophagus against the spinal column, and avoids air insufflation of the stomach and/or regurgitation and aspiration of stomach contents.

Bag-valve masks are excellent but require some practice to get a good seal between the face and the mask. The seal and head position is maintained with one hand; the other hand squeezes the self-inflating bag. If you are comfortable with this technique, use it. Otherwise, the mouth-to-mask technique is much simpler to do correctly.

Positive-pressure ventilation is successful in the vast majority of patients with airway problems. It will fail if the airway is blocked due to acute laryngeal edema, laryngospasm, or aspirated food contents in the trachea.

For those who possess intubation skills, endotracheal or nasotracheal intubation may be an option if airway clearance and positive-pressure ventilation do not result in an acceptable oxygen saturation. However, most gynecologists and obstetricians have little recent experience with intubation skills. They would be more skilled and successful creating a surgical airway.

Surgical Airway

Cricothyroidotomy is the surgical airway of choice in adults. The cricothyroid membrane is 5–10 mm below the skin in adults. There are no overlying large arteries or veins, thyroid isthmus, strap muscles, or nerves. The membrane is 10–20 mm inferior to the vocal cords. The posterior wall of the trachea is protected from the esophagus by the "signet ring" of the cricoid cartilage (Figure 7.4).

The cricothyroid membrane is usually located easily by (1) extension of the neck if there is no suspicion of cervical spine injury; (2) location of the thyroid cartilage via palpation of the thyroid notch, the midline prominence on the anterior neck; (3) palpation of the cricoid cartilage immediately inferior to the thyroid cartilage; and (4) palpation of a 9-mm concavity between the inferior border of the thyroid cartilage and the cricoid cartilage. This concavity is the cricothyroid membrane (Figure 7.5).

Necessary instruments for a surgical cricothyroidotomy are 10 cc of local anesthetic in a syringe, scalpel with No. 11 or No. 15 blade, a Trousseau dilator or Kelly clamp, a curved Mayo scissors, Cryle clamps, free ties, and a standard-sized tracheostomy tube or endotracheal tube with a maximum *outside* diameter of 9 mm.

Infiltration of the skin and subcutaneous tissues with local anesthetic is necessary in the awake patient. Adding an injection of local anesthetic into the trachea through the cricothyroid membrane will decrease the cough reflex during tube placement. After standard skin preparation, the thyroid cartilage is stabilized between the thumb and

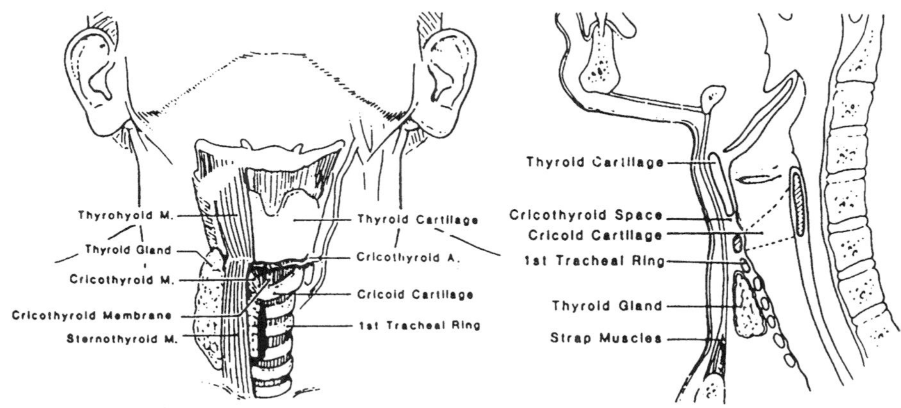

Figure 7.4 Anatomy of cricothyroid space and associated structures. Reproduced with permission from: Feinberg SE, Peterson JL: Use of cricothyroidostomy in oral and maxillofacial surgery. *Oral and Maxillofacial Surg* 45:874, 1987.

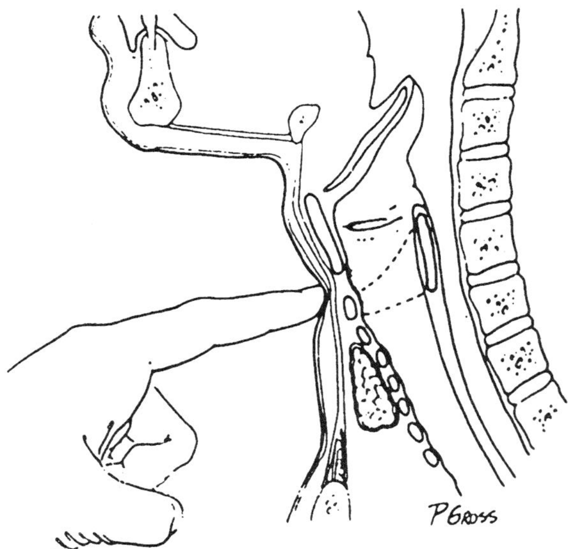

Figure 7.5 Identification of cricothyroid space by palpation with index finger. Reproduced with permission from: Feinberg SE, Peterson JL: Use of cricothyroidostomy in oral and maxillofacial surgery. *Oral Maxillofacial Surg* 45:875, 1987.

middle finger of the operator's nondominant hand. The cricothyroid membrane's position is verified by palpation by the free index finger of the same hand (Figure 7.5).

The cricothyroidotomy incision may be placed transversely or vertically over the cricothyroid membrane. A 2-cm transverse skin and platysma incision over the cricothyroid membrane is standard when the anatomy is clearly identified. However, a 2-cm incision may be difficult for the inexperienced clinician to work with; a transverse extension increases the likelihood of lacerating superficial jugular veins. A vertical skin incision is simpler if the anatomy is not clear, the neck cannot be extended, or the operator is inexperienced. It will also avoid superficial bleeding.

Blunt dissection exposes the cricothyroid membrane, which is usually 5–10 mm deep to the skin. The membrane is divided with the No. 11 blade 2 cm *transversely*. Using the Trousseau dilator or Kelly clamp, dilate the tracheal opening *vertically* and place the tracheostomy/endotracheal tube. If the opening is too small, remove the dilator and extend the cricothyroidotomy transversely bluntly with the Mayo tips or sharply with the scalpel. Remember, the *transverse* incision in the cricothyroid membrane must be extended to enlarge the cricothyroidotomy *vertically* without fracturing the cricoid cartilage (Figure 7.6).

Most authors agree that an airway with an outside diameter of less than 9 mm is optimal. The cricothyroid membrane marks the narrowest portion of the trachea in the adult at an average dimension of 9 × 36 mm. Tight fits correlate with tracheal stenosis. Remember to note the *outside* diameter of tracheostomy tubes; it can be 3–4 mm larger than the tracheostomy (inside diameter). This author suggests using a Protex No. 4 or No. 6 or a Shiley No. 4.

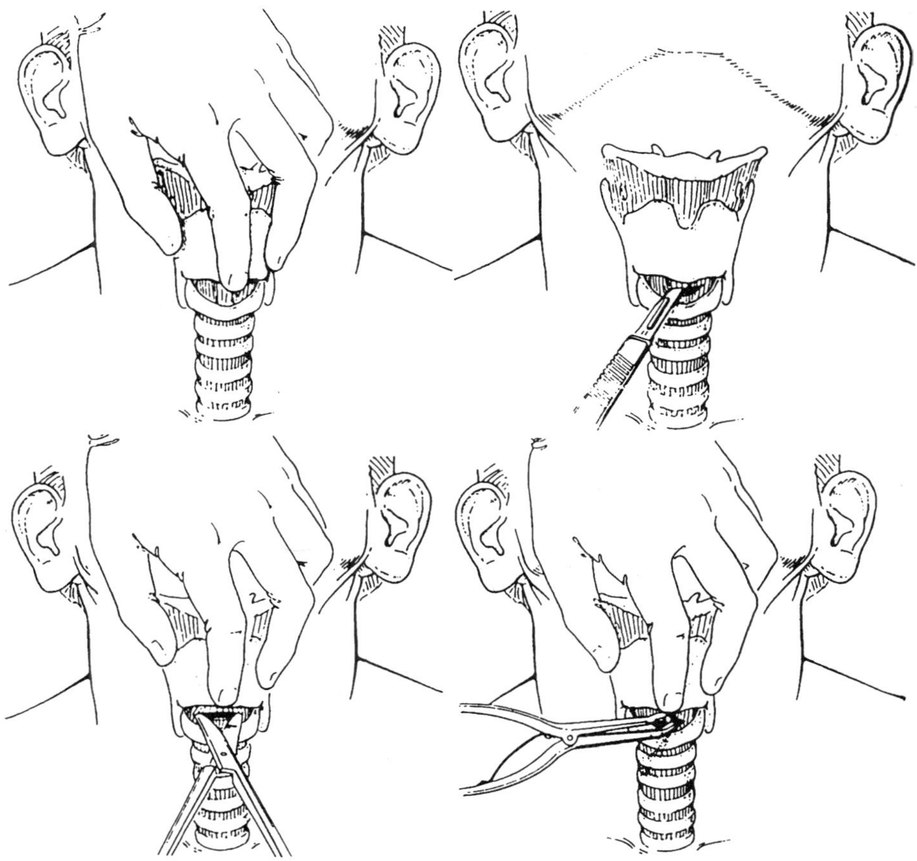

Figure 7.6 *Top left:* Surgeon stabilizes the thyroid cartilage between the thumb and middle finger of the nondominant hand and identifies the cricothyroid space with the index finger. *Top right:* The cricothyroid membrane is incised with a short, stabbing stroke with a No. 11 blade, parallel to the skin incision, and perpendicular to the long axis of the trachea. *Bottom left:* Using a curved Mayo scissor to enlarge the perforation through the cricothyroid membrane by opening the beaks in a horizontal direction. *Bottom right:* Opening is enlarged with a Trousseau dilator spread at right angles to the incision. Reproduced with permission from: Feinberg SE, Peterson JL: Use of cricothyroidostomy in oral and maxillofacial surgery. *Oral Maxillofacial Surg* 45:876, 1987.

CIRCULATION

After you have ensured a patent airway with good ventilation, it is necessary to assess the adequacy of the circulation.

Blood Pressure

1. Try to palpate the pulses; the radial, femoral, and carotid arteries are most easily accessed. A palpable radial pulse usually means that the patient has a blood pressure of at least 90 systolic. Record time, rate, regularity of pulse.

2. Take a blood pressure using a standard blood pressure cuff or whatever equipment your office uses. Record the time and results.
3. If there is no palpable or audible blood pressure, begin cardiopulmonary resuscitation (CPR) according to BLS techniques. Establish intravenous access if you can while someone continues CPR. Check a fingerstick glucose; if less than 60, give one ampule of $D_{50}W$. If glucose is normal, give 500 cc of normal saline or Ringer's lactate solution. If possible, obtain an ECG.
4. If the blood pressure is audible or palpable but less than 90 systolic, establish an intravenous access and give 500 to 1000 cc of isotonic fluid (normal saline or lactated Ringer's solution) over 10–15 min. Sometimes leg elevation can raise the blood pressure temporarily while intravenous fluids are being infused. The intravenous catheter should be as large as possible—preferably 18 gauge or larger. Monitor the blood pressure and pulse every 5 min and record. Get an ECG if possible.
5. You have infused 1000 cc of isotonic fluid and the blood pressure has not changed. If you suspect blood loss, continue rapid fluid resuscitation at the rate of 500 cc every 15 min. If the patient's past history, cardiac rhythm, ECG, or clinical exam (rales on chest auscultation) suggest a cardiac origin, consider starting advanced cardiac life support (ACLS) or beginning an intravenous infusion of dopamine (40 mg/250 cc D_5W). Titrate the dopamine to a blood pressure of over 100 systolic. Few offices have the equipment or training to do ECGs, titrate dopamine drips, or begin ACLS. If you and your staff are not trained in using these intervention, it is safer to stay with BLS protocols.
6. If the blood pressure is above 90 systolic, establish intravenous access and start isotonic fluids at an appropriate maintenance rate (usually around 80 cc/hr).

WHAT CAUSED THE PROBLEM

Fainting and Vaso/Vagal Reactions

Typically, this patient is anxious. He or she may report feeling faint before the event. The patient is breathing well as long as the airway remains patent. Usually the patient has a *slow* pulse and low blood pressure that responds to a supine position, intravenous fluids, and smelling salts.

Hypovolemia

Profound hypovolemia generally does not characterize the patient seen in the office. However, there are some gynecologic and obstetric conditions that can cause hypovolemia: a ruptured ectopic pregnancy, prolonged menometarrhagia with severe anemia, acute uterine bleeding after or during procedures, or a ruptured placenta previa.

Good airway management with high supplemental oxygen and rapid fluid resuscitation while obtaining rapid transport to a hospital is the cornerstone of care. Few offices are equipped to perform the interventions needed to stop active bleeding.

Anaphylaxis

Anaphylaxis is an acute allergic reaction. Symptoms usually begin within 30 min of exposure to the antigen. If the antigenic substance has been administered intravenously, the reaction tends to be more severe and rapid in onset. Patients often have premonitory symptoms of pruritus on the hands and feet, tingling of the tongue and lips, a lump in the throat, chest tightness, or a feeling of impending doom. Pay attention to these complaints. They may be the only clue you get.

Individual signs and symptoms, as well as severity, vary. The most common symptoms involve the skin—angioedema and/or urticaria. Urticaria are raised, reddened, pruritic welts covering most of the body. Angioedema does not itch and is not erythematous. It consists of nonpitting edema of the lips, face, and hands. Gastrointestinal cramping, diarrhea, nausea, and vomiting are other common symptoms. Mild wheezing is also frequent.

Although these symptoms may be disturbing, laryngeal edema is the principal cause of death in anaphylaxis. The second most frequent cause is intractable hypotension. Complaints of hoarseness or a lump in the throat, with or without angioedema of the oropharynx, are signs of impending laryngeal edema and airway loss. Immediate treatment should be started (Table 7.1).

Treatment of Anaphylaxis

1. Give supplemental oxygen and be prepared to secure a surgical airway.
2. Give epinephrine, 0.3–0.5 mg (0.3–0.5 mL of a 1:1000 solution) IM.
3. Establish intravenous access. If the blood pressure is below 90 systolic infuse 1 L of isotonic solution over 15 min.
4. If shock or incipient airway obstruction occurs, start an epinephrine drip (1 mg of a 1:1000 solution of epinephrine in 250 cc D_5W) at a rate of 1 mg/min and increase to 4 mg/min as needed.
5. Give diphenhydramine (Benadryl), 50 mg, IV or IM.
6. Give methylprednisolone, 125 mg, or hydrocortisone, 500 mg IV push (Table 7.1).
7. Continue to check the ABCs and call for help.
8. If you cannot maintain good ventilation and oxygenation, it is necessary to establish an airway (see the discussion of the surgical airway).

Insulin Shock

Hypoglycemia can produce different alterations in consciousness—confusion, coma, or focal neurologic signs. It is necessary to treat the patient for low blood sugar if you find no other reason for the collapse.

Treatment consists of the ABCs—control the airway, ensure adequate breathing, and start an IV plus one ampule of $D_{50}W$ given IV.

If the patient's unconsciousness is due to hypoglycemia, there is usually rapid improvement after $D_{50}W$ is given. When the patient is awake, give some juice with two packets of sugar mixed in.

TABLE 7.1 Treatment of Anaphylaxis

1. Remove antigen, delay absorption.
2. Maintain an adequate airway.
3. Epinephrine
   - If a mild episode:
     - 0.3 cc subcutaneously (0.01 cc/kg in a child) 1/1000
     - Repeat at 10- to 20-minute intervals.
   - If more severe episode:
     - 0.3–0.5 mL intramuscularly 1/1000
     - Repeat at 5- to 10-minute intervals
   - If in shock or incipient airway obstruction:
     - 1/100,000 dilution intravenously, 1–2 cc per minute up to a total of 10 cc (0.1 mg)
     - If persistent shock, may repeat dose or start a drip: 1 mg in 250 cc D_5W, 1–4 μ per minute.
   - If patient is elderly (over 50) or has a cardiac history, and life-threatening symptoms exist:
     - Test dose of 0.1–0.15 cc subcutaneously or IM.
     - If shock is resistant to other measures or there is imminent airway closure, consider a drip as noted previously.
4. Volume expansion with saline or lactated Ringer's
   - Shock:
     - Adult: 1 L over 15 minutes, then reassess
     - Child: 20 cc/kg bolus
5. Methylprednisolone
   - 125 mg IV push, may repeat every 4 hours if persistent symptoms. (or hydrocortisone 500 mg)
   - If discharging home, prednisone 40 mg per day, for 2 to 3 days.
6. Diphenhydramine
   - 25–50 mg IV push, IM, or by mouth, depending on severity; repeat every 2–4 hours as needed.
   - If patient is being discharged, 50 mg q6hr pm for 3 days
7. If resistant hypotension
   - A. MAST suit, Trendelenburg position
   - B. Dopamine infusion
   - C. Naloxone, 0.4–0.8 mg IV
   - D. Cimetidine, 300 mg IV
8. If beta blocker accentuated anaphylaxis (epinephrine-resistant)
   - A. Glucagon, 1–2 mg IV over 2 minutes, then drip
   - B. Terbutiline 0.25 mg subcutaneously
   - C. Isoproterenol drip

Source: Reproduced with permission from: Schwartz GR, Cayten CG, Mangelson MA (eds): *Principle and Practice of Emergency Medicine*, ed 3. Philadelphia, Lea and Febiger, p. 1925.

Most offices do not have glucometers. If you do, use it, but don't delay the administration of $D_{50}W$ while waiting for results.

Seizures

The first goals of treatment for the seizure victim are to control the airway, ensure adequate oxygenation, and protect the patient from self-injury.

1. If possible, place a bite block between the patient's teeth. An oral airway can be used. Bite blocks are commercially available or can be made simply by wadding some 4 × 4-in. gauze packets over one end of two tongue depressors placed together. Wrap tightly with tape. Often you cannot place a bite block. In these cases, place a nasopharyngeal airway and give 100% oxygen.
2. Start an IV simultaneously or when the airway has been secured. This is your route for IV therapy. Monitor blood pressure and oxygen saturation.
3. Is this seizure eclamptic? If so, the first-line treatment is magnesium sulfate (M_gSO_4), 4 g IV over 2–6 min, followed by a continuous infusion of 2g/h. Mix 40 g M_gSO_4 in 1000 cc of D_5W or D_5RL. Run at 50 cc/h to deliver 2 g/h. If seizures continue, give an additional 2 g of M_gSO_4 IV. If they still persist, continue a continuous infusion of M_gSO_4 and give valium (Diazepam), 5 mg IV. Repeat the IV valium every 3–5 min if the seizures do not stop.
4. For noneclamptic seizure activity, secure a patent airway and good oxygenation, protect the patient from injury, start an IV, and give valium, 5 mg IV. Repeat every 3–5 min until the seizures stop or 30 mg has been given. Valium can depress respiratory function; be sure to reassess and check the ABCs. The effects of valium may disappear after 30 min. You may need to repeat the dosing.

The usual additional treatment is to load with phenytoin (Dilantin), 20 mg/kg, but few offices stock this drug. Infusion must be given slowly in normal saline at a rate of 50 mg/min.

SUMMARY

Most patients who require office resuscitation can be treated adequately by remembering the ABCs—airway, breathing, and circulation—and using BLS techniques to assess and treat the ABCs. Some basic supplies are enumerated in the following appendix. If you are able to deliver effective BLS treatment, you are serving your patient in the best possible way.

APPENDIX: EQUIPPING THE OFFICE

All of the equipment mentioned in this chapter can be stocked and/or hung on a portable crash cart. It is a good idea to label the drawers and keep equipment designed to deal with the airway separate from the circulatory equipment. Here is what you need:

Crash cart—on wheels, with multiple drawers and compartments
Oxygen tank
Tank holder to attach to crash cart
Flow regulator
Oxygen wrench
Oxygen supply tubing
Adult Ambu bag with reservoir tubing
High-concentration O_2 mask (nonrebreathing mask)

Nasal cannula
Portable pulse oximetry (Novametrics, Nonin, Ohmeda, CSI, and Nellcor are some companies)
Portable suction with tubing and Yankaeur catheters
Oral airways (small, medium, large)
Nasal airways (32–36 French)
Bite blocks on stick
Surgilube
Cricothyroidotomy equipment
- No. 4 and No. 6 tracheostomy tubes
- Scalpel, No. 11 blade, No. 15 blade
- Kelly clamp
- Trousseau dilator
- 10-cc syringe
- 1% lidocaine

Mouth-to-mask ventilation units with one-way valve
Liter bags of D_5 Ringer's lacate, normal saline, D_5W
IV tubing (unfiltered)
No. 20, 18, 16, and 14 angiocaths
$D_{50}W$ (50-cc) amps
Magnesium sulfate, 50% solution (5 g/10 cc)
Selection of syringes (3, 5, 10 cc)
Selection of needles (No. 18, 20, 25)
Alcohol packets
Tourniquet
Blood pressure cuff (adult cuffs: small, regular, and large sizes) and manometer or Doppler
Betadine solution
Packets of 4 × 4-in. gauze
Sterile gloves
epinephrine (1:1000)
epinephrine (1:100,000)
diphenylhydramine (25 or 50 mg)
methylprednisolone (125 mg)
or hydrocortisone (500 mg)
diazepam (5 mg)

BIBLIOGRAPHY

Textbook of Advanced Cardiac Life Support, Dallas, American Heart Association, 1987, pp 27–39.

Feinberg SE, Peterson JL: Use of cricothyroidostomy in oral and maxillofacial surgery. *Oral Maxillofacial Surg* 45:873–878, 1987.

Merrick, C (ed): *Basic and Advanced Pre-Hospital Trauma Life Support,* ed 3. New York, Mosby–Year Book, 1994, pp 74–121.

Schwartz GR, Cayten CG, Mangelsen MA (eds): *Principles and Practice of Emergency Medicine,* ed 3. Philadelphia, Lea and Febiger, 1992, pp 1920–1926.

Chapter 8

Common Skin Problems

Rachelle A. Scott
Jonathan D.K. Trager

There are over 50 million visits to physicians each year related to skin complaints; less than half of these are to the dermatologist. With an expanding primary care role, the obstetrician-gynecologist will be called upon to recognize both common and serious skin disorders and to provide appropriate first-line care and timely referral. In this chapter, we discuss these common and serious skin disorders which may present in primary care.

BASIC ANATOMY AND PHYSIOLOGY OF THE SKIN

The skin is the largest organ of the body and is easily accessible for examination of both primary dermatologic conditions and cutaneous signs of internal disease. The outer layer is the *epidermis,* which provides a barrier against fluid losses, infection, and the damaging effects of ultraviolet (UV) light. Keratinocytes proliferate in the basal layer of the epidermis then migrate up through the spinous layer toward the granular layer. The cells then flatten, lose their nuclei, and form the stratum corneum, the major physical barrier of the skin. The epidermis contains melanocytes, which impart pigment to the skin and protect it from UV light, and Langerhans cells which serve as the first line of immunologic defense in the skin. Beneath the epidermis is the *dermis*. Made up of collagen and elastic fibers, fibroblasts, and ground substance, the dermis gives strength and elasticity to the skin. In the dermis are blood vessels, lymphatics, nerves, and skin appendages—hair follicles, sebaceous glands, apocrine and eccrine sweat glands, and the matrices of nails. The underlying *subcutis* contains mainly fat cells and serves as a protective cushion and thermal insulator.

The skin reacts to insult, injury, or disease in several ways. Scaling may occur due to overproliferation of epidermal cells. Blisters may form from thermal or chemical injury or from bacterial or viral infection. Skin breaks caused by trauma, excessive dryness or moisture, or infection may elicit an inflammatory response with erythema, migration of inflammatory cells, and induration. Wheals may form due to release of histamine from mast cells after antigenic stimulation.

Skin Lesions

Primary skin lesions are those most representative of a particular skin disease. These include *macules* (flat lesions up to 1 cm), *patches* (flat lesions greater than 1 cm), *papules* (raised lesions up to 1 cm), *plaques* (raised lesions greater than 1 cm), *vesicles* (blisters up to 1 cm), *bullae* (blisters greater than 1 cm), *pustules* (elevated collections of leukocytes), *nodules* (solid, dome-shaped lesions greater than 1 cm), and *wheals* (solid elevations caused by localized edema). *Secondary skin lesions* represent evolutionary changes that occur during the course of a cutaneous disease. These include *crusts* (dried serum, blood, pus), *scales* (accumulation of layers of stratum corneum), *fissures* (linear cleavage), *erosions* (areas of denuded epidermis), *excoriations* (traumatized or abraded areas), *ulcers* (areas of necrosis of epidermis and part or all of dermis), *atrophy* (loss of dermis and/or subcutaneous fat), and *scars* (permanent fibrotic changes).

ACNE

Acne is a common disorder and involves the pilosebaceous unit, which is composed of the hair follicle and the sebaceous gland. Individuals of all ages are affected, but acne is most prevalent during the teenage and young adult years. Lesions begin at sebarche, when sebum production in sebaceous glands increases; this may occur as early as 8 to 10 years of age and may precede menarche by over a year. Approximately 85% of Americans between the ages of 12 and 24 are affected by acne; 8% of those aged 25 to 34 and 3% of those aged 35 to 44 are affected.

Important historical questions concerning the patient with acne relate to the possibility of underlying endocrinologic disease, the relationship of acne to the menstrual cycle, and factors which may exacerbate acne such as medications and local trauma (Table 8.1).

There are two types of acne lesions, which may coexist in the same patient: *noninflammatory* and *inflammatory*. The lesions of noninflammatory acne are closed comedones (whiteheads) and open comedones (blackheads), while the lesions of inflammatory acne are papules, pustules, cysts, and nodules (Figure 8.1).

Four factors are thought to lead to the production of acne lesions: (1) increased androgen-dependent sebum production; (2) abnormal keratinization (terminal differentiation) and desquamation of the epithelium of hair follicles; (3) proliferation of *Propionibacterium acnes,* a bacterium contained within hair follicles; and (4) inflammation. A rational treatment approach will address several or all of these factors: (1) reduce sebum production; (2) curtail abnormal keratinization and desquamation of the follicular epithelium; (3) reduce the population of *P. acnes;* and (4) reduce the inflammation.

The pathogenesis of acne involves the pilosebaceous unit. Comedone formation is caused by abnormal shedding of the cells lining the hair follicles. The impaction and distention of the follicles with tightly packed keratinocyte debris results in the

TABLE 8.1 Factors Important in the Patient with Acne

Historical Factor	Importance
Irregular menstrual periods Hirsutism	Endocrinopathies associated with androgen excess may cause acne
Premenstrual flare-up	Caused by greater obstruction of sebum flow between days 15 to 20 of the menstrual cycle; these women may benefit greatly from anovulatory drugs
Use of oral contraceptives (OCPs)	Acne may flare after starting OCPs; postpill acne may also occur; OCPs differ widely in their effects on sebaceous glands; OCPs with androgenic and antiestrogenic progestogens may provoke acne
Seasonal changes	Humid environment may lead to sebaceous gland duct obstruction
Exposure to heavy oils, greases, polyvinyl chloride, or tars	These are comedogenic agents
Use of occlusive or tight clothing Mechanical trauma from clothing or behavioral habits	These initiate or aggravate acne lesions
Medications	Many medications, including steroids, isoniazid, lithium, and vitamin B_{12}, may exacerbate acne
Rapid onset of acne with fever, elevated white blood cell count	Known as *acne fulminans;* patients are systemically ill
Prior treatment?	Was the prior treatment appropriate? What over-the-counter or prescription medications have been used?
Stress or emotional upset	These may exacerbate, but not cause, acne

Source: Manual of Dermatologic Therapeutics, ed 5., Arndt KA, copyright 1995. Published by Little, Brown and Company.

formation of a solid plug, the closed comedone. If this comedone protrudes from the follicle, it is seen as an open comedone. The dark color of the open comedone is not due to dirt but probably results from the presence of melanin or the oxidation of lipids.

At the same time, sebaceous glands, under androgen control, enlarge and secrete sebum into the now blocked and dilated hair follicles; this condition contributes to an increase in the quantity of *P. acnes.* This bacterium produces chemotactant factors for neutrophils and acts on sebum to produce free fatty acids, the primary irritant in inflammatory acne. An inflammatory cascade is thus initiated, leading to the lesions of inflammatory acne.

Most patients have this common type of acne, known as *acne vulgaris.* Other types of acne are *steroid acne,* caused by oral or topical steroids, in which the inflammatory papules and pustules appear fairly uniform; *pomade acne,* caused by pomade applied to the scalp and forehead, resulting in multiple, closed, closely packed comedones close to the hairline; *nodulocystic acne,* a severe form of inflammatory acne; and *acne conglobata,* a highly inflammatory form of acne in which there are comedones, nodules, abscesses, and draining sinus tracts. Patients with the last two types of acne should be referred to a dermatologist since they are difficult to manage and will most certainly scar.

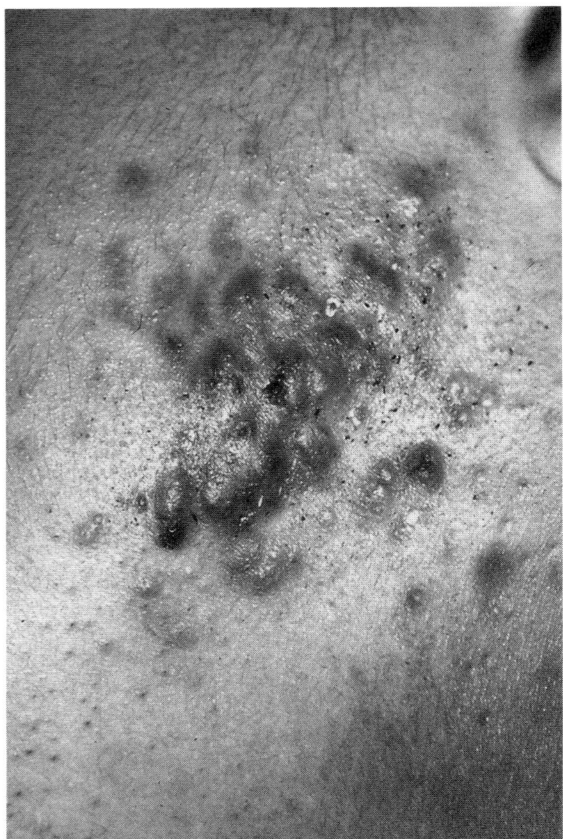

Figure 8.1 Acne: noninflammatory (open and closed comedones) and inflammatory (papules, pustules, cysts, nodules) on the face of a young woman.

The differential diagnosis of acne includes *rosacea* and *gram-negative folliculitis.* In rosacea, there is redness of the facial skin associated with telangiectasia but no plugged sebaceous follicles or comedones. Rosacea usually presents later in life (middle age), occurs gradually, and may be exacerbated by cold, stress, hot or spicy foods, and sunlight. Gram-negative folliculitis is an infection of hair follicles by gram-negative bacteria such as *Enterobacter, Klebsiella,* or *Proteus,* and is characterized by papules and pustules. It is usually seen in patients who are taking long-term antibiotics for acne and have a sudden flare.

The therapy of acne involves topical and systemic medications and addresses the factors involved in its pathogenesis (Table 8.2). Combination therapy (two or three topical agents, with or without systemic therapy) will enhance the likelihood of success. Patients should be informed that improvement is slow and that 2 to 4 months are necessary to determine the efficacy of a particular treatment plan.

TABLE 8.2 Common Treatment Options in Acne

Agent	Usual Regimen	Mechanism	Problems/ side effects
Topical			
Antibiotics		Reduces *P. acnes* population; decreases free fatty acids, which lead to comedone formation and inflammation	Skin irritation, dryness; potential pseudo-membranous colitis with clindamycin (rare)
Erythromycin 2% (solution, gel, pledget, wipe)	Twice a day		
Clindamycin phosphate 1%(solution, pledget, lotion, gel)	Twice a day		
Benzoyl peroxide 2.5% to 10% (gel, cream, lotion, wash)	Once a day (may start qod)	Reduces *P. acnes* population; decreases free fatty acids,which lead to comedone formation and inflammation	Skin irritation, dryness; contact dermatitis; may bleach clothing and carpet
Tretinoin (*Retin-A®*) 0.01%, 0.025%, 0.05%,0.1% (solution, cream, gel)	Once a day (may start qod)	Normalizes desquamation of follicular epithelium; inhibits comedone formation	Skin irritation, dryness
Systemic			
Antibiotics			
Tetracycline	1 g/day (divide bid-qid); decrease to maintenance dose or eliminate	Reduces *P. acnes* population	Poor compliance; gastrointestinal upset; cannot be taken with dairy products and iron
Erythromycin	1 g/day (divide tid); decrease to maintenance dose or eliminate	Reduces *P. acnes* population	Gastrointestinal upset; *P. acnes* may become resistant
Minocycline	50 mg/day; slowly increase to maximum of 100 mg bid	Reduces *P. acnes* population at a low dose; penetrates sebaceous gland	Vertigo, nausea, vomiting; expensive
Isotretinoin (*Accutane®*)	0.5 to 1.0 mg/kg/day for 4 to 5 months	Reduces size of sebaceous gland; decreases sebum production; reduces *P. acnes* population	Teratogenic; absolutely contraindicated prior to or during pregnancy; hypertriglyceridemia

Source: Adapted from Bergfeld WF: Evaluating and managing acne. *Skin* 1:17–21, 1995.

Topical Acne Therapy

Topical therapy is used for patients with noninflammatory (comedonal) acne or mild to moderate inflammatory acne. These agents include topical antibiotics, benzoyl peroxide, and tretinoin.

Topical antibiotics are used both for their bacteriostatic action on *P. acnes* and for their anti-inflammatory effect. The agents used most commonly are *erythromycin* and *clindamycin,* which are applied twice a day. Erythromycin (2%) is available as a solution, gel, pledget, and wipe. An ointment may be used for especially irritated skin. Clindamycin phosphate (1%) comes as a solution, pledget, lotion, and gel. The lotion is best for sensitive skin. Topical antibiotics are safe and effective in the treatment of mild to moderate acne. There have been rare reports of pseudomembranous colitis with the use of topical clindamycin.

Benzoyl peroxide is used for its potent bactericidal effect, and is useful for both inflammatory and noninflammatory lesions. It is available as a gel, cream, lotion, and wash, and in concentrations from 2.5% to 10%. The choice of formulation depends on the degree of drying desired, with gels being most drying. Since benzoyl peroxide can initially irritate the skin, starting at a lower dose every other or every third day and gradually increasing the frequency of application to once a day can be helpful. A small percentage of patients may develop a contact hypersensitivity to this agent. Benzoyl peroxide may bleach the color out of clothing or carpets.

Tretinoin (trans-retinoic acid, Retin-A®) causes increased epidermal cell turnover and decreased "stickiness" of the cells in the stratum corneum, the top layer of the epidermis. This inhibits the formation of new comedones and helps existing ones to loosen and become expelled. Tretinoin is available as a solution, cream and gel in concentrations from 0.01% to 0.1%. Tretinoin may cause transient erythema, burning, peeling, and exacerbation of inflammatory acne; thus, patients should start with a mild cream (0.025%) and increase the dose or frequency of application (to once a day) as tolerated. Tretinoin should be applied lightly to the entire face except around the eyes, lips, and neck. It should be applied to skin which is thoroughly dry—at least 15 min after washing.

A combination of topical agents will help ensure effective treatment. A regimen for comedonal acne might include Retin-A® 0.025% cream in the morning and benzoyl peroxide 2.5% or 5% gel at bedtime.

For mild to moderate inflammatory acne, one may use erythromycin 2% solution or clindamycin 1% lotion twice a day and benzoyl peroxide 2.5% or 5% gel at bedtime.

Tretinoin and benzoyl peroxide should *not* be applied simultaneously, as they will inactivate each other.

Systemic Acne Therapy

Systemic therapy is used when acne fails to respond adequately to topical therapy, for more severe inflammatory acne, and for extra-facial areas such as the back or chest. The two modalities most widely used are systemic antibiotics and isotretinoin.

Systemic antibiotics used for acne include tetracycline, erythromycin, and minocycline. These agents are bactericidal, reducing the amount of *P. acnes* within the follicle, and anti-inflammatory. Antibiotics are used daily for 4 to 6 months, usually in combination with topical agents. While all antibiotics are effective in treating inflammatory acne, each has its own side effects which must be considered in individualizing treatment. For example, tetracycline may cause gastrointestinal distress, vaginal candidiasis, phototoxicity, and decreased efficacy of oral contraceptives. It should not be used in younger children or given to pregnant women. Erythromycin, useful for women who take oral contraceptives or who have photosensitivity, may cause greater resistance in *P. acnes* than tetracycline. Minocycline is expensive and may occasionally cause blue discoloration of the skin.

Isotretinoin, (13-cis-retinoic acid, Accutane®) is used for severe, recalcitrant cystic acne. This agent reduces sebaceous gland size, production of sebum, and consequently the amount of *P. acnes*. Isotretinoin is very effective but is teratogenic, and adequate contraception *must* be ensured. It is *absolutely contraindicated in pregnancy*. It may also cause hypertriglyceridemia. Patients treated with isotretinoin should be under the care of a dermatologist.

BIBLIOGRAPHY

American Academy of Dermatology: Guidelines of care for acne vulgaris. *J Am Acad Dermatol* 22:676–680, 1990.

Arndt KA: Acne. In *Manual of Dermatologic Therapeutics,* ed 5. Boston, Little, Brown, 1995, pp 3–15.

Bergfeld WF: Evaluating and managing acne. *Skin* 1:17–21, 1995.

Cunliffe W, Gollnick H: Sebaceous gland science, clinical description, and therapies. In Arndt KA, Leboit PE, Robinson JK, et al (eds): *Cutaneous Medicine and Surgery.* Philadelphia, WB Saunders, 1996, pp 461–480.

Pochi PE: The pathogenesis and treatment of acne. *Annu Rev Med* 41:187–198, 1990.

Redmond GP, Bergfeld WF: Diagnostic approach to androgen disorders in women: Acne, hirsutism, and alopecia. *Cleve Clin J Med* 57:423–427, 1990.

Redmond GP, Bergfeld WF: Treatment of androgenic disorders in women: Acne, hirsutism, and alopecia. *Cleve Clin J Med* 57:428–432, 1990.

Rothman KF, Pochi PE: Use of oral and topical agents for acne in pregnancy. *J Am Acad Dermatol* 19:431–442, 1988.

Straus JS: Sebaceous glands. In Fitzpatrick TB, Eisen AZ, Wolff K, et al (eds): *Dermatology in General Medicine.* New York, McGraw-Hill, 1993, pp 709–726.

Taylor MB: Treatment of acne vulgaris: Guidelines for primary care physicians. *Postgrad Med* 89:40–42, 45–47, 1991.

HAIR LOSS

Hair loss is a problem many women will face during their lifetime. There is great anxiety associated with hair loss, and the physician must be mindful of the significant psychological impact of this symptom.

Alopecia is defined as any abnormal hair loss and has many causes. There are four main categories of hair loss based on clinical findings: *scarring, nonscarring, diffuse,* and *focal* (Table 8.3). Although most patients will have a single type of hair loss, multiple factors may play a role in a particular patient. A thorough history (Table 8.4) and a

TABLE 8.3 Differential Diagnosis of Hair Loss Based on Clinical Presentation

Nonscarring		Scarring	
Diffuse	**Pathcy/Focal**	**Diffuse**	**Patchy**
Telogen effluvium	Alopecia areata	Burns, thermal or chemical	Prolonged trauma
Female pattern baldness	Trichotillomania	Infectious	Pseudopelade
Thyroid disease	Syphilis		Sarcoidosis
Chemotherapy	Tinea capitis		Metastatic cancer
	Pressure or traction		

Reprinted by permission of the publisher from Kois JM, Phelan ST: *Hair loss in women. Prim Care Update Ob/Gyn*. Vol. 1, p. 131, Copyright 1994 by Elsevier Science, Inc.

TABLE 8.4 History Taking in Patients with Hair Loss

Present
1. Which areas of the scalp are involved?
2. Are other body areas involved?
3. When did it start?
4. Is it worsening, staying the same, or improving?
5. Have you experienced this before?
6. Is there any change in skin and nails?
7. Have you changed your hairstyle?
8. Do you pick, pull, or twist your hair?

Health history
1. List past illnesses, operations, or hospitalizations, especially in the last year.
2. Current health problems?
3. Any major stresses such as major life change, weight loss?
4. Medication for 6 months prior to hair change.
5. Last pregnancy.
6. Use of oral contraceptives.
7. Menstrual history.
8. Endocrine disorders, especially thyroid.
9. Unusual dietary habits or changes.
10. Exposure to radiation therapy

Hair care
1. Brands of current shampoos, conditioners, etc.
2. Last permanent and/or hair coloring, with type and frequency.
3. Hair setting—use of curlers, hot combs, hair straighteners, etc.
4. Hair styling—especially tight ponytails, plaits, braids.

Family history
1. Describe any illnesses that run in the family.
2. Sytematically describe the condition of hair and age of each first- and second-degree relative.

Reprinted by permission of the publisher from Kois JM, Phelan ST: *Hair loss in women. Prim Care Update Ob/Gyn*. Vol. 1, p. 131, Copyright 1994 by Elsevier Science, Inc.

physical examination are the first steps in obtaining an accurate diagnosis and will enable the clinician to distinguish between causes that are genetically based, physiologic, externally related, or associated with underlying systemic disease.

The most common cause of hair loss in Caucasian women is *diffuse, nonscarring, androgenetic alopecia.* This occurs in up to 30% of the population prior to age 50. Together with *telogen effluvium (acute or persistent),* these two categories account for up to 90% of the cases of hair loss in women. *Alopecia areata, traumatic alopecia,* and *scarring alopecia* account for most of the remaining cases.

Anatomy and Physiology

The average scalp has approximately 100,000 hairs; approximately 100 hairs are shed daily. Hair grows at a rate of 1 cm per month. Hairs are designated as *vellus hairs,* which are short, fine, light-colored hairs, and *terminal hairs,* which are coarser and darker. *Lanugo hairs* are fine hairs found on the body of the fetus. Scalp hairs are terminal hairs. There are three phases of hair growth: *anagen (growing), catagen (transitional),* and *telogen (resting).* Anagen hairs account for about 85% of scalp hairs. The anagen phase of the growth cycle lasts for approximately 1000 days. The catagen phase lasts for approximately 1 to 2 weeks as hair follicle cells cease to divide. The telogen phase lasts for about 100 days as hairs move to the upper dermis, are shed, and are replaced by growing hairs below.

Androgenetic Alopecia

Androgenetic alopecia, also known as *androgen-dependent alopecia, androgenic alopecia, common baldness, diffuse hair loss, genetic hair loss,* and *female hair loss,* is a form of common progressive hair loss in women. Patients have diffuse hair loss over the crown. This condition occurs early in genetically predisposed women. The frontal hair line is characteristically retained. The clinical presentation of androgenetic alopecia has been classified by Ludwig as follows:

Grade 1—perceptible thinning of the hair on the crown limited in the front by a line situated 1 to 3 cm behind the frontal hair line
Grade 2—progression of grade 1 with decreased density of hair
Grade 3—full baldness within the crown areas seen in grades 1 and 2

Androgenetic alopecia associated with virilizing signs such as acne, hirsutism, and irregular menses should prompt laboratory investigation for virilizing syndromes.

Androgenetic alopecia is genetically based. Its pathogenesis is not clearly understood, but may involve increased androgen receptor activity and increased enzymatic activity regulating gene expression in susceptible hair follicles.

The genetic predisposition of susceptible hair follicles cannot be altered in androgenetic alopecia. *Minoxidil 2%* was approved by the Food and Drug Administration (FDA) in 1991 for the treatment of frontal alopecia in premenopausal women, but the efficacy of this drug in the treatment of this condition has not yet been completely confirmed. Treatment with antiandrogen medications such as *cyproterone acetate, spironolactone,* and *flutamide* has also been tried; these are often used in combination with oral contraceptive agents. *Dexamethasone* has also been used. Flutamide is not yet FDA approved in the United States. It is important for the clinician to know that even a moderate improvement in hair growth potentially results in great patient satisfaction.

Senescent Alopecia

Senescent alopecia is the diffuse thinning of the hair and decreased hair density found in elderly women. It usually begins in the 70s; there is no genetic predisposition. Early onset of senescent alopecia may be confused with other diffuse hair-thinning conditions such as androgenetic alopecia, telogen effluvium, and alopecia areata.

Telogen Effluvium

Telogen effluvium is hair loss due to an aberration of the hair cycle that results in an increased loss of hairs in the telogen or resting phase. The causes include *infectious agents, metabolic disturbances, medications, pregnancy, high fever,* and *psychosocial stressors.* An important cause of chronic telogen effluvium is iron deficiency anemia. Hair loss is due to shedding of the resting hairs with the initiation of a new hair cycle approximately 3 months after the initial insult. The thinning is noticeable to the patient but not always to the physician. Hair plucks show that the percentage of telogen hairs is 30% or more. In postpartum patients, an abrupt drop in estrogen levels causes up to 50% of the hairs to enter telogen; these hairs are pushed out 3 months later.

In most cases, the prognosis is excellent and the patient should be assured that the condition is self-limiting. Identification of any underlying or precipitating cause is necessary, as is psychological support and patient education.

Anagen Effluvium

Anagen effluvium is an abrupt loss of hairs that are in their growth phase. Drugs such as chemotherapeutic agents (antimetabolites, alkylating agents, mitotic inhibitors) and radiation are frequently the cause. These drugs cause an abrupt insult to the metabolic and follicular apparatus. Since only the rapidly dividing cells of the hair matrix and cortex are affected, permanent hair damage does not result. The entire hair is shed intact, and full regrowth is expected once the drug is discontinued. In patients with anagen effluvium, about 10–20% of the hair remains. Applying pressure cuffs to the scalp during chemotherapy may help to avoid this condition.

Alopecia Areata

Alopecia areata is a T-cell-mediated autoimmune disorder, but the specific antigenic cause is unknown. Clinically, there are round, smooth, bald patches measuring 1–5 cm in diameter or larger (Figure 8.2); there may be complete or nearly complete absence of hair. The most common site is the scalp, but other areas may also be involved. Complete loss of scalp hairs is called *alopecia totalis.* Complete loss of body hair, including scalp hair, is termed *alopecia universalis.* "Exclamation point hairs" are classically seen at the edges of the bald areas. These hairs are tapered at the distal end; the tapering is caused by the underlying inflammatory process. Nail abnormalities may be seen in patients with alopecia areata and include erythema of the lunula, pitting, and

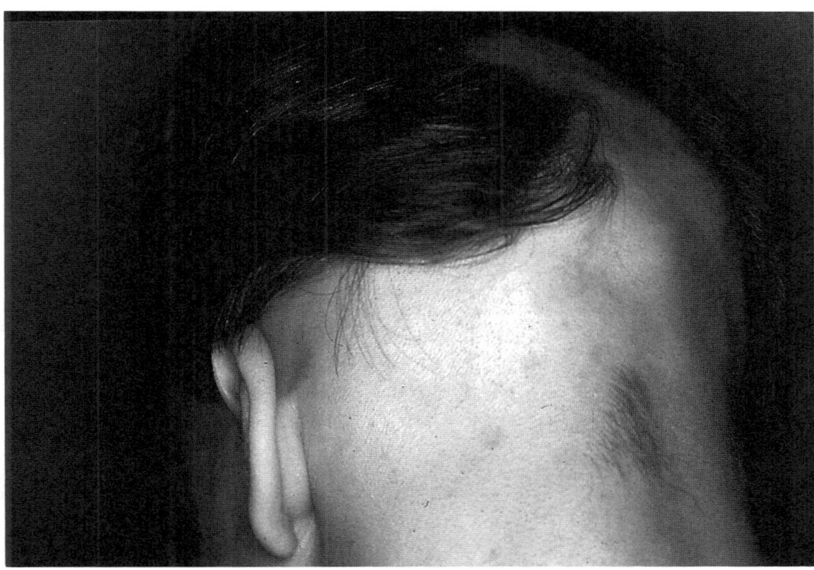

Figure 8.2 Alopecia areata.

longitudinal ridging. Alopecia areata is often associated with other diseases such as atopic dermatitis and autoimmune disorders such as vitiligo, Hashimoto's thyroiditis, and connective tissue diseases. There may be antithyroid, antithyroglobulin, anti-adrenal, or antiparietal cell antibodies. A poor prognosis is associated with early onset (before puberty) and an ophiasis pattern (snaking of hair loss involving the temporal, parietal, and occipital areas).

Emotional stress can be a precipitating factor in alopecia areata and may play a role in stimulating the autoimmune process. The lymphocytes surrounding the hair follicles in alopecia areata are predominantly T-helper cells. Anti-hair follicle antibodies may also play a role.

The differential diagnosis of alopecia areata includes trichotillomania, traumatic hair loss, tinea capitis, secondary syphilis, sarcoidosis, systemic lupus erythematosus, and telogen effluvium. However, the smooth, circumscribed bald patches and the presence of exclamation point hairs usually make this diagnosis straightforward.

It is often difficult to assess the efficacy of treatment modalities due to spontaneous regrowth and the high recurrence rate. Treatment of alopecia areata includes topical, intralesional, or systemic corticosteroids and topical agents such as anthralin, minoxidil 2%, and contact sensitizing agents such as dinitrochlorobenzene. Side effects of topical sensitizing agents include eczematous dermatitis, burning, and itching. More recalcitrant cases of alopecia have been treated with PUVA (psoralen, a photosensitizer, plus UV A light).

Trichotillomania

Trichotillomania is the manual removal of hair patches by the patient. This may be a conscious or subconscious habit and is most often seen in children, adolescents, and women. In contrast to alopecia areata, the borders of hair loss in trichotillomania are often angular and irregular. The clinical hallmark of this condition is uneven, broken hairs within a patch of hair loss. This disorder may represent a simple habit such as a tic or may be symptomatic of a deeper psychological problem. Treatment consists of identifying the precipitating factors and making the patient aware of this habit. Psychiatric referral may be necessary.

Traumatic Alopecia

Traumatic alopecia may be caused by traction, pressure, and cosmetic manipulation. Traction alopecia is most commonly located in the frontotemporal areas and is due to excess traction caused by certain hairstyles. Pressure alopecia usually results from prolonged pressure at a particular site on the scalp during a surgical procedure. Traumatic hair loss due to various hair styling techniques, particularly in black women, should be identified. Treatment is based on identifying the underlying cause. The prognosis is usually excellent once the patient has been advised to avoid the precipitating factor. Early intervention is important since prolonged traumatic hair loss can eventually lead to scarring and permanent loss of hair follicles.

Scarring Alopecia

Scarring alopecia has many causes. These may include developmental defects such as aplasia cutis congenita; hereditary disorders; inflammatory conditions such as connective tissue disorders; sarcoidosis; underlying neoplasms; metastatic disease; and infectious diseases such as syphilis and tinea capitis. Treatment depends upon identification of the underlying cause. Dermatologic referral and scalp biopsy may be necessary.

BIBLIOGRAPHY

Arnold HL Jr, Odom RB, James WD: *Andrews' Diseases of the Skin,* ed 8. Philadelphia, WB Saunders, 1990, pp 879–887.

Baden HP: *Diseases of the Hair and Nails.* Chicago, Year Book Medical, 1987.

DeVillez RL, Jacobs JP, Szpunar CA: Androgenetic alopecia in the female: Treatment with 2% topical minoxidil solution. *Arch Dermatol* 130:303–307, 1994.

Habif TP: *Clinical Dermatology. A Color Guide to Diagnosis and Therapy,* ed 3. St Louis, CV Mosby, 1990, pp 739–757.

Headington JT: Telogen effluvium. New concepts and review. *Arch Dermatol* 129:356–363, 1993.

Jacobs JP, Szpunar CA, Warner ML: Use of topical minoxidil therapy for androgenetic alopecia in women. *Int J Dermatol* 32:758–762, 1993.

Kligman AM: Pathologic dynamics of human hair loss I: Telogen effluvium. *Arch Dermatol* 83:175–198, 1961.

Kois JM, Phelan ST: Hair loss in women. *Prim Care Update Ob/Gyn* 1:130–136, 1994.

Rooh A, Dawber RS: *Diseases of the Hair and Scalp,* ed 2. Oxford, Blackwell Scientific, 1991, pp 113–166.

Rushton DH: Management of hair loss in women. *Dermatol Clin* 11:47–53, 1993.

Tobin DJ, Orentreich N, Fenton DA: Antibodies to hair follicles in alopecia areata. *J Invest Dermatol* 102:721–724, 1994.

SKIN INFECTIONS

Skin infections caused by bacteria, fungi, and viruses are commonly seen in primary care. Prompt recognition and treatment are necessary to reduce the likelihood of serious complications.

Bacterial Skin Infections

Bacterial skin infections may be caused by organisms which normally inhabit the skin and mucous membranes or may arise from exogenous sources such as other people, the environment, or contaminated objects. Factors which disrupt the integrity of the skin such as trauma, inflammatory skin diseases, and excess hydration predispose to infection.

Gram-Positive Organisms

Two common gram-positive bacteria causing skin infections are *Staphylococcus aureus* and *Streptococcus pyogenes*. *S. aureus* is located mainly in the anterior nares and colonizes about 30% of the normal population. It is present on normal skin in less than 5% of healthy people, but in disorders such as atopic dermatitis and diabetes mellitus its prevalence is markedly increased. The organism may spread to cutaneous locations and cause infection, colonize or infect others, and spread to inanimate objects. *S. pyogenes* is also often located in the nasopharynx of normal individuals. It may contaminate the skin from that site, become inoculated during trauma, and produce clinical infection.

Impetigo is a superficial bacterial infection which may be caused by both *S. pyogenes* and *S. aureus*. It usually occurs in children but may occur in adults as well. Factors which predispose to infection are poor hygiene, preceding varicella and scabies, and preexisting skin conditions such as atopic dermatitis. The initial lesions are red papules which become vesicles and pustules; these quickly rupture and form honey-colored crusts on an erythematous base. Treatment may be topical *mupirocin*, three times a day for 1 week, or oral administration of antibiotics effective against gram-positive organisms such as *erythromycin*. Alternatively, *dicloxacillin*, *cephalexin*, or *cephadrine* can be used in erythromycin-resistant cases (about 25%). Antibacterial cleansers such as Phisohex or Hibiclens should be recommended. Some cases of impetigo are caused by nephritogenic strains of *S. pyogenes* and may result in subsequent acute glomerulonephritis; treatment with antibiotics does not protect against this complication.

Bullous impetigo is a type of impetigo seen mainly in children (Figure 8.3) and is caused by certain strains of *S. aureus* which elaborate an exfoliative toxin. The toxin causes an intraepidermal split and results in blister formation. Treatment is the same as for impetigo.

Staphylococcal scalded skin syndrome is caused by the same toxin-producing strains of *S. aureus* and is characterized by widespread blistering and sloughing of the skin; this

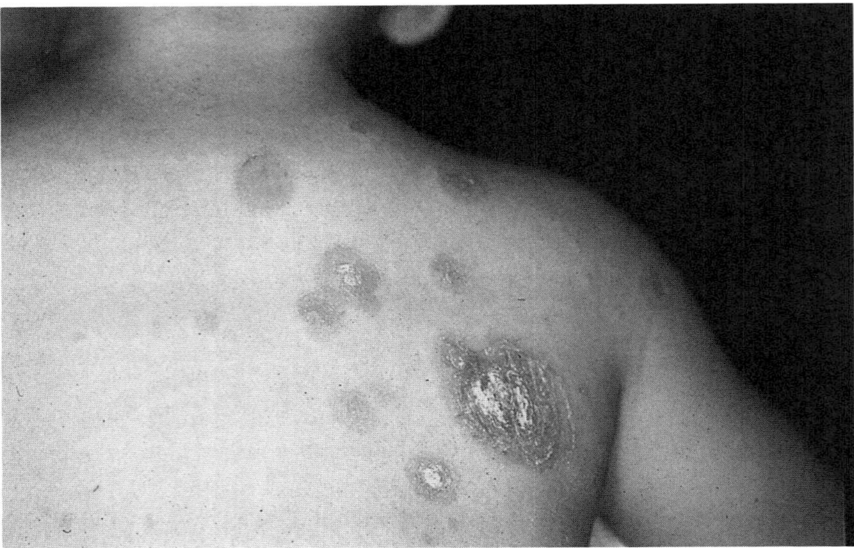

Figure 8.3 Bullous impetigo in a child.

disorder is seen mainly in infants and children. Treatment is with antimicrobial agents and supportive measures.

Infection within hair follicles is called *folliculitis*. Clinical findings are erythematous papules and pustules surrounding hair follicles singly or in clusters, most commonly located on the scalp, face, thighs, or buttocks. Predisposing factors are follicular occlusion, excess skin hydration, and surrounding inflammatory processes such as chemical or mechanical injury. Lesional cultures may grow *S. aureus* or normal skin flora or may be sterile. Treatment consists of good local hygiene and a systemic antistaphylococcal antibiotic; topical antibiotics may be sufficient for localized disease.

If staphylococcal infection of the hair follicle occurs at a deeper level, *furuncles* and *carbuncles* may develop. A furuncle is a deep-seated papule or boil and is found most often in hair-bearing areas subject to friction such as the scalp, face, axillae, thighs, and buttocks. A carbuncle is a staphylococcal abscess which is larger and deeper and usually drains at several sites. Carbuncles are more common in individuals with diabetes mellitus. Moist, warm compresses and topical antibiotics usually suffice for furuncles. Larger furuncles and carbuncles should be incised and drained, followed by application of topical antibiotics. Systemic antibiotics are used if there is surrounding cellulitis or fever.

Cellulitis is an acute, rapidly spreading infection of the skin and underlying subcutaneous tissue (deep dermis and subcutaneous fat) but not involving the muscle. It is caused most frequently by *S. pyogenes* and most commonly involves the extremities. Local trauma, which may go unrecognized, often precedes the infection. Local erythema and tenderness are present; there may be systemic symptoms such as fever and chills. Infection spreads rapidly to contiguous skin. The margin of infected skin is irregular, and there may be accompanying vesicles, bullae, petechiae, and purpura. Lymphangitis may be present. Cultures of needle-aspirated material and blood have low yields; consequently, the diagnosis is usually made clinically, and therapy is guided by the patient's response to antimicrobial agents. Skin biopsy may be necessary if the diagnosis is in doubt. *Erysipelas* is a more superficial type of cellulitis. It is caused almost exclusively by *S. pyogenes* and, in contrast to cellulitis, has a well-demarcated, raised, indurated border. It commonly involves the face. There may be a several-hour prodrome of malaise, chills, fever, headache, vomiting, and arthralgias. Vesicles and bullae may be present. Both erysipelas and cellulitis may progress to septicemia. Treatment is similar for both cellulitis and erysipelas. Oral agents such as erythromycin, dicloxacillin, clindamycin, cephalexin, or cephadrine may be used. Penicillin may be used for erysipelas since this condition is nearly always of streptococcal origin. For patients who are very ill, intravenous administration of appropriate antibiotics is indicated. Local measures such as elevation of the infected area are helpful.

In patients with recurrent cellulitis in the same location, predisposing factors such as tinea pedis and preexisting skin conditions should be explored. Antibiotic prophylaxis may be necessary.

Ecthyma is an ulcerative streptococcal infection which usually affects the shins or dorsa of the feet and is caused by *S. pyogenes*. The lesion starts as a vesicle or vesicopustule which enlarges and in a few days becomes crusted (Figure 8.4). Beneath the crust is a superficial ulcer which usually heals in a few weeks and leaves a scar. Gangrene may ensue in a debilitated patient. Treatment is with an intravenous antibiotic effective against *S. pyogenes*. In addition, cleaning with soap and water followed by application of a topical antibiotic such as mupirocin is performed.

Gram-Negative Organisms

Gram-negative folliculitis, described earlier in the section on acne, is characterized by erythematous papules and pustules. Treatment is with oral antibiotics based on the results of lesional cultures and sensitivity tests.

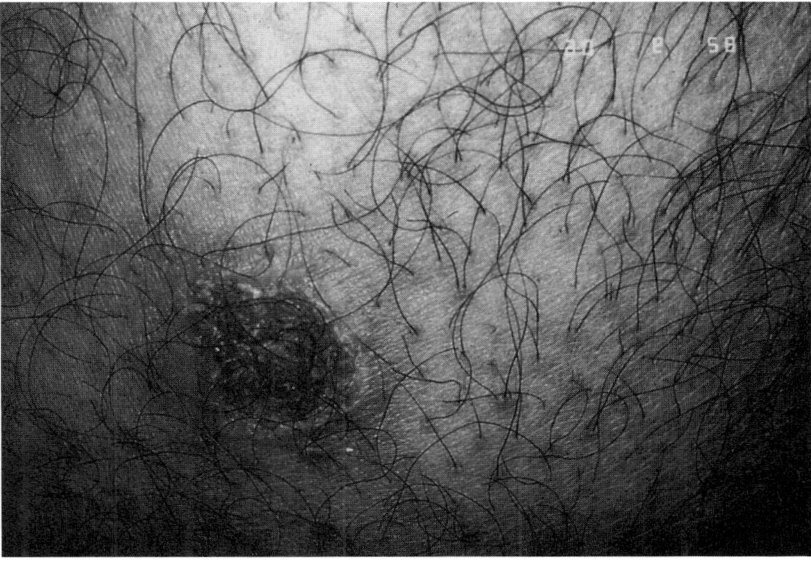

Figure 8.4 Ecthyma.

Pseudomonas folliculitis may be seen 1 to 4 days after bathing in a hot tub, whirlpool, or public pool. Clinically, there are pruritic, follicle-based macules, papules, vesicles, or pustules. Typical sites of infection are the trunk, axillae, buttocks, and proximal extremities. This infection is usually self-limited and resolves within 1 to 2 weeks.

Lyme Disease

Lyme disease is currently the most common tick-borne illness in the United States, with over 40,000 cases reported to the Centers for Disease Control (CDC) from 1982 to 1991. The illness is caused by infection with the spirochete *Borrelia burgdorferi,* which is transmitted to humans by the Ixodes tick (Ixodes scapularis in the Northeast and Ixodes pacificus in the West), whose two main hosts are the white-footed mouse (nymphal and larval ticks) and the white-tailed deer (adult ticks). Although the clinical manifestations of Lyme disease are well described and effective treatment is available, the disease is often overdiagnosed and overtreated. The reasons include lack of physician knowledge concerning the illness, problems with laboratory testing, and intense public anxiety. Patients and physicians are often quick to suspect Lyme disease when confronted with vague symptoms and various skin findings. The best strategy for overcoming these obstacles is to obtain a careful history and pay close attention to the clinical findings; laboratory investigations are useful in certain settings.

The clinical manifestations of Lyme disease occur in stages defined as early infection and late infection (Table 8.5). Early infection occurs during the first few months and includes stage 1, localized infection (erythema migrans), and stage 2, disseminated infection (secondary annular lesions, meningitis, seventh nerve palsy, and carditis). Late infection or stage 3, persistent infection (chronic arthritis, chronic neurologic abnormalities, and acrodermatitis chronica atrophicans), occurs months to years into the illness. Not all patients with Lyme disease have all of these manifestations or this characteristic progression.

Erythema migrans, the pathognomonic skin lesion of Lyme disease, is seen in 60–80% of patients at the site of the tick bite. Many patients do not recall being bitten by a tick. An erythematous macule or papule is seen 3 to 32 days after the bite (median, 7 days); this expands gradually (over days to 1–2 weeks) to form a large, erythematous, annular patch with central clearing and a bright border (Figure 8.5). The center of the lesion may in some cases be vesicular or necrotic. The CDC surveillance definition of erythema migrans requires that the lesion be at least 5 cm in diameter. The lesion is usually larger (median diameter, 15 cm). It is usually painless and resolves within several weeks. Erythema migrans may lack central clearing. During stage 2 (disseminated disease), secondary annular lesions may occur; no central papules are present, since these lesions are not at the site of the original tick bite.

The differential diagnosis of erythema migrans includes bacterial cellulitis, contact dermatitis, fixed drug eruption, tinea corporis, tick bite reaction, and insect or spider bite reaction. Tick bite reactions occur within hours after a bite and expand over hours. Insect or spider bite reactions usually occur minutes to hours or days after the bite and expand over a similar time period.

Diagnosis of Lyme disease is based on the characteristic clinical manifestations, exposure in an endemic area, and a serologic response to *B. burgdorferi.* The

TABLE 8.5 Manifestations of Lyme Disease by Stage

	Early Infection		
System*	**Localized**	**Disseminated**	**Late Infection**
Skin	Erythema migrans	Secondary annular lesions, malar rash, diffuse erythema or urticaria, evanescent lesions, lymphocytoma	Acrodermatitis chronica atrophicans, localized scleroderma-like lesions
Musculoskeletal system		Migratory pain in joints, tendons, bursae, muscle, bone; brief arthritis attacks; myositis,† osteomyelitis,† panniculitis†	Prolonged arthritis attacks, chronic arthritis, peripheral enthesopathy, periostitis or joint subluxations below lesions of acrodermatitis
Neurologic system		Meningitis, cranial neuritis, Bell's palsy, motor or sensory radiculoneuritis, subtle encephalitis, mononeuritis multiplex, myelitis,† chrorea,† cerebellar ataxia†	Chronic encephalomyelitis, spastic paraparesis, ataxic gait, subtle mental disorders, chronic axonal polyradiculopathy, dementia†
Lymphatic system	Regional lymphadenopathy	Regional or generalized lymphadenopathy, splenomegaly	
Cardiovascular system		Atrioventricular nodal block, myopericarditis, pancarditis	
Ocular system		Conjunctivitis, iritis,† choroiditis,† retinal hemorrhage or detachment,† panophthalmitis†	Keratitis
Gastrointestinal system		Mild or recurrent hepatitis	
Respiratory system		Nonexudative pharyngitis, nonproductive cough, adult respiratory distress syndrome†	
Genitourinary system		Orchitis;† microscopic hematuria or proteinuria	
Constitutional	Minor	Severe malaise and fatigue	Fatigue

Source: Reprinted by permission of *The New England Journal of Medicine*. Steere AC: Lyme Disease. *New Engl J Med* 321:589, copyright 1989, Massachusetts Medical Society.

*Systems listed from most to least commonly affected.

†Based on one or a few cases.

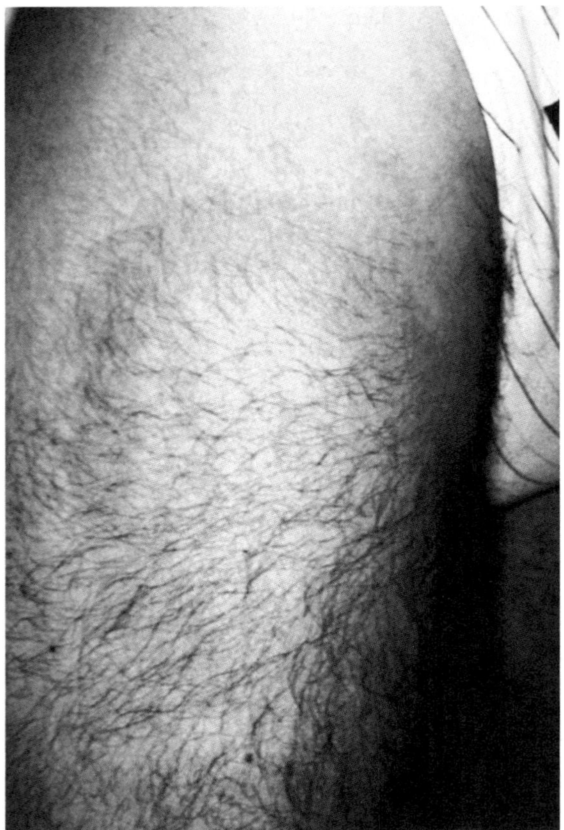

Figure 8.5 Erythema migrans.

enzyme-linked immunosorbent assay for detecting IgM and IgG to this organism is, however, not standardized, and false-negative and, more commonly, false-positive results may occur. In the absence of typical clinical symptoms or exposure in an endemic area, one should consider other diagnostic possibilities even if the serologic test is positive. Polymerase chain reaction may become useful in detecting the organism in patients with suspected Lyme disease.

First-line treatment of Lyme disease is doxycycline, 100 mg po bid. The optimal duration of treatment is not established; 10–30 days have been recommended. For children less than 9 years old, amoxicillin, 250 mg tid, is used. In the pregnant or lactating woman, amoxicillin, 500 mg tid, is given. Infectious disease specialists should be consulted for up-to-date treatment guidelines.

Maternal-fetal transmission of Lyme disease was described in 1985 and has been documented in over 40 pregnancies worldwide. Fetal damage and wastage may occur secondary to intrauterine infection; however, providing an accurate prognosis for the fetus may be difficult based on the limited amount of information available. Treatment of erythema migrans during pregnancy is with amoxicillin or erythromycin in the penicillin-allergic patient.

Fungal Skin Infections

Fungal skin infections may be due to *dermatophytes, Candida albicans,* and the *superficial mycoses.* The dermatophytes are fungi which invade the stratum corneum and its appendages. *Candida* is a yeast-like fungus which normally inhabits the skin, mucosa, gastrointestinal tract, and vagina, and which, under certain conditions, becomes pathogenic. The superficial mycoses infect only the superficial layers of the stratum corneum; the most important of these infections is pityriasis (tinea) versicolor, caused by *Pityrosporum orbicularis.*

Dermatophytes

Dermatophyte infections are described according to the site affected: *tinea capitis* (head), *tinea facei* (face), *tinea corporis* (body), *tinea manuum* (hands), *tinea cruris* (groin), *tinea pedis* (feet), and *tinea unguim* (nails). The three genera of dermatophytes are *Epidermophyton, Microsporum,* and *Trichophyton.* Infection may be acquired from three sources: soil, animals, and other humans. Although some species of dermatophyte cause specific clinical infections, it may be difficult to differentiate among them clinically. Predisposing factors for infection include poor nutrition, tropical climate, skin injuries, and underlying debilitating disease.

Tinea capitis is seen most frequently in children. There is infection of the hair shaft, with resultant patchy hair loss and broken hairs, scaling, and inflammation. There may be an accompanying hypersensitivity reaction with a boggy, inflammatory mass known as a *kerion.* Tinea corporis, infection of nonhairy skin, is seen in all age groups. There may be a history of contact with puppies or kittens. The initial lesion is an erythematous macule or papule which spreads outward to form circular patches with sharp, scaling, or vesicular borders; healing occurs centrally and is seen as central clearing

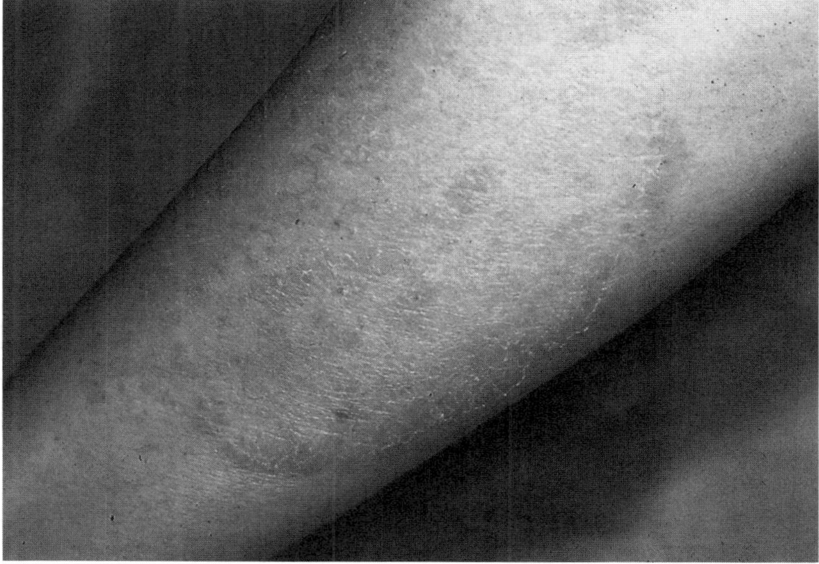

Figure 8.6 Tinea corporis, partially treated.

(Figure 8.6). Tinea manuum presents with mild erythema, hyperkeratosis, and scaling over the palmar surfaces. Tinea pedis or "athlete's foot" almost always accompanies tinea manuum. Tinea pedis may be seen as interdigital scaling and maceration, widespread scaling in a "moccasin foot" distribution, or as a vesicular or bullous eruption. Tinea cruris or "jock itch" is an infection of the groin and upper inner thigh; there are sharply demarcated, bilaterally symmetrical, scaly, erythematous patches which may extend into the gluteal folds and buttocks. This condition is more frequent in hot, humid climates and in athletic individuals. Tinea ungium, fungal infection of the nail plate, is seen in about 40% of patients with fungal infections in other areas. Toenails are more commonly involved than fingernails. There is thickening and distortion of the nail, which may be lifted up by subungual debris.

Diagnosis of dermatophyte infection rests on demonstration of hyphae and spores in potassium hydroxide (KOH) preparations; the specific infecting organism is identified by fungal culture.

Topical therapy is usually sufficient for infection of the face, body, and groin and for superficial infections of the palms and soles; numerous effective preparations are available for this purpose, including the imidazoles (e.g., clotrimazole, econazole, ketoconazole, sulconazole) and the allylamines (naftifine, terbinafine). Treatment is generally given twice a day and should continue for at least 4 weeks to decrease the rate of relapse. Systemic therapy is needed for tinea ungium and tinea capitis. Recently, itraconazole and terbinafine were approved for oral treatment of onychomycosis. Griseofulvin remains the mainstay of treatment for tinea capitis in children.

Candidiasis

There are many factors which predispose to infection with *Candida:* systemic antibiotics; local moisture, warmth, and maceration; diabetes; pregnancy; Cushing's disease; debilitating illness; and immunosuppression.

Clinical infections may occur as *paronychia, perleche, intertriginous lesions, thrush,* and *vulvovaginitis.* Diagnosis involves the demonstration of budding yeasts, with or without hyphae or pseudohyphae, on direct examination with KOH. Gram stain will show yeast forms producing germ tubes. Culture may also be used, especially for nonmucosal infections.

In candidal paronychia there is chronic inflammation of the nail fold. The area surrounding the nail is tender, and the nail itself becomes thickened, with brownish discoloration, development of transverse ridges, and erosion of the lateral borders. Pus may be expressible. Usually only the fingernails are affected, often only one nail. This condition is seen frequently in patients with diabetes mellitus and in those whose hands are frequently moist—food handlers, cooks, dishwashers, bartenders, nurses, canners, and laundry workers. Treatment is with topical anticandidal solutions or creams such as *miconazole, clotrimazole,* or other *imidazoles* and must be continued for 2 to 3 months to prevent recurrences. In addition, all wet work should be stopped, and gloves and cotton liners must be worn to protect the hands.

Perleche (angular cheilitis), manifests as erythema, maceration, and transverse fissuring of the oral commissures. This entity is a symptom and may be caused by infection (candidal as well as bacterial) and by drooling in persons with ill-fitting dentures. It may be seen in the elderly with atrophy of the alveolar ridges, resulting in the upper

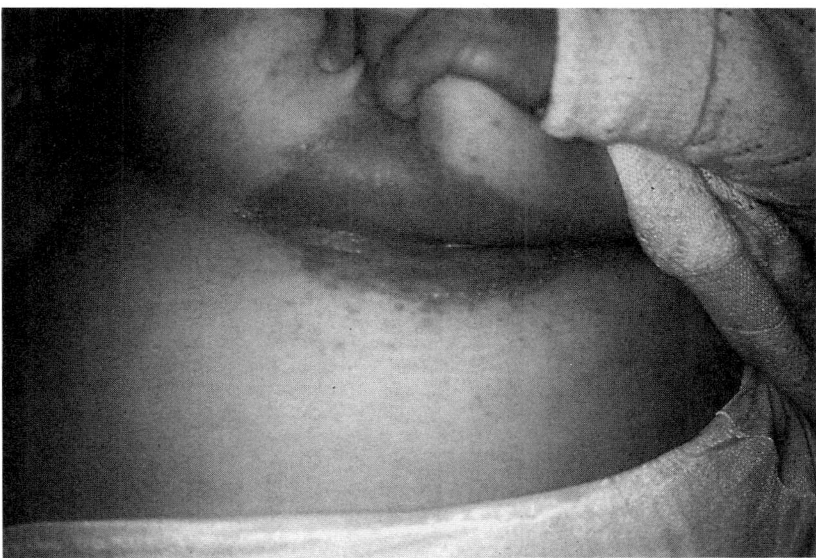

Figure 8.7 Candidal intertrigo.

lip overhanging the lower lip at the commissures, and in children who lick their lips, drool, or suck their thumbs. Candidal perleche is treated with topical anticandidal agents.

The intertriginous lesions of candidal infection occur in areas predisposed to maceration: inframammary folds (Figure 8.7), axillae, groin, perianal area, and interdigital areas. There are moist, erythematous papules and plaques, occasionally with scaling, often causing pruritus and discomfort. Satellite papules or pustules are characteristic. Topical agents are applied indefinitely until resolution occurs.

Thrush is seen as white plaques loosely attached to the oral mucosa, which is bright red and moist. Nystatin oral suspension 3 to 4 times a day until resolution or clotrimazole troches 5 to 10 times a day for 2 weeks are highly effective. Oral fluconazole may also be used.

Candidal vulvovaginitis presents with vulvar erythema and pruritus, with or without vaginal discharge. The degree of erythema and edema parallels the severity of the infection. Treatment is with anticandidal tablets, suppositories, or creams.

Pityriasis (Tinea) Versicolor

Pityriasis versicolor, also known as *tinea versicolor,* is a common superficial fungal infection caused by *Pityrosporum orbicularis.* This is the pathogenic, filamentous form of *P. ovale,* a normal skin inhabitant. Factors which predispose to transformation from the yeast to the filamentous form, and thus to infection, are increased humidity, sweating, use of systemic corticosteroids, Cushing's syndrome, immunodeficiency, malnutrition, and pregnancy. Infection may be chronic because of inadequate treatment, reinfection, or a genetic predisposition to infection. There is no racial or sex predominance. Most patients develop the disease in the summer months.

Figure 8.8 Pityriasis (tinea) versicolor.

Infection typically occurs on the trunk and proximal upper extremities. One sees slightly scaly, hypopigmented, and/or hyperpigmented, erythematous, salmon-colored patches (Figure 8.8). Initially, the lesions are discrete, scaly macules which later coalesce into large patches. Patients are usually asymptomatic and present for cosmetic reasons. Occasionally there may be pruritus. Infection often becomes noticeable in the summertime after the affected areas fail to tan.

The diagnosis rests on the clinical appearance and the characteristic findings on microscopic examination of scale with KOH, which shows both hyphae and yeast forms, likened to "spaghetti and meatballs." Fungal cultures are seldom used for diagnosis. The differential diagnosis include pityriasis alba, vitiligo, seborrheic dermatitis, and postinflammatory hyper- or hypopigmentation.

Treatment is generally topical, with selenium sulfide or antifungal azole creams. Systemic medications such as ketoconazole, fluconazole, and itraconazole may be used in severe or extensive cases or in those patients who do not respond to topical agents. Topical agents should be applied to the entire torso from neck to waist, since the lesions may be widespread or clinically inapparent. Pigmentary changes may take several months to resolve.

Viral Skin Infections and Viral Exanthems

Viruses may cause primary skin infections as well as exanthems, which are acute, generalized, cutaneous eruptions.

Herpes simplex virus (HSV) is a member of the human herpesvirus family, which includes HSV types 1 and 2, varicella-zoster virus, Epstein-Barr virus, cytomegalovirus,

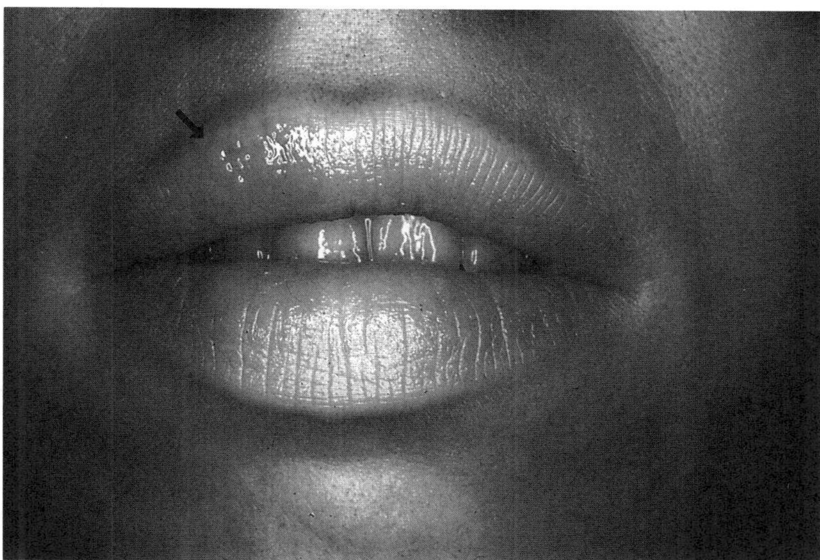

Figure 8.9 Herpes labialis (arrow).

human herpesvirus 6, and human herpesvirus 7. HSV type 1 usually causes nongenital herpes, while HSV type 2 usually causes genital lesions. Infection with HSV is extremely common; in the United States, orolabial herpes affects an estimated one-third of the U.S. population, while an estimated 25 million adults have serologic evidence of prior infection with HSV type 2. While effective immunity may develop in some individuals after primary infection, 20–45% of individuals will have recurrent disease. Genital HSV infection recurs six times more frequently than orofacial HSV infection.

Clinical lesions of *primary orofacial herpes* occur about 5 to 10 days after exposure. Lesions may occur on the face, lips, tongue, and buccal mucosa. There are painful, grouped vesicles which progress to erosions and ulcers. Systemic symptoms vary from mild to severe and include fever, lymphadenopathy, and pharyngitis. In *primary genital herpes,* lesions appear 3 days to 2 weeks after exposure. There are painful grouped vesicles which progress to ulcers on the vulva, labia, and surrounding skin. Inguinal lymphadenopathy may be present.

A *herpetic whitlow* is caused by primary inoculation of the paronychial area of the fingers. This may occur in children with concurrent herpes gingivostomatitis and in physicians and nurses. There is a sudden appearance of vesicles and extreme pain; lesions may last for up to 28 days. This entity is often misdiagnosed as a bacterial infection and mistreated with incision and drainage.

Recurrent herpes occurs upon reactivation of latent virus and may be precipitated by factors such as stress, trauma, menstruation, fatigue, and exposure to sunlight. Recurrent lesions are preceded by a premonitory sensation of burning or tingling. *Recurrent orofacial herpes* ("cold sores") may occur on the lips (Figure 8.9), perioral area, cheeks, and nose and may manifest as multiple small, grouped, clear vesicles on an erythematous base. The vesicles become cloudy and purulent; and then they dry, crust, and heal

TABLE 8.6 Treatment of HSV Infections with Acyclovir

Host	Dose of Acyclovir
Immunocompetent	
First episode, genital only	Acyclovir ointment q2h
First episode, genital or nongenital	200 mg po 5×/day × 10 days
Recurrences (<6/yr)	200 mg po 5×/day × 5 days
Recurrences (≥6/yr)	200 mg po tid-5×/day or 400 mg po bid
Immunocompromised	
First episode	Acyclovir ointment q2h or 200 mg po 5×/day × 10 days
Recurrence	400 mg po 5×/day × 15 days then 400 mg po tid × 1–2 months then 400 mg po bid
Severe infection	5 mg/kg q8h IV × 7 days (given over 1h q8)

Source: Scheman AJ, Severson DL: *Pocket Guide to Medications Used in Dermatology*, ed 4. Baltimore, Williams & Wilkins, 1994, pp 70–71.

in 7 to 10 days. There is accompanying regional lymphadenopathy. In *recurrent genital herpes* there is also a cluster of painful vesicles which progress to ulceration and crusting. Recurrent *erythema multiforme* may be associated with recurrent HSV infection.

Diagnosis of HSV infection is usually made on clinical grounds. A Tzanck preparation is a cytologic smear used to detect the multinucleate giant cells characteristically seen in infection with HSV and varicella-zoster virus. A vesicle is unroofed with a No. 15 scalpel blade; the base of the vesicle is scraped with the blade, and the contents are rubbed on a glass slide and stained with Wright-Giemsa stain. One sees multinucleate giant cells in about 75% of cases of culture-positive, recurrent orofacial herpes but in only 40% of genital lesions. Viral culture can be done to confirm the infection; HSV will easily grow from up to 90% of typical lesions.

Treatment of HSV infection with acyclovir, a guanosine analogue which inhibits viral DNA synthesis (Table 8.6). Acyclovir may be used to treat primary HSV infections, individual recurrent episodes, and as prophylaxis against recurrent outbreaks. Oral acyclovir therapy will promote resolution of primary orofacial and genital herpes if begun within 3 days of onset. Early treatment of recurrent genital herpes (<48 h duration) may shorten the healing time and reduce the formation of new lesions. Daily prophylaxis with acyclovir will also decrease the number of episodes of recurrent orofacial and genital herpes. Topical acyclovir may be of modest benefit for the first outbreak of genital herpes in the immunocompetent host or for orofacial herpes in the immunocompromised host. The antiviral agents Valacyclovir (Valtrex®, 500 mg po bid × 5 days) and famciclovir (Famvir®, 125 mg po bid × 5 days) were recently approved for treatment of recurrent genital herpes in the immunocompetent host.

Varicella-zoster virus (VZV) causes primary infection in the form of *varicella (chicken pox)* and secondary disease in the form of *herpes zoster (shingles)*. More than 90% of adults in the United States have serologic evidence of prior VZV infection. As in HSV infections, cytologic smears and viral cultures may assist in the diagnosis, as may direct immunofluorescence assays of lesional scrapings for VZV antigens.

Varicella is acquired through the respiratory tract after exposure to an infected individual. The incubation period is 10 to 21 days. Infected persons are contagious for 1 to 2 days before lesions develop until all lesions have crusted over, usually about a week. The lesions begin as erythematous macules and papules which quickly evolve to vesicles with an erythematous halo ("dewdrop on a rose petal"). Lesions first appear on the head, trunk, or mucous membranes and then extend centripetally for 2 to 4 days. The vesicles quickly become umbilicated; the fluid then changes from clear to cloudy, and the vesicles become crusted and heal. A characteristic finding in varicella is that lesions in all stages are seen simultaneously. Systemic symptoms such as fever, malaise, anorexia, and pruritus are usually present.

In the normal host, varicella is usually a benign, self-limited illness. Acyclovir may be used to decrease the number and healing time of lesions. In the immunosuppressed host, acyclovir is given since the severity of disease may be greater, with more lesions, longer healing time, visceral complications, and increased mortality. In any host, supportive measures such as Aveeno® oatmeal baths and antihistamines are helpful. The nails should be kept short and the hands clean to help prevent bacterial superinfection in excoriated lesions. Complications of varicella include bacterial superinfection (impetigo, erysipelas, cellulitis, myositis), varicella pneumonia, acute cerebellitis, optic neuritis, transverse myelitis, and Guillain-Barré syndrome. Reye's syndrome (encephalopathy with liver dysfunction) has been associated with varicella infection and aspirin use.

A live-attenuated varicella vaccine (Varivax, Oka/Merck) was recently approved for use in the United States for vaccination against varicella in individuals 12 months of age and older; its use is contraindicated during pregnancy.

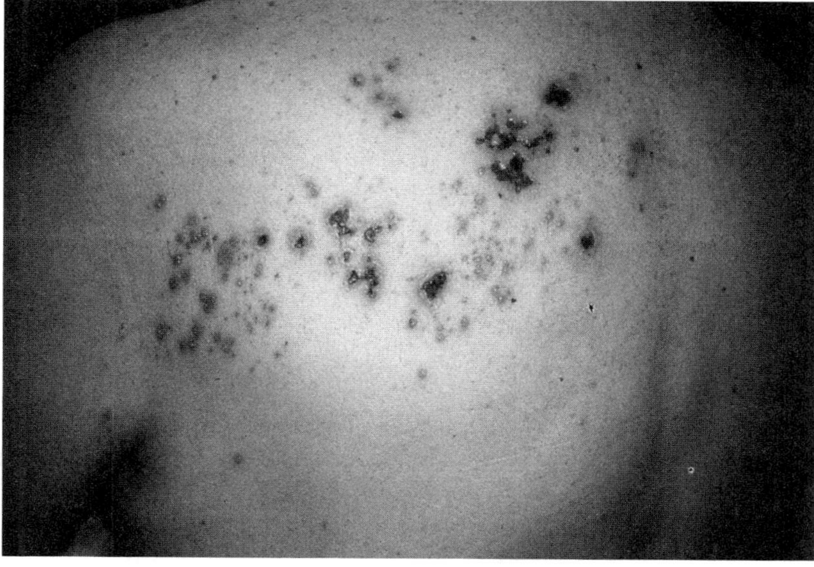

Figure 8.10 Herpes zoster.

Herpes zoster is caused by reactivation of latent VZV. Patients present with radicular pain followed by an eruption of vesicles on an erythematous base in a dermatomal distribution (Figure 8.10). The lesions crust and heal, as in varicella. The rash may involve one to three dermatomes; if widespread lesions are present, this condition is said to be disseminated or generalized herpes zoster, occurring most often in patients with malignancies or immunosuppression and in the aged. The dermatomes most often involved are the thoracic ones, followed by the lumbar, trigeminal, cervical, and sacral ones. If lesions involve the ophthalmic branch of the trigeminal nerve, an ophthalmologist should be consulted. Ramsay-Hunt syndrome occurs when herpes zoster involves the geniculate ganglion; patients have a polycranial neuropathy involving cranial nerves VI and VII. Vesicles may appear on the tympanic membrane, and there may be a peripheral facial nerve palsy.

The lesions of herpes zoster heal in 1 to 2 weeks. In the immunocompetent host, acyclovir (800 mg po five times a day for 7 to 10 days) hastens healing and decreases acute pain. Postherpetic neuralgia—debilitating pain at the site of the previous zoster infection—may occur in up to half of patients over age 50. Traditional analgesics are used. Famciclovir (500 mg po tid for 7 days) reduces the symptoms of postherpetic neuralgia. Valacyclovir (1 g po tid for 7 days), may also shorten the duration of postherpetic neuralgia, but as of this writing, the reduction has not been statistically significant.

Molluscum contagiosum is a poxvirus infection which commonly occurs in children but which may also affect normal and immunocompromised adults. Transmission is from person to person; genital lesions in adults may be sexually transmitted. In immunosuppressed hosts, the disease is more severe and difficult to treat. It is also more common in children with atopic dermatitis.

The characteristic lesions are grouped, umbilicated, flesh-colored or pearly papules a few millimeters in diameter. They are usually asymptomatic but may be pruritic. The diagnosis is usually made clinically, but it can be confirmed by skin biopsy or by cytologic examination for molluscum bodies. The contents of a papule are expressed and smeared on a glass slide; stained with Wright, Giemsa, or Gram stain; and examined microscopically for molluscum bodies, which are ovoid, smooth cytoplasmic masses containing incomplete virions and cellular debris.

The lesions usually resolve spontaneously in 6 to 9 months but, if untreated, may last for years. Treatment options include curettage, light electrodessication, or cryotherapy with liquid nitrogen.

Measles (rubeola) is caused by a paramyxovirus for which humans are the only reservoir. Recent epidemics underscore the need for ensuring immunization in all children and for considering this disorder in the differential diagnosis of viral exanthems. Recent reports indicate that 10–20% of women of childbearing age are serosusceptible to rubella. Currently, the initial vaccination is given at 12 to 15 months of age as part of the MMR (measles, mumps, rubella) vaccine, followed by a second vaccination at ages 4 to 6 or 11 to 12 to protect against primary vaccine failure. Young adults should be asked if they have received their second vaccination.

The illness begins with a prodrome which lasts for 2 to 4 days. There is fever, cough, coryza, and conjunctivitis. There may be a transient macular or urticarial rash early in the prodrome. The enanthem of measles are Koplik spots—tiny white or bluish-gray

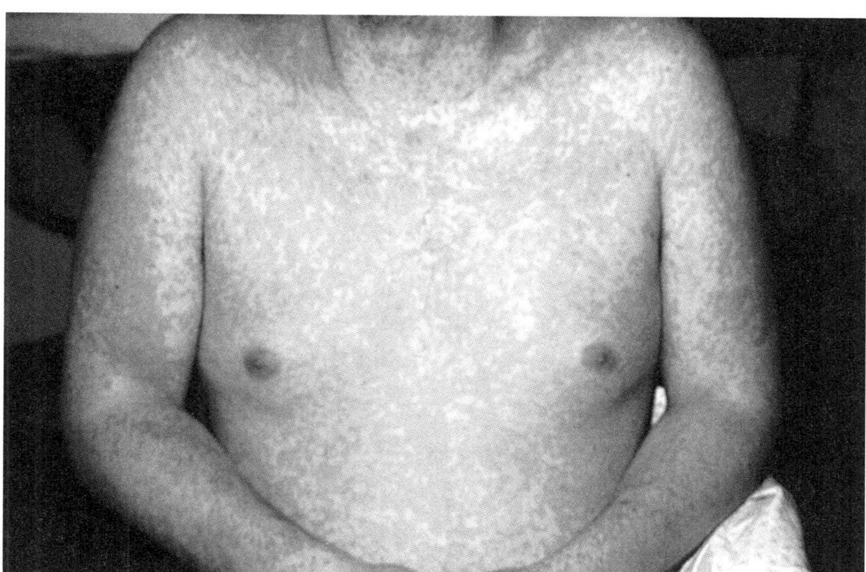

Figure 8.11 Measles.

papules on an erythematous base on the buccal mucosa and palate. The exanthem of measles starts behind the ears, spreads from head to toe, and involves the whole body by the third day. There are discrete, erythematous macules and papules which initially blanch (Figure 8.11). The rash fades in the order of its appearance. Complications of measles are related to the viral infection itself, such as encephalitis, or are due to secondary bacterial infections, such as otitis media and pneumonia. The diagnosis is made on clinical grounds; the rash of measles may be confused with drug eruptions and other exanthems. Care is supportive; antibiotics are used for secondary bacterial infections.

Erythema infectiosum (fifth disease) is caused by parvovirus B19. Infection with this virus may cause an exanthem, an acute arthritis in adults, and an aplastic crisis in patients with underlying hereditary hemolytic anemias. Hydrops fetalis or fetal death may occur if it is acquired during pregnancy.

The infection spreads via the respiratory route. The prodrome of erythema infectiosum includes fever, malaise, and headache for 1 to 2 days prior to the exanthem. The classic exanthem initially manifests as fiery red erythema on the cheeks ("slapped cheek" appearance). This is followed within days by erythematous macules and papules on the proximal extremities and sometimes the trunk; the rash may be lacy or reticulate. Finally, there is a waxing and waning of the rash, which lasts from 1 to a few weeks.

The diagnosis is made clinically but can be confirmed by serologic testing. There is no specific treatment. The individual is generally no longer contagious when the rash appears. There is no specific therapy, and treatment is supportive.

BIBLIOGRAPHY

Arndt KA: Bacterial skin infections. In *Manual of Dermatologic Therapeutics,* ed 5. Boston, Little, Brown, 1995, pp 24–29, 75–89, 90–97, 98–104.

Arnold HL Jr, Odom RB, James WD: *Andrews' Diseases of the Skin,* ed 8. Philadelphia, WB Saunders, 1990, pp 268–317, 318–374, 436–485.

Baddour LM: Primary skin infections in primary care: An update. *Infect Med* 10:42–48, 1993.

Baker DA: Herpes simplex virus infections. *Curr Opin Obstet Gynecol* 4:676–681, 1992.

Berger RS, Seifert MR: Whirlpool folliculitis: A review of its cause, treatment, and prevention. *Cutis* 45:97–98, 1990.

Bisno AI, Stevens DL: Streptococcal infections of skin and soft tissues. *N Engl J Med* 334:240–245, 1995.

Borelli D, Jacobs PH, Nall L: Tinea versicolor: Epidemiologic, clinical, and therapeutic aspects. *J Am Acad Dermatol* 25:300–305, 1991.

Elewski BE, Hazen PG: The superficial mycoses and the dermatophytes *J Am Acad Dermatol* 21:655–673, 1989.

Elewski BE: Common superficial mycoses. In Arndt KA, Leboit PE, Robinson JK, et al (eds): *Cutaneous Medicine and Surgery.* Philadelphia, WB Saunders, 1996, pp 1037–1042.

Elewski BE: The dermatophytoses. In Arndt KA, Leboit PE, Robinson JK, et al (eds): *Cutaneous Medicine and Surgery.* Philadelphia, WB Saunders, 1996, pp 1043–1059.

Gulick R: Herpesvirus infections. In Arndt KA, Leboit PE, Robinson JK, et al (eds): *Cutaneous Medicine and Surgery.* Philadelphia, WB Saunders, 1996, pp 1074–1092.

Hirschmann JV: Skin infections caused by staphylococci, streptococci, and the resident cutaneous flora. In Arndt KA, Leboit PE, Robinson JK, et al (eds): *Cutaneous Medicine and Surgery.* Philadelphia, WB Saunders, 1996, pp 919–929.

Horowitz BJ: Giaquinta D, Ito S: Evolving pathogens in vulvovaginal candidiasis: Implications for patient care. *J Clin Pharmacol* 32:248–255, 1992.

Jacobs PH: Treatment of fungal skin infections: State of the art. *J Am Acad Dermatol* 25:549–551, 1990.

Nadelman RB, Wormser GP: Erythema migrans and early Lyme disease. *Am J Med* 98:15S–23S, 1995.

Nocton JJ, Steere AC: Lyme disease. *Adv Intern Med* 40:69–115, 1995.

Smith LG Jr, Pearlman M, Smith LG, et al: Lyme disease: A review with emphasis on the pregnant woman. *Obstet Gynecol Surv* 46:125–130, 1991.

Sobel JD: Individualizing treatment of vaginal candidiasis. *J Am Acad Dermatol* 23:572–576, 1990.

PAPULOSQUAMOUS DISORDERS

Papulosquamous disorders are those in which papules and scales occur. These are common disorders which share many clinical features. Prompt and accurate diagnosis may be challenging but is necessary for appropriate treatment of these often distressing conditions.

Psoriasis

Psoriasis, a chronic inflammatory skin disorder involving increased turnover of epidermal cells, affects 2 to 8 million people in the United States. The usual age of onset is in the third decade, although it may develop at any age from birth on. A family history of psoriasis is seen in 30% of patients. The cause of psoriasis is unknown but may involve various immunologic factors. What is known is that the time necessary for an epidermal cell to travel from the basal layer to the skin surface is 3 or 4 days compared with 26–28 days in normal skin. The disease is characterized by exacerbations and remissions, is unpredictable, and, when severe, may be disabling.

There are several types of psoriasis, the most common being *plaque-type psoriasis,* in which there are well-demarcated, erythematous plaques with silvery scale. These lesions may appear anywhere on the body but are most common on the elbows, knees, scalp, genitalia, and intergluteal cleft. Localized plaque-type psoriasis may also be seen just on the palms and soles. The plaques may be pruritic; subsequent scratching may exacerbate the disease. The plaques may last for months or years, and there may be periodic flares of other types of psoriasis, such as pustular or erythrodermic psoriasis.

An important phenomenon in psoriasis is the *Koebner phenomenon,* in which new psoriatic lesions develop in previously normal-appearing skin after local injury. Such injuries may include scratching, surgical or laparoscopic wounds, sunburn, contact dermatitis, or chemical irritation. The Koebner phenomenon is not specific for psoriasis but may be seen in other disorders such as lichen planus. Another phenomenon seen in psoriasis is the *Auspitz sign,* in which pinpoint bleeding occurs after a psoriatic plaque is scraped away; this occurs because of disruption of capillaries lying close to the epidermis.

Other types of psoriasis are *pustular psoriasis,* which may be generalized or localized. The prominent features are erythematous plaques covered with pustules. Patients with *generalized pustular psoriasis of von Zumbusch* may be quite ill, with painful, tender skin, fever, malaise, arthralgias, diarrhea, and electrolyte abnormalities. *Guttate psoria-*

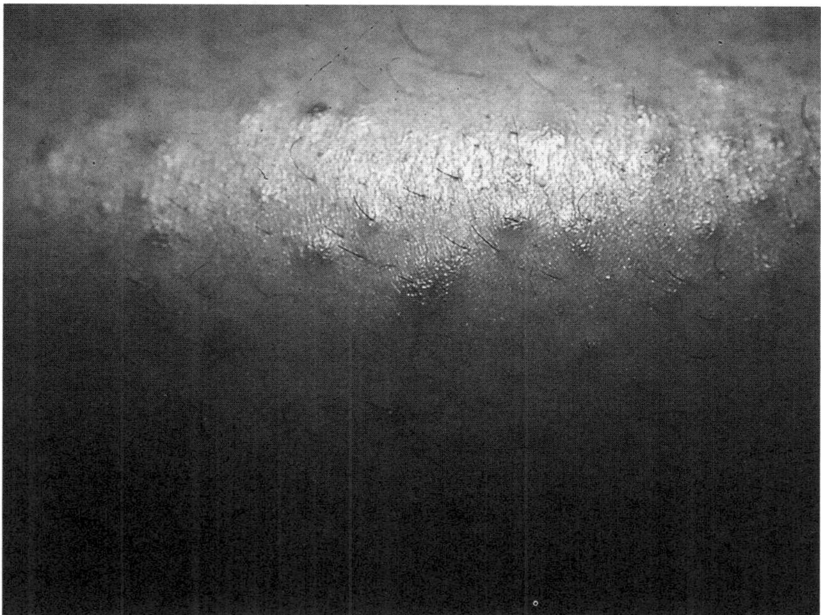

Figure 8.12 Guttate psoriasis.

sis is most common in children and young adults. There is an acute onset of numerous erythematous, raindrop-like, scaly papules (Figure 8.12). A frequent antecedent to guttate psoriasis is streptococcal infection, and this must be searched for (throat culture, antistreptolysin O titer) and treated. *Inverse psoriasis* involves intertriginous areas such as the axillae, groin, submammary area, navel, and intergluteal fold. *Erythrodermic psoriasis* is a severe form of psoriasis in which there is generalized erythema and scaling. Accompanying signs and symptoms include fever, chills, pruritus, malaise, and fatigue; there may also be lower extremity edema, hypothermia from excessive heat loss, and high-output cardiac failure in those with underlying heart disease.

The scalp and nails are often involved in psoriasis. In the scalp there are well-demarcated, erythematous plaques with scaling. This condition may be difficult to distinguish from seborrheic dermatitis. However, in seborrheic dermatitis the scaling is more diffuse, dry, and powdery. In addition, psoriatic plaques often extend onto the forehead and bald areas, while seborrheic dermatitis spares bald areas and the forehead adjacent to the hairline. Characteristic nail changes in patients with psoriasis are *nail pitting, onycholysis* (separation of the distal nail plate), and *oil spots,* which are yellow-brown subungual discolorations.

Arthritis may occur in approximately 20–30% of patients with psoriasis; this condition, termed *psoriatic arthritis,* is a seronegative spondyloarthropathy. Skin lesions usually occur before the onset of arthritis.

The differential diagnosis of plaque-type psoriasis includes seborrheic dermatitis, eczematous dermatitis, and mycosis fungoides (cutaneous T-cell lymphoma). For guttate psoriasis one should consider secondary syphilis and pityriasis rosea. Inverse psoriasis may look like candidal infection or erythrasma (skin infection with *Corynebacterium minutissimum*). Erythrodermic psoriasis should be differentiated from drug eruptions, eczematous dermatitis, and mycosis fungoides. A skin biopsy should be done to confirm the diagnosis of psoriasis, and other diagnostic studies should be performed, such as a serologic test for syphilis.

There are many treatment modalities for psoriasis. These include topical agents (corticosteroids, tar preparations, vitamin D analogues), oral agents (methotrexate, cyclosporine, retinoids), and UV light. Patients with psoriasis should be under the care of a dermatologist.

Pityriasis Rosea

Pityriasis rosea is a common, self-limited papulosquamous disorder seen mainly in adolescents and young adults. The cause of this disorder is unknown, but a viral etiology is suspected.

The initial lesion is the "herald patch"; noted in 70–80% of cases, this is a round, erythematous, 2–6 cm plaque with scale that may occur anywhere on the body. After several days to 2 weeks, multiple 1–2 cm, round to oval red macules and papules with a rim of fine scales appear on the trunk and proximal extremities. A characteristic finding in pityriasis rosea is the arrangement of the long axis of these lesions along the planes of cleavage in a Christmas tree–like pattern. Most patients are asymptomatic, but some may have intense pruritus.

The disorder is usually diagnosed clinically. All patients with suspected pityriasis rosea should have a serologic test for syphilis, since secondary syphilis may mimic pityriasis rosea. The differential diagnosis includes psoriasis, tinea corporis, and tinea versicolor.

The lesions usually resolve in 6 to 8 weeks; if they do not, a skin biopsy should be performed to obtain a tissue diagnosis. In general, no treatment is required. For pruritus, antipruritic lotions, emollients, or antihistamines may be used. Topical corticosteroids are rarely helpful. UVB light may be used to decrease the pruritus and the extent of the eruption.

Dermatitis

Seborrheic dermatitis is an erythematous, scaling rash that occurs on sebaceous gland–rich skin of the scalp, face, and trunk. It occurs with a bimodal distribution in early infancy and in adulthood, usually in the third decade or later. The cause of this disorder is unknown, but an etiologic role for *Pityrosporum ovale,* a normal yeast inhabitant of the skin, has been hypothesized. The incidence of seborrheic dermatitis is increased in patients with AIDS and in those with Parkinson's disease.

The lesions of seborrheic dermatitis are erythematous, scaling plaques; the scales may be either dry or greasy. Typical lesions show erythema and scaling of the hair-bearing areas of the scalp. The eyebrows, nasolabial creases, and posterior auricular areas may have well-defined pink plaques with powdery scale. There may be a seborrheic blepharoconjunctivitis. Other areas which may be involved are the inframammary folds, groin, gluteal crease, and umbilicus. In scalp involvement, pruritus is almost always present.

The differential diagnosis of seborrheic dermatitis can be approached regionally. On the scalp, one should also consider psoriasis, tinea captitis, atopic dermatitis, head lice, and dandruff. Facial dermatitis may also be caused by atopic dermatitis, rosacea, and perioral dermatitis. Seborrheic dermatitis on the trunk or in intertriginous areas may resemble tinea corporis, candidiasis, psoriasis, atopic dermatitis, and contact dermatitis.

Several agents are effective in treating seborrheic dermatitis. The goals of treatment are to remove scale, reduce yeast colonization, and reduce erythema and pruritus. Shampoos containing zinc pyrithione, selenium sulfide 1% to 2.5%, coal tar, or ketoconazole 2% can be used daily; the shampoo must be left in contact with the skin for at least 5 min to be effective. Maintenance therapy can be given to the face and groin with ketoconazole 2% cream. Topical corticosteroids are also used when required: low- or mid-potency corticosteroid solutions for the scalp; low-potency corticosteroids for the face, groin, or axillae; and midpotency corticosteroids for the trunk.

Atopic dermatitis, commonly known as *eczema,* is an intensely pruritic, chronic eruption which may be seen at all ages. The family history is usually significant for atopy, and about half of the children with atopic dermatitis will develop allergic rhinitis or asthma. The most significant symptom is pruritus; this leads to itching and rubbing, which cause many of the secondary signs of the disease. The precise cause of atopic dermatitis is not known; immunologic mechanisms likely play a major role. Known triggers for atopic dermatitis are extremes of heat or cold, rapid changes in temperature, sweating, irritating clothing such as wool, fragrances, greases, oils, soaps, and detergents. Inhaled antigens may also play a role.

The assessment of the patient with atopic dermatitis should include elicitation of a detailed personal, family, and environmental history. The psychological impact of the disorder should be assessed, as this condition may cause severe emotional stress. One should elicit a history of precipitating factors. One should also inform the patient with atopic dermatitis that she has lowered resistance to certain viral infections including HSV, which may result in eczema herpeticum; human papilloma virus (HPV), which may result in warts; and molluscum contagiosum.

Atopic dermatitis may manifest as acute, subacute, and chronic lesions. Acute lesions are highly pruritic, erythematous papules and vesicles. Commonly involved areas are the neck, antecubital and popliteal fossae, wrists, and ankles. Scratching of these lesions leads to excoriation and exudation; secondary infection is common. Subacute lesions are characterized by excoriated, erythematous papules and plaques with scaling. In the chronic phase of atopic dermatitis one sees dry, lichenified, hyperpigmented plaques on the flexor surfaces and around the eyes. A hand dermatitis may be the only manifestation. Additional skin findings may be ichthyosis vulgaris (dry skin with fish-like scale), keratosis pilaris (hyperkeratotic papules on the outer extremities), and Dennie-Morgan lines (extra skin folds below the eyes).

The differential diagnosis of atopic dermatitis includes allergic contact dermatitis, seborrheic dermatitis, nummular eczema, dermatophyte infections, various immunodeficiencies and metabolic disorders, and neoplastic diseases such as mycosis fungoides and Sézary's syndrome. When atopic dermatitis does not respond to conventional treatment or involves unusual sites (groin, axillae), these other diagnoses should be entertained.

The mainstay of treatment of acute atopic dermatitis is topical corticosteroids, which decrease inflammation and pruritus. Hydration of skin enhances their penetration, so they are best applied after bathing. Mid- to high-potency agents can be used for severe acute flares on the body and low-potency agents for mild flares. Treatment of secondarily infected skin with an oral antistaphylococcal agent is often necessary. Liberal use of emollients, limitation of long, hot showers, avoidance of irritating clothing, and judicious use of antihistamines are all helpful in managing this disease.

Contact dermatitis may be caused by irritants or allergic sensitizers. *Irritant contact dermatitis* is a nonallergic reaction to various irritating skin substances. The reaction depends on the amount and duration of the exposure. Irritants which are mild and require prolonged exposure include soaps, detergents, and most solvents; strong ones such as strong acids and alkalis cause immediate injury to the skin. *Allergic contact dermatitis* is due to a delayed hypersensitivity response to an antigen to which the patient has become sensitized. The dermatitis resolves with avoidance of the antigen. The most common cause of allergic contact dermatitis in North America is nickel sulfate (in earrings, bracelets, hairpins, rings, wristwatches, clasps, eyelash curlers, glasses, brassiere cups, pants buttons). Other common allergens include thimerosal (a preservative), neomycin sulfate (a topical antibiotic, present in numerous ointments, creams, and lotions), formaldehyde (in fabrics, toilet paper, facial tissues, and various papers), and paraphenylenediamine (seen in furriers, hairdressers, and those in the rubber vulcanization and photographic industries). Plant dermatitis, such as to poison ivy and poison oak, is also common. Latex and rubber hypersensitivity are important problems affecting health care workers. Contact dermatitis may be caused by topical corticosteroids; this should be suspected if treatment with a topical steroid causes worsening

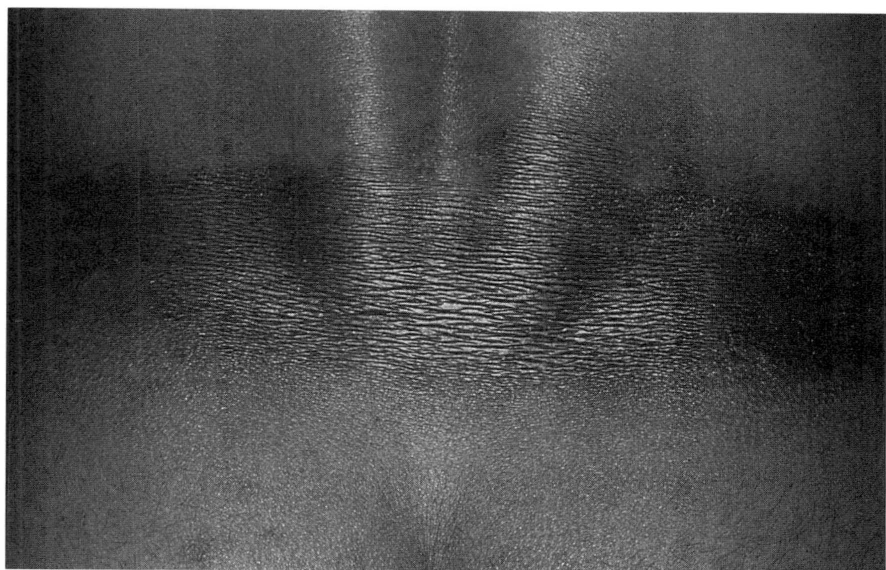

Figure 8.13 Contact dermatitis from waistband with postinflammatory hyperpigmentation.

of symptoms. Sunscreen containing para-aminobenzoic acid and its derivatives may cause contact as well as irritant dermatitis. Eyelid dermatitis is often caused by nail lacquers. Phototoxic and photoallergic contact dermatitis are special forms of contact dermatitis which are caused by an interaction involving the offending agent and UV light.

Mild irritant dermatitis may present with erythema, microvesicles, and weeping; chronic exposure may cause thick, dry, fissured skin. Strong irritants can produce extensive skin damage including blistering, erosions, and ulcers. In allergic contact dermatitis there are erythematous,edematous plaques; vesicles and bullae are common. Linear lesions result from exposure to plants such as poison ivy. Phototoxic and photoallergic reactions occur in sun-exposed areas.

A thorough history to identify the offending agent is necessary in both irritant and allergic contact dermatitis. Occupational exposures, exposures during household duties, and exposures to cosmetics should be asked about specifically. In allergic contact dermatitis, the location is often an important clue (eyelid dermatitis—nail polish dermatitis; circumferentially around the wrist—nickel dermatitis from a bracelet or watchband; circumferentially around the waist—rubber dermatitis; Figure 8.13). Patch testing with a panel of common antigens is often necessary to identify the offending agent in allergic contact dermatitis.

A key issue in the treatment of contact dermatitis is avoidance of the offending irritant or allergen. This may require modification of work or household practices, wearing of protective gloves with cotton liners, and use of hypoallergenic cosmetics.

For treatment of irritant dermatitis, emollients and intermittent courses of mild topical steroids are used. For allergic contact dermatitis, emollients and moderate to potent topical corticosteroids are used. For the vesicular and weeping lesion of contact dermatitis, cold compresses with Burow's solution, diluted 1:20, are helpful.

Lichen Simplex Chronicus

Lichen simplex chronicus is common disorder characterized by extreme pruritus, with rubbing, scratching, and consequent thickening of the skin. There are well-circumscribed, erythematous plaques and accentuated skin markings. The plaques may be dry and scaly, and scratch marks may be present. Commonly involved areas are the wrists, ankles, neck, and extensor forearms. The predominant symptom is pruritus; scratching and rubbing are both intense and pleasurable. The disorder is maintained by repetitive rubbing and itching. The initial trigger may be other pruritic dermatoses such as atopic dermatitis, stasis dermatitis, insect bites, or allergic contact dermatitis. Other patients may have an idiopathic form. The underlying itch hypersensitivity has been called a *neurodermatitis,* but this term is probably overused. Treatment includes potent topical corticosteroids, sometimes under occlusion. Sometimes just occlusion of the area to prevent rubbing or itching is sufficient. Contributing factors such as stress or anxiety should be addressed. Underlying disease states causing pruritus should be ruled out (psoriasis, mycosis fungoides, atopic dermatitis, contact dermatitis, lichen planus, underlying metabolic disorder).

BIBLIOGRAPHY

Arndt KA: *Manual of Dermatologic Therapeutics,* ed 5. Boston, Little, Brown, 1995, pp 43–56, 142–143, 149–159, 164–167.

Bernhard JD: Lichen simplex chronicus, prurigo nodularis, and notalgia paresthetica. In Arndt KA, Leboit PE, Robinson JK, et al (eds): *Cutaneous Medicine and Surgery.* Philadelphia, WB Saunders, 1996, pp 205–210.

Christophers E, Sterry W: Psoriasis. In Fitzpatrick TB, Eisen AZ, Wolff K, et al (eds): *Dermatology in General Medicine.* New York, McGraw-Hill, 1993, pp 489–514.

Cropley TG: Seborrheic dermatitis. In Arndt KA, Leboit PE, Robinson JK, et al (eds): *Cutaneous Medicine and Surgery.* Philadelphia, WB Saunders, 1996, pp 214–217.

Fitzpatrick TB: Effective treatment of psoriasis. *Skin* 1:6–9, 1995.

Trozak DJ: Topical corticosteroid therapy in psoriasis vulgaris. *Cutis* 46:341–350, 1990.

Hanifin JM: Atopic dermatitis: New therapeutic considerations. *J Am Acad Dermatol* 24: 1097–1101, 1991.

Nethercott JR, Nield G, Holness DL: A review of 79 cases of eyelid dermatitis. *J Am Acad Dermatol* 21:223–230, 1989.

Nethercott JR: Contact dermatitis and occupational dermatology. In Arndt KA, Leboit PE, Robinson JK, et al (eds): *Cutaneous Medicine and Surgery.* Philadelphia, WB Saunders, 1996, pp 173–183.

REACTIVE ERYTHEMAS

The reactive erythemas are a group of disorders characterized by erythematous patches, plaques, and nodules of varying size, shape, and distribution. These are not specific dermatoses but rather cutaneous reaction patterns triggered by various endogenous and exogenous agents.

Erythema Multiforme

Erythema multiforme (EM) is a cutaneous reaction pattern characterized by variable erythematous lesions ranging from macules and papules, to more characteristic target

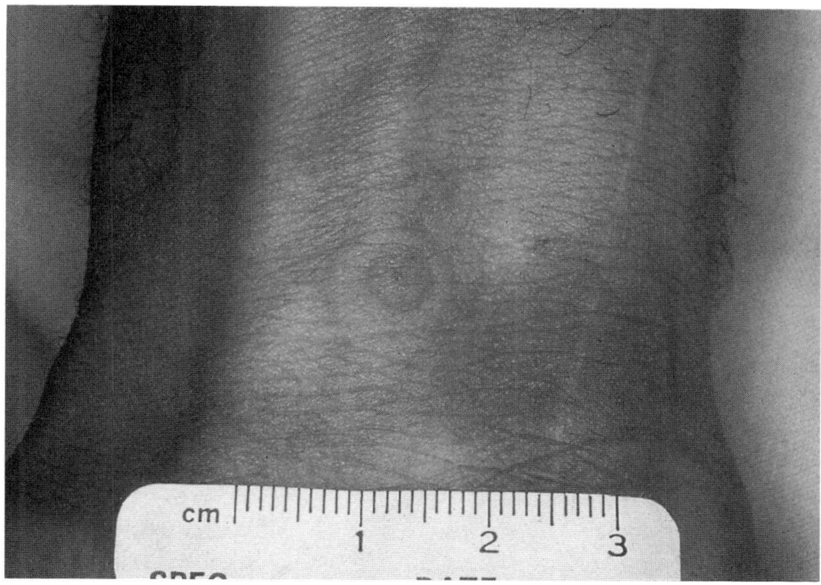

Figure 8.14 Erythema multiforme—target lesion.

lesions (Figure 8.14) or red, annular plaques with dusky centers, to vesicles and vesicobullae. EM is thought to have an immunologic basis and to result from various antigenic stimuli such as drugs and infectious agents.

EM is clinically divided into two major categories: EM minor and EM major. Included in this cutaneous reaction pattern are Stevens-Johnson syndrome or EM major with severe mucous membrane involvement, and toxic epidermal necrolysis (TEN). The nosology of these conditions remains controversial, but many authors feel they represent a clinical spectrum. In addition, a rarer EM subtype, a chronic persistent type with continuously appearing lesions, has been reported. These lesions can be atypical and include papular, necrotic, and purpuric lesions.

EM minor tends to have a benign clinical presentation with acrally distributed lesions and is most often linked with HSV infection. Active herpes labialis can precede this eruption by several days. This form of EM is self-limited.

The lesions of EM major are symmetric, sometimes sparing the trunk but in more severe forms occurring throughout the integument. A prodrome of fever and malaise may occur. Bullous lesions occur in the more severe form. In Stevens-Johnson syndrome, involvement of two mucous membrane surfaces is required for diagnosis. The onset is often abrupt, with painful, burning lesions which quickly evolve into bullae. The lesions may become confluent, with the appearance of confluent epidermal necrolysis on some parts of the body.

In TEN there is widespread detachment of the full thickness of the epidermis, which is partially or totally necrotic. Mucous membrane involvement (conjunctival, genital, and oral) occurs in nearly all patients. Internal organ involvement (lungs, gastrointestinal tract, and kidneys) occurs in TEN, as well as in EM major and Stevens-Johnson syndrome. Severe electrolyte disturbances and susceptibility to infection are major complications that contribute to morbidity and mortality.

A rarer form of chronic or persistent EM has been reported. This entity has been associated with underlying inflammatory disorders such as inflammatory bowel disease. In this variant, lesions are chronic and uninterrupted and can have a more atypical appearance.

The pathogenesis of EM is not known. IgM and complement are deposited around dermal blood vessels. Circulating immune complexes have been reported in some patients, although a histologic vasculitis has not been found. EM probably represents a hypersensitivity syndrome or immunologic reaction pattern involving the skin and mucous membranes which results from various antigenic stimuli. In recurrent EM minor, which is most often associated with HSV infection, chronic suppression with antiviral agents such as acyclovir can be helpful. Treatment with systemic steroids, particularly early in the course of a clear-cut drug reaction, may also be beneficial. However, the use of systemic steroids in EM major, Stevens-Johnson syndrome, and TEN remains controversial. The mainstay of care in these situations is supportive. This involves maintaining the skin barrier to prevent secondary infection and managing fluid and electrolyte disturbances.

The differential diagnosis of EM includes delayed hypersensitivity reactions, particularly those precipitated by drugs; vasculitis; idiopathic bullous disorders such as bullous pemphigoid and pemphigus vulgaris; and severe contact dermatitis. Diseases with extensive desquamation or superficial blisters may mimic TEN. These include severe drug reactions, toxic shock syndrome, staphylococcal scalded skin syndrome, acute pustular psoriasis, and severe bullous drug eruptions.

Erythema Nodosum

Erythema nodosum (EN) is also thought to be an immunologic reaction pattern in the skin precipitated by various antigens. It is most commonly seen in young adult women and is characterized by the sudden onset of tender, erythematous subcutaneous nodules, primarily over the extensor aspects of the legs. Although lower extremity involvement is most common, lesions can be found on other sites such as the trunk and upper extremities. A prodrome of fever, malaise, and arthralgia may be present. Various agents known to be associated with EN are infectious agents (bacteria such as streptococci and *Mycobacterium tuberculosis;* viruses such as Epstein-Barr virus and hepatitis B virus; dermatophytes and other fungi; and protozoa such as *Toxoplasma gondii*), drugs (sulfonamides, bromides, oral contraceptives, and many others), malignant diseases (Hodgkin's disease, non-Hodgkin's lymphoma, leukemia), and miscellaneous conditions (e.g., sarcoidosis, ulcerative colitis, pregnancy).

Patients with EN present with an acute onset of painful red nodules, usually on the legs and occasionally on the thighs or upper extremities. These nodules have a bruised or contused appearance, with no overlying epidermal changes. The lesions often occur in crops. A significant prodrome of fever, malaise, and neuralgia may occur. Lofgren's syndrome is EN occurring with sarcoidosis. Sarcoidosis presenting in the setting of EN is felt to have a better long-term prognosis than sarcoidosis appearing alone. Laboratory evaluation should be guided by a search for the underlying cause and may include a complete blood count with differential, erythrocyte sedimentation rate, chest x-ray, and anti-streptolysin O titer. Other studies to identify an underlying infectious etiology are guided by the clinical presentation. Supportive care such as anti-inflammatory agents, bed rest, and leg elevation is recommended.

The differential diagnosis of EN includes other panniculitides such as erythema induratum, connective tissue panniculitis, polyarteritis nodosa, vasculitis, and syphilitic gumma. The lack of surface ulceration and the recurrent nature of the nodules in EN help distinguish it from these other entities.

BIBLIOGRAPHY

Bondi EE, Lazarus GS: Panniculitis. In Fitzpatrick TB, Eisen AZ, Wolff K, et al (eds): *Dermatology in General Medicine.* New York, McGraw-Hill, 1993, pp 1338–1340.

Fritsch PO, Elias PM: Erythema multiforme and toxic epidermal necrolysis. In Fitzpatrick TB, Eisen AZ, Wolff K, et al (eds): *Dermatology in General Medicine.* New York, McGraw-Hill, 1993, pp 585–600.

Gordon H: Erythema nodosum: A review of 115 cases. *Br J Dermatol* 73:393–409, 1979.

Howland WW, Golitz LE, Weston WL, et al: Erythema multiforme: Clinical, histopathologic, and immunologic study. *J Am Acad Dermatol* 10:438–446, 1984.

Huff JC, Weston WL, Tonnesen MG: Erythema multiforme: A critical review of characteristics, diagnostic criteria, and causes. *J Am Acad Dermatol* 8:763–775, 1983.

Huff JC: Acyclovir for recurrent erythema multiforme caused by herpes simplex. *J Am Acad Dermatol* 18:197–199, 1988.

Salvatore MA, Lynch PJ: Erythema nodosum, estrogens, and pregnancy. *Arch Dermatol* 116: 557–558, 1980.

VULVAR DISORDERS

Vulvar diseases are complex conditions which require astute clinical and history-taking skills for successful diagnosis and treatment. Women may present with symptoms of persistent vaginal discharge, burning, itching, and pain. Often these patients are sent to the dermatologist for consultation. Due to the persistent nature of these complaints, many of these women may have sought previous medical attention, which involved only partial or unsuccessful diagnostic and therapeutic intervention. These patients are often anxious and frustrated. An understanding and considerate approach to these patients is important while instilling confidence that their problem can be resolved with a rational diagnostic method.

A thorough history and a search for precipitating factors are important. Inquiries regarding the duration of symptoms, previous treatments, topical contactants, medication history, and coexistent dermatologic conditions are important. Examination of the external genitalia for signs of rubbing, swelling, erythema, or infestation should be done. The appearance of primary cutaneous lesions, such as papules, nodules, or vesicles, should be noted. Any abnormal vaginal discharge should be examined for diagnostic clues. Finally, examination of the entire skin and mucous membrane surfaces for primary dermatologic conditions can be helpful.

A number of disorders may cause vulvar symptoms; we will focus on two common categories of disease: infectious and inflammatory.

Infectious Conditions

Various infections may cause vaginal and vulvar burning and itching. These include HSV infection, condyloma acuminata, molluscum contagiousum, scabies, and pediculosis pubis. Candidiasis, bacterial vaginosis, and trichomoniasis are also common causes. Differentiation among *Candidiasis,* bacterial vaginosis, and trichomoniasis can be made by direct examination of a vaginal smear with either KOH (pseudohyphae of *Candida*) or saline (clue cells of bacterial vaginosis or motile trichomonads in trichomoniasis).

In HSV infection, vulvar erosions or vesicles are present. Tzanck smear will demonstrate the characteristic multinucleated keratinocytes; viral culture can be used for confirmation. If, after treatment, any erosions persist, a biopsy should be performed to rule out a vulvar malignancy.

Condyloma acuminata present as flesh-colored verrucous papules. They are caused by HPV which has at least 50 subtypes. HPV 16 and 18 are associated with vulvar carcinoma. Eradication of HPV from the genitalia is important to decrease this risk and to avoid transmission to infants in future pregnancies.

Molluscum contagiosum presents as flesh-colored to slightly pink umbilicated papules. Scabies is often seen as a nonspecific, extremely pruritic dermatitis with areas of excoriation elsewhere, such as the axillae and abdomen. Direct examination of lesional scrapings with either KOH or oil will reveal the mite, eggs, or feces.

Treatment of vulvar and vaginal infectious depends, of course, on the etiologic agent. Candidal vulvovaginitis is treated with topical or oral anticandidal agents. In HSV infection, acyclovir is used (200 mg five times a day for 10 days; see Table 8.5). Lindane (Kwell®) shampoo or lotion is the treatment of choice for pediculosis pubis. The shampoo is applied to the perineum for 4 min; the treatment is repeated in 1 week. Treatment for scabies involves the entire integument, using either 5% permethrin cream (Elimite®) or lindane lotion. It is important to treat all household members and to follow guidelines regarding environmental cleaning. Both bacterial vaginosis and trichomoniasis are treated effectively with oral metronidazole.

Inflammatory Conditions

Findings of primary dermatologic conditions such as psoriasis, seborrheic dermatitis, or atopic dermatitis are helpful clues in the diagnosis of associated vulvar diseases. One should be familiar with the clinical findings of common inflammatory skin disorders affecting the vulva and perineum.

Psoriasis of the vulva usually presents as a sharply demarcated, erythematous plaque with a moist, macerated surface. Lesions on other parts of the body have the more characteristic appearance of a well-defined, erythematous plaque with heaped-up white scale. Psoriasis of the perineum presents with classic scaly, erythematous plaques.

Atopic dermatitis may present in the vulva with erythematous patches which are ill-defined; often there are secondary changes such as lichenification and excoriations. Superinfection with *Candida* and *S. aureus* is common.

A history of an intermittent course associated with exposure to a contactant is a diagnostic clue for *allergic contact dermatitis.* Possible agents include spermacides, various topical medications, condoms, diaphragms, and lubricants.

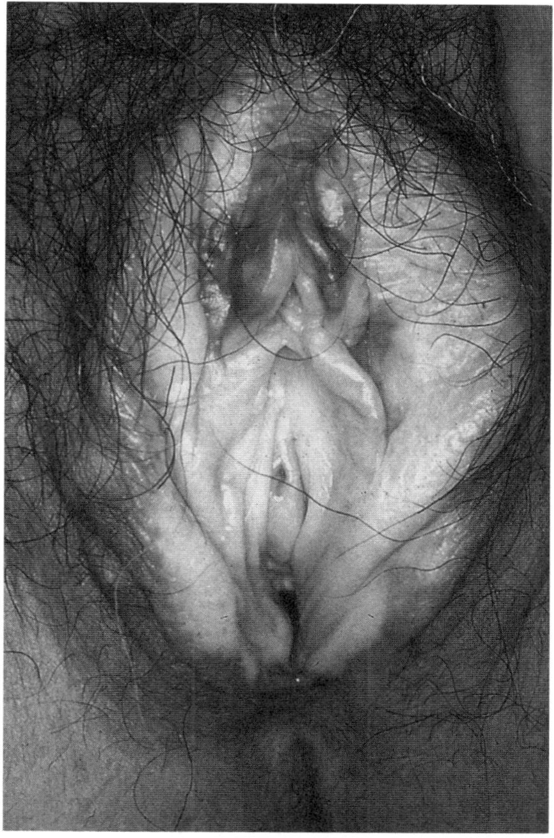

Figure 8.15 Lichen sclerosus, genital.

Seborrheic dermatitis can occur on the vulva and external genitalia. The clinical appearance can be similar to that of either psoriasis or atopic dermatitis, but the characteristic findings in seborrheic dermatitis of oily, scaly patches on the scalp, face, and chest are differentiating features.

Intertrigo may be caused by irritant factors such as sweat and friction. Infectious agents such as staphylococci, streptococci, *Candida,* and *Corynebacterium* (erythrasma) also commonly cause intertrigo. In erythrasma, the lesions are noninflammatory; on Wood's light examination there is a characteristic coral red fluorescence. This diagnosis is easily missed without a Wood's light examination.

Treatment regimens are based on the specific dermatologic diagnosis. In atopic dermatitis in particular, decreased frequency of washing, avoidance of harsh soaps and detergents, and use of emollients are the key to successful long-term management. In contact dermatitis, allergens should be removed and completely avoided in the future. Mid- to low-potency topical corticosteroids are useful in resolving the initial pruritic symptoms in noninfectious inflammatory dermatoses. Dermatologic referral may be needed, especially if lesions fail to respond to the prescribed course of treatment.

Lichen sclerosus is an inflammatory disorder of unknown cause primarily affecting women of all ages, from childhood to old age. Symptoms of itching and burning are

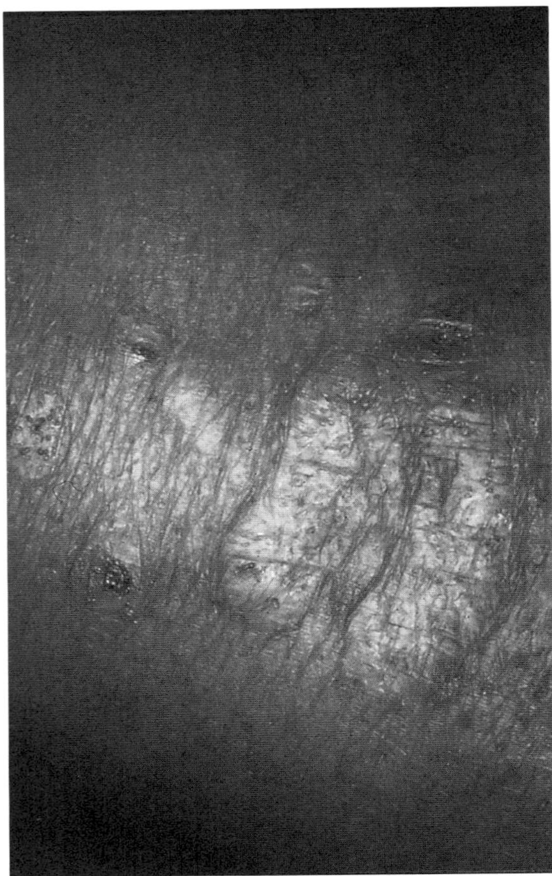

Figure 8.16 Lichen sclerosus, extragenital.

common. Early in the course, primary lesions are white to violaceous, polygonal papules which eventually coalesce into plaques. Later, typical features include textural changes such as atrophy and loss of pigment (Figure 8.15). In advanced stages, scarring with absorption of clitoral tissue, lichenification or thickening, fissuring, erosions, and blistering can occur. The vulva is the most commonly affected area, and when the perianal area is involved, a characteristic keyhole or figure-of-eight pattern is seen. Extragenital lesions on the neck, shoulders, or trunk, with similar-appearing violaceous or white-colored polygonal papules, may be present (Figure 8.16).

In 1986, the International Society of Gynecological Pathologists recommended that lichen sclerosus be classified as a nonneoplastic disorder of the vulva. However, an increased incidence of vulvar squamous cell carcinoma, up to 5%, has been associated with lichen sclerosis, particularly at sites of long-standing erosions. Any persistent erosions in this disorder should be biopsied to rule out vulvar carcinoma, which necessitates regular, long-term follow-up.

Lichen sclerosus in children is felt to be a subset of this disorder in which spontaneous resolution is more likely to occur. The clinical presentation is similar to that in adults.

The pathogenesis of lichen sclerosus is not known. Various infectious agents including spirochetes have been studied, without conclusive evidence of their pathogenic role. Patients with lichen sclerosus are known to have associated autoimmune disorders and increased frequency of certain human leukocyte antigen types. Current research regarding the role of infectious, genetic, and immunologic factors should more clearly elucidate the pathogenesis of this disorder.

The treatment of choice in highly symptomatic patients is initially mid-potency topical corticosteroids. Low-potency corticosteroids are useful for long-term control of symptoms. Patients should be monitored for side effects of topical corticosteroids such as thinning of the skin and increased vascularization. Oral retinoids may be useful; topical retinoids are also efficacious. Bland emollients are safe, useful adjunctive agents. Topical testosterone ointment or cream, popular in the past, is less desirable now; if used, side effects such as vocal changes should be monitored closely.

The differential diagnosis of lichen sclerosis includes morphea and lichen planus. Erosive vulvar lesions are seen in lichen planus and closely mimic those of lichen sclerosus. However, examination of the oral mucosa in patients with lichen planus should demonstrate the characteristic lacy white plaques on the buccal mucosa. In cases with prominent features of lichenification, other skin conditions such as psoriasis or atopic dermatitis may be considered.

Lichen planus is a chronic, pruritic dermatosis of unknown etiology. *Erosive lichen planus* of the vulva is the most common cause of desquamative vaginitis. Clinical symptoms include vaginal itching, burning, and pain. Physical findings are erosive lesions with whitish macules often arranged in a laciform or reticulate pattern. Chronic involvement can lead to scarring and loss of pigment. It is important that patients with erosive vulvar lichen planus undergo close inspection of the oral mucosa. Vulvar disease accompanied by mucous membrane involvement in lichen planus is a syndrome called *vulvar-vaginal-gingival syndrome of lichen planus*. Patients may not mention the oral lesions since they may not associate them with the vulvar lesions. Additionally, the characteristic finding on glabrous skin in lichen planus—violaceous, polygonal, scaly papules—may not been seen in this syndrome. Biopsy is necessary for diagnosis.

Potent topical corticosteroids are the treatment of choice. Other topical treatments include retinoic acid, intralesional steroids, and cyclosporine. Anecdotal reports have shown that oral prednisone, griseofulvin, cyclopsorine, doxycycline, dapsone, and etretinate give temporary relief in some patients. Unfortunately, most patients obtain only partial relief despite various forms of therapy. Long-term control of symptoms in erosive vulvar lichen planus often proves unsatisfactory.

The differential diagnosis includes primarily lichen sclerosus, which morphologically can be confused with erosive lichen planus. Idiopathic blistering disorders such as bullous pemphigoid, cicatricial pemphigoid, and pemphigus vulgaris can cause erosive lesions of the vulva and sometimes precede involvement of other sites. Erosive squamous cell carcinoma should also be considered.

Several *immunobullous diseases* or idiopathic bullous disorders can present with vulvar involvement. Occasionally, vulvar erosions are the first clinical finding in a given patient; other sites later become involved. These diseases include bullous pemphigoid, cicatricial pemphigoid, linear IgA bullous dermatosis of childhood, and pemphigus vulgaris. Each of these disorders has diagnostic findings on direct immunofluorescence studies of perilesional skin; skin biopsy must be done to confirm the diagnosis. As in the vulvar-vaginal-gingival syndrome of lichen planus, oral mucosal involvement accompanies most of these disorders. Since widespread blistering can occur throughout the integument, dermatologic referral is in order.

Treatment of immunobullous disorders generally requires high doses of oral prednisone or other immunosuppressive agents.

It is important for the gynecologist to think of other inflammatory disorders, such as erythema multiforme, Stevens-Johnson syndrome, and lupus erythematosus, in the context of vulvar erosions. With few presenting signs other than the erosive vulvar lesions, diagnosis is often challenging. Close inspection of the remainder of the skin and a thorough history will be helpful in diagnosis and referral for biopsy and management.

BIBLIOGRAPHY

Chanco Turner ML: Genital disorders. In Arndt KA, Leboit PE, Robinson JK, et al (eds): *Cutaneous Medicine and Surgery*. Philadelphia, WB Saunders, 1996, pp 1378–1440, 1996.

Eisen DE: The vulvo-vaginal-gingival syndrome of lichen planus. The clinical characteristics of 22 patients. *Arch Dermatol* 130:1379–1382, 1994.

Meffert JJ, Davis BM, Grimwood RC: Lichen sclerosus. *J Am Acad Dermatol* 32:393–415, 1995.

Ridley CM: Lichen sclerosus. *Dermatol Clin* 10:309–318, 1992.

Pincus SH: Vulvar dermatoses and pruritus vulvae. *Dermatol Clin* 10:297–308, 1992.

Sobel JD: Vulvovaginitis. *Dermatol Clin* 10:339–359, 1992.

NEOPLASTIC SKIN DISEASES

Melanoma and nonmelanoma skin cancers are the most common cancers worldwide. One in three of all cancers are of the skin. An estimated 900,000 to 1.2 million skin cancers are diagnosed each year. The rates of melanoma and nonmelanoma skin cancer rose between 1960 and 1986 by 400% and 200%, respectively. The incidence of melanoma is rising faster than that of any other skin cancer. Excessive sunlight exposure and phenotypic susceptibility (fair skin, blue eyes, blonde or red hair, poor tanning ability) are major risk factors. Increased susceptibility to UVB light (290–320 nm) is directly related to the increased risk of developing skin cancer, particularly the nonmelanoma skin cancers, basal cell carcinoma and squamous cell carcinoma. Ninety percent of all skin cancers occur in sun-exposed skin. The role of UVB light exposure in the development of melanoma is more complicated. Other factors such as genetics and the presence of precursor marker lesions are also important. Most skin cancers can be cured if detected and treated early.

Basal cell carcinoma usually occurs on highly sun-exposed areas such as the face, ears, hands, lips, and upper trunk. Initial lesions are flesh-colored to pink, waxy, translucent papules. As their size progresses, the papules coalesce around a central depression, producing a "rolled border" appearance. Lesions go through cycles of

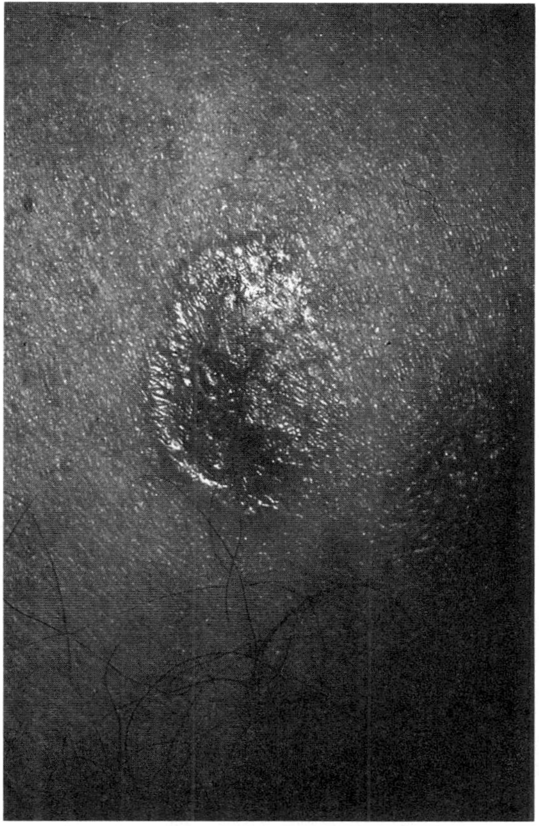

Figure 8.17 Basal cell carcinoma.

crusting, bleeding, and healing. Several variants can be seen: (1) pigmented basal cell carcinoma (black or brown and can mimic melanoma), (2) morpheic-type basal cell carcinoma (have ill-defined borders and prominent telangiectases), (3) cystic basal cell carcinoma (appear as dome-shaped, blue-gray nodules), and (4) superficial basal cell carcinoma (Figure 8.17) (can have a dry, scaly, flat appearance with a telltale thread-like, rolled border).

The course of basal cell carcinomas is chronic. These carcinomas rarely metastasize but, when long-standing, can significantly invade local tissues.

The treatment of choice is simple, elliptical excision for lesions less than 5 to 7 mm in diameter. Mohs micrographic surgery yields the least incidence of recurrence for larger lesions and for those located on areas with typically higher recurrence rates (nose, nasolabial fold). Skin grafting may be needed for larger lesions. Other treatments include electrosurgery, ionizing radiation, and cryosurgery; these are often used when patients are unable to tolerate a surgical procedure. Major emphasis should be placed on prevention, with proper measures for decreasing daily UV light exposure in the most susceptible patients.

Squamous cell carcinoma occurs in patients with excessive UV light exposure who are fair-skinned and tan poorly—similar risk factors for the development of basal cell carcinoma. However, squamous cell carcinoma more frequently occurs in darker-pig-

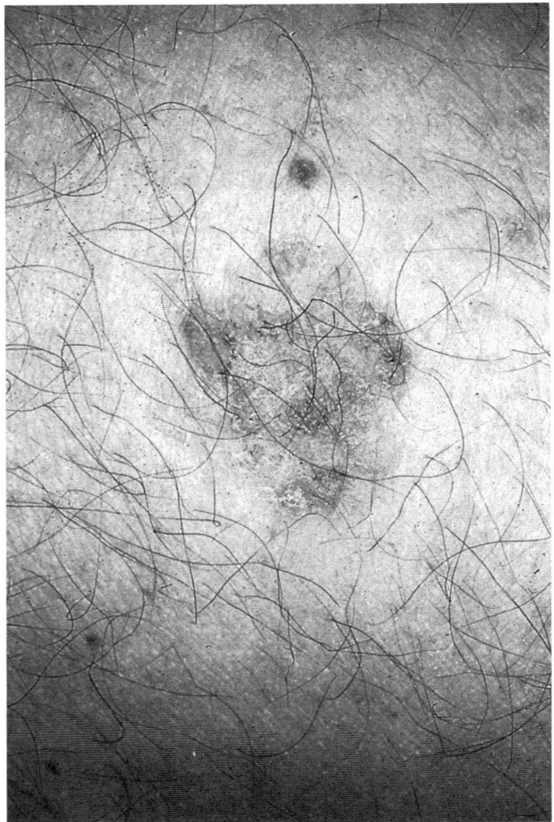

Figure 8.18 Squamous cell carcinoma.

mented individuals and can occur in non-sun-exposed areas such as the mucous membranes, with a resulting poorer outcome. Unlike basal cell carcinoma, which rarely metastasizes, squamous cell carcinoma can metastasize; this is seen more frequently in lesions arising in non-sun-exposed skin. Other risk factors for metastasis are lesions arising in areas of a previous burn, irradiation, or a chronic scarring process.

Initial lesions in squamous cell carcinoma are red, scaly plaques which often crust (Figure 8.18). Lesions on the lower lip often develop in the midst of severe sun-damaged skin. Lesions on the mucous membranes, lip, and scalp have a higher incidence of metastases and should be treated decisively.

The differential diagnosis of squamous cell carcinoma includes keratoacanthoma, a benign lesion. This lesion grows rapidly and has a central keratotic plug, features which, in general, differentiate it from squamous cell carcinoma.

The ideal treatment of squamous cell carcinoma is elliptical excision with margin control. Mohs micrographic surgery should be used for larger lesions and lesions in areas with higher recurrence rates.

Preventive measures for decreasing daily UV light exposure, particularly in the phenotypically susceptible host, especially in early childhood and adolescence, can play a significant role in preventing the occurrence of this skin cancer.

Malignant melanoma is the most deadly of all skin cancers. It is a neoplasm arising in the melanocytes, the skin cells producing the pigment melanin. Approximately 35,000 patients develop malignant melanoma each year, resulting in 6500 deaths annually. The incidence of melanoma has risen 4–6% per year since 1973 in the United States. Malignant melanoma is the most common cancer in women between the ages of 25 and 29 and is second only to breast cancer in women between ages 30 and 35. Malignant melanoma is now the eighth most common type of cancer and is an increasingly important neoplasm in clinical practice today as early detection and treatment improve its outcome and prognosis.

The role of UV light and the development of cutaneous melanoma are not correlated as directly as are chronic sun exposure and nonmelanoma skin cancer. However, epidemiologic studies suggest that UV light exposure in the phenotypically at-risk patient does play a minor role. Melanomas are relatively uncommon in darker-pigmented individuals and, when diagnosed, most commonly occur in acral locations. The role of precursor lesions such as dysplastic nevi is also important, as it is in the familial dysplastic mole syndrome. Intermittent, intense sun exposure may play a more important role in cutaneous melanoma than chronic UV light exposure.

The initial stages of melanoma involve proliferation in the basal cell layer of atypical melanocytes. Melanomas expand by horizontal proliferation during the horizontal growth phase of the malignant melanocytes. This stage may last for periods ranging from years to months prior to onset of the vertical growth phase or invasion of the dermis. With deeper invasion, metastases occur.

Clark's levels is a system developed to correlate tumor thickness and survival. Another system, introduced by Breslow in 1979, measures the actual tumor thickness with an ocular micrometer as the distance between the granular layer and the deepest part of the melanoma. Using the Breslow level, the survival rate for melanoma with a thickness of less than 0.75 mm is nearly 96%; 0.76 to 1.49 mm, 87%; 1.50 to 2.49 mm, 75%; 2.50 to 3.00 mm, 66%; and above 4.00 mm, 47%. There is a definite correlation between poor prognosis and tumor thickness which underscores the importance of early detection and management.

Initial clinical signs of malignant melanoma include itching, bleeding, ulceration, or tenderness. A family history of melanoma, features of phenotypic susceptibility, a history of frequent sunburns, and a history of atypical moles should be elicited. The cardinal cutaneous signs of malignant melanoma, established by the American Cancer Society, are the ABCD rules (Figure 8.19): asymmetry, border irregularity, color variation, and diameter above 6 mm. Although the ABCD rules are *not* completely inclusive of all malignant melanomas, they remain very useful in the detection of most early lesions.

There are generally four types of melanoma: (1) superficial spreading malignant melanoma, (2) nodular melanoma, (3) lentigo maligna melanoma, and (4) acral lentiginous melanoma.

Superficial spreading malignant melanoma is the most common cutaneous melanoma (75% of cases). It tends to have initial slow growth in the horizontal phase. This growth phase may last for years. However, some lesions may have an unexpectedly rapid conversion from the horizontal to the vertical growth phase, with invasion of the dermis. These lesions are often minimally raised, round or oval, with polycyclic, finger-like projections (Figure 8.20). The maximum incidence of superficial spreading malignant

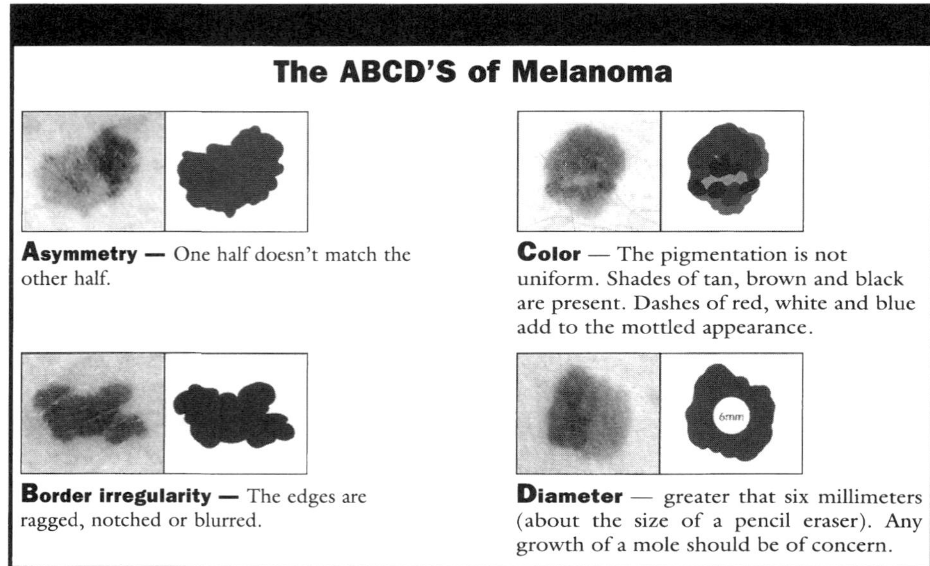

Figure 8.19 The ABCDs of melanoma. Reprinted with permission of the American Academy of Dermatology.

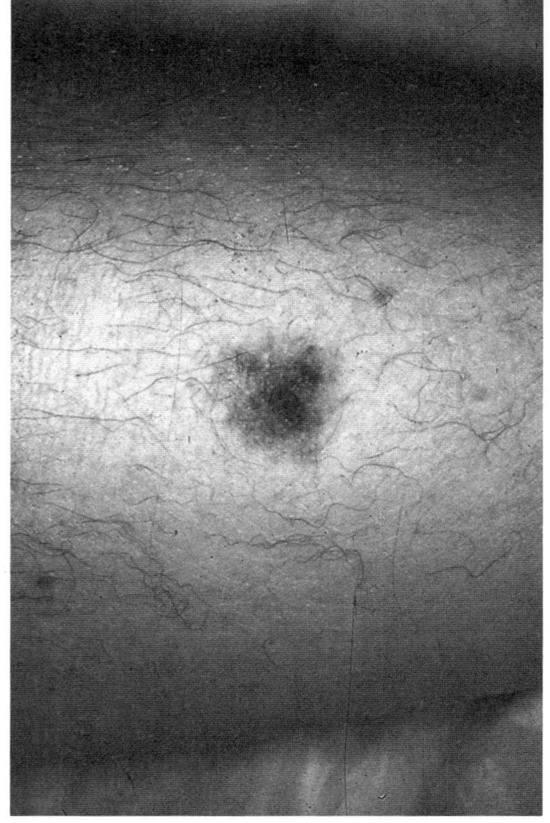

Figure 8.20 Superficial spreading malignant melanoma.

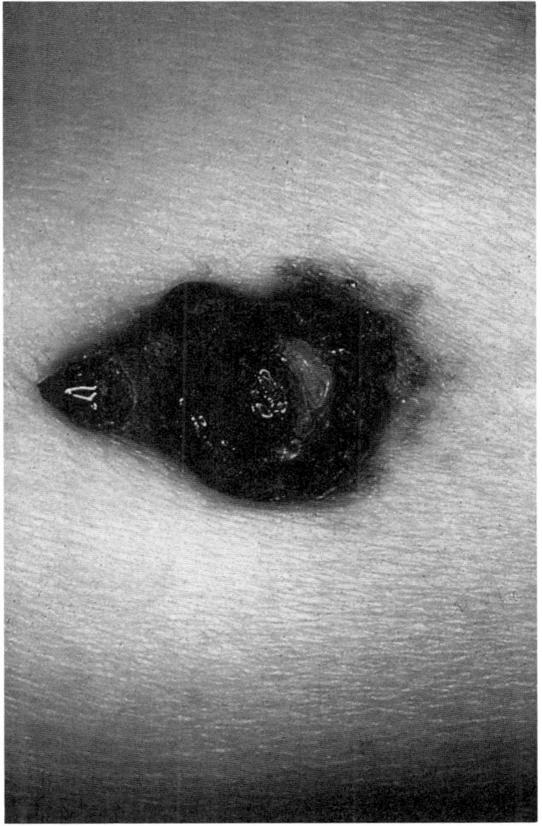

Figure 8.21 Nodular melanoma.

melanoma occurs in middle age in persons with very fair complexions. It arises most commonly on the trunk, forearms, lower extremities, and, rarely, on the face and thighs. In more advanced stages there may be red, white, or blue areas within the lesion. Gray-white areas are often correlated with histologic regression.

Nodular melanoma accounts for approximately 14% of all malignant melanomas. These melanomas may appear as dark nodules which may or may not have surface ulcerations (Figure 8.21). This tumor also occurs less commonly on sun-exposed areas. It has a vertical growth phase from its initial development. These lesions can have a blue-black color and occasionally are nonpigmented. The differential diagnosis includes various nonpigmented tumors.

Lentigo maligna melanoma is the least common cutaneous melanoma. An older term for it is *Hutchinson's melanotic freckle.* Of all the cutaneous melanomas, this melanoma is distinguished by the fact that long-term cumulative UVB light exposure is a widely accepted risk factor in its development. It occurs most commonly in chronically sun-exposed skin such as that on the head and neck, and it has a strong predilection for the cheeks. It usually occurs in older patients, with a mean age of 65. The clinical presentation is of a slowly growing, pigmented macule which may be present for many years (Figure 8.22). There is often some variation in color, with areas of tan, brown, pink, or white. Occasionally these lesions are amelanotic and easily confused with superficial

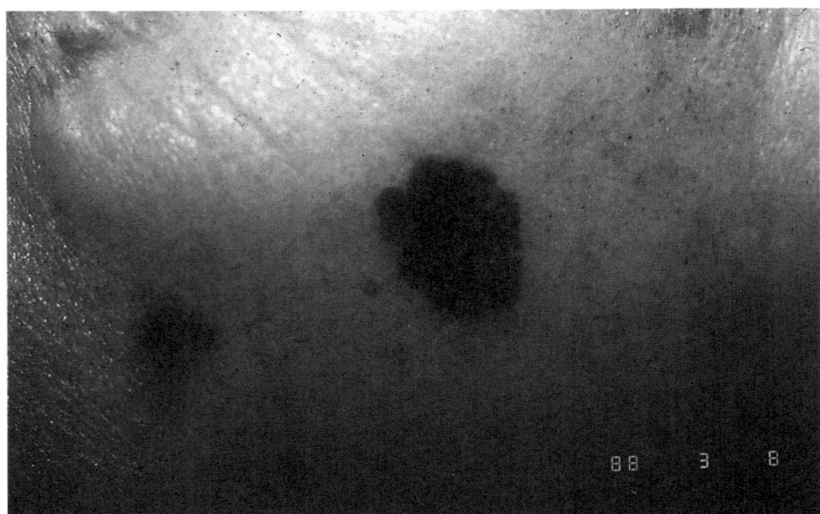

Figure 8.22 Lentigo maligna melanoma.

basal cell carcinomas, actinic keratoses, or solar lentigos. Histologic diagnosis can be difficult, as areas of melanocytic hyperplasia can occur within the lesion and may not be clearly diagnostic. Several biopsies may be required for accurate diagnosis. As noted, an important distinguishing feature is that lentigo maligna melanoma develops in chronically sun-damaged skin.

Acral lentiginous melanoma accounts for 2–8% of melanomas occurring in whites but up to 50–70% of those occurring in Asians and blacks. Acral lentiginous melanoma most often occurs in darker-pigmented individuals. This tumor arises on the soles, palms, fingernail and toenail beds, and on the mucocutaneous skin of the mouth, genitalia, and anus. Clinical features are more subtle in this tumor. Often a delay in diagnosis is the reason for its poorer prognosis. Initial features may be a linear brown-black macule with little variation in the pigment. Subungual melanomas often occur in the nail beds; the telltale sign may be spread of the pigment beyond the nail plate into the nailfold proper (Figure 8.23). Lesions of the mucous membranes may show a dark brown macule with blue-gray tinges. Nodules develop in this condition in the late phase.

The differential diagnosis of melanoma includes dermatofibroma, seborrheic keratosis, atypical nevus, and hemangioma. Wide local excision is the treatment of choice for primary melanoma. For tumors less than 0.75 mm in thickness, 1-cm surgical margins are recommended. Lesions measuring 0.76 to 1.49 mm require 1- to 2-cm surgical margins while thicker lesions require margins of up to 3 cm; elective lymph node dissection is recommended in some cases.

Other treatment modalities currently used or in clinical trials include adjuvant immunotherapy with agents such as tumor necrosis factor, gamma interferon, and granulocyte-macrophage stimulating factor, all in an effort to induce tumor regression. Other treatment modalities include gene therapy, chemotherapy, monoclonal antibody therapy, and combinations of these therapies.

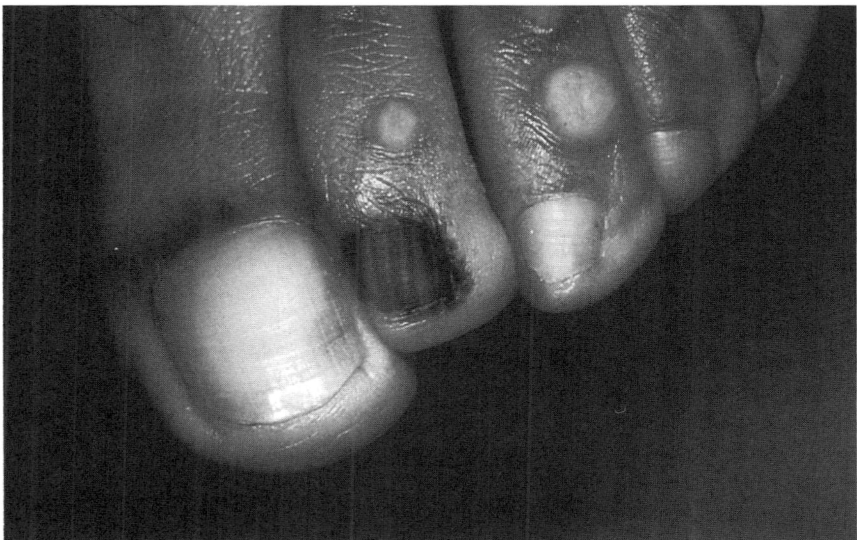

Figure 8.23 Acral lentiginous melanoma.

Since cutaneous malignant melanoma is a clearly visible lesion, it is amenable to early diagnosis and management, presently the only effective curative intervention. Throughout the country, the American Academy of Dermatology, in conjunction with the American Cancer Society, provided free skin cancer screenings for more than 750,000 Americans from 1985 to 1994. This is a helpful public service and provides a forum for patient education. Public information campaigns have encouraged skin self-examination on a routine basis to aid in early detection. Since approximately 85% of the U.S. population see a physician every 2 years, all physicians should play a role in patient education and detection of melanoma in its early stages in order to help reduce the mortality caused by this condition.

BIBLIOGRAPHY

Barnhill RL, Fitzpatrick TB, Fandray KL: *Color Atlas and Synopsis of Pigmented Lesions.* New York, Mcgraw-Hill, 1995, pp 145–198.

Cohen LM: Lentigo maligna and lentigo maligna melanoma. *J Am Acad Dermatol* 33:923–933, 1995.

Fitzpatrick TB, Rhodes AR, Sober AJ, et al: Seven deadly melanomas. A photographic compendium. *Fitzpatrick's J Clin Dermatol* 3:12–21, 1995.

Johnson TM, Smith JW, Nelson BR, et al: Current therapy for cutaneous melanoma. *J Am Acad Dermatol* 32:689–706, 1995.

Koh HK, Geller AC, Miller DR: The current status of melanoma, early detection, and screening. *Dermatol Clin* 13:623–632, 1995.

Leshin B, White WL: Malignant neoplasms of keratinocytes. In Arndt KA, Leboit PE, Robinson JK, et al (eds): *Cutaneous Medicine and Surgery*. Philadelphia, WB Saunders, 1996, pp 1378–1440.

Preston DS, Stern RS: Nonmelanoma cancers of the skin. *N Engl J Med* 327:1649–1662, 1992.

Chapter 9

Basic Bedside Cardiac Examination and Easy Principles of ECG Interpretation

Brendan Phibbs

CARDIAC HISTORY

There are only two major symptoms of heart disease—*dyspnea and pain.* Consider dyspnea first. The dyspnea of heart disease is always caused by congestive heart failure. By definition, this means that the lungs are congested with blood; the left ventricle is not pumping the blood out of the lungs as fast as the right ventricle is pumping it in. This excess blood volume in the lungs causes water to ooze out of the pulmonary capillaries into the perialveolar tissues. In severe cases, the alveoli will fill with fluid. In simple terms, there's too much water in the lungs; the air passages are compressed and there isn't enough room for the exchange of oxygen.

Dyspnea of congestive heart failure is therefore always characterized by rapid, shallow breathing because there isn't enough mechanical room for the air to move into and out of the lungs. When a patient complains of dyspnea, count the respirations per minute and note the depth of breathing. The diagnosis will be obvious.

There are only two other causes of dyspnea. One is chronic obstructive lung disease—emphysema, bronchiolitis, or both. The productive chronic cough, the long, agonized expiration, the history of smoking or asthma, and the general appearance of the patient are easy to recognize. The other—and much more common—cause is hysterical hyperventilation—"I keep taking deep breaths because I'm not getting enough air in my lungs." The isolated deep breath of hysterical hyperventilation is totally different from the rapid, uncontrollable, shallow breathing of congestive heart failure; it's almost impossible to confuse the two. (Useful tip: when a patient complains of "trouble breathing," demonstrate hyperventilation with one deep, exaggerated breath and ask if that's how the patient feels. The answer will usually establish the diagnosis.)

PAIN

For practical purposes, the only kind of heart trouble that causes pain is coronary artery disease. This is, of course, very rare in menstruating females, but after the menopause it increases apace. Be prepared to recognize it. Here are some rules.

1. *The pain of angina pectoris.* Discomfort with effort, which is relieved by rest, should always raise the suspicion of angina pectoris. The problem lies in defining what you and the patient mean by discomfort. The discomfort may be the classic heavy pressure in the chest, neck, shoulders, or arms. It may also appear in the form of sudden, inappropriate dyspnea, with or without pain. In most cases, the pain of angina is preceded by dyspnea if you ask the patient. (Angina pectoris is in fact a transient episode of left heart failure, hence the dyspnea.) Various paresthesias are common, including "burning," a "full, pounding sensation in the head," and "feeling funny and weak all over." In every case, they are provoked by exertion and relieved by rest.

Apprehension is a surprisingly common manifestation of angina. It may accompany any of the other symptoms or may appear alone. When walking or working, the patient is aware of a sudden sense of impending disaster; the foreboding disappears with rest. Be prepared to recognize the constellation of discomfort caused by exertion and relieved by rest, and remember that the term *discomfort* includes many different symptoms.

2. *The pain of myocardial infarction.* Published descriptions of this pain would probably fill a small encyclopedia; there's no need to repeat them. Here are some rules to help you decide that the pain is *not* caused by myocardial infarction.

1. Pain that arises in the myocardium is never pleuritic. If the pain is affected by breathing, it has nothing to do with the myocardium. Have the patient inhale, exhale, and hold the breath without straining, and see what effect this has on the pain. If the pain is provoked by inhaling and if there's no pain while the patient holds the breath, you have ruled out myocardial infarction.
2. Myocardial ischemic disease never produces tenderness on the chest wall. If you reproduce the pain by touching or pressing on the chest wall, it's not myocardial.
3. Always ask the patient how long the pain lasts. The pain of myocardial ischemia is never quick or stabbing. If the patient tells you that the pain felt "like a needle" or "like a knife stabbing, quick and then gone," you can be sure you're not dealing with a myocardial infarct.
4. Myocardial pain is never reproduced by motion of the arms, neck, or torso. If the patient tells you that the pain comes on with motion of the arm or shoulder muscles, it's not cardiac.

SEMANTICS IN THE CLINIC (LIFE AND HEALTH DEFINITIONS)

Be sure you know what the patient means by the word *pain*. Many people think of pain only as the sensation that comes with a burn, contusion, or laceration. It doesn't occur to them that a sense of pressure in the chest is the very pain you're asking about.

Tell the patient what you mean by the word "pain" when you're asking about heart disease. Pericarditis produces pain in the anterior chest, but it's totally different from the pain of myocardial ischemia. Two or three questions will almost always establish the diagnosis. First, there is a pleuritic component. Tell the patient to breathe in, and you'll hear that the pain is worse, clearly related to breathing. This rules out myocardial pain. Second, there is a steady, nonpleuritic component. As the heart beats, the diseased pericardium rubs against the epicardium, producing pain. Tell the patient to hold the breath with the mouth open to rule out the Valvsalva effect. The patient will always report that there's still some pain, but that it's not nearly as severe as the pain with inspiration. You have now established the diagnosis of pericarditis.

There are two minor symptoms of heart disease—syncope and vertigo. There are two cardiac causes of these symptoms. One is aortic stenosis. You make this diagnosis with the fingertip and stethescope (see below). The other is an abnormally slow heart rate caused by an inadequate sinus node or by some type of atrioventricular block (see the section on the electrocardiogram).

PHYSICAL EXAMINATION

Start with the obvious: rate of respiration? deep or shallow? pulse rate? color?

Now the not-so-obvious: Always begin your cardiac examination in the neck. Put one finger on a carotid artery and allow it to rise and fall like a small recording device. Try palpating your own carotid and note the brisk upstroke. Base to peak, it takes about 1 s. You'll feel the same swift, smooth upstroke in your radial pulse or anywhere you palpate the arteries. This is normal.

When you palpate the carotid, you gain two critical bits of information. First, you identify the first heart sound. When the heart is rapid or irregular, this may not be easy with the stethescope, but you can always do it with your index finger. *The heart sound that comes with the carotid upstroke is the first heart sound.* If the upstroke is normal and brisk, there is no deformity in the stroke and the aortic valve is normal. Second, if there is any slurring, slowing or deformity of that arterial upstroke, or if you feel an actiual thrill, you have made a life-and-death diagnosis with 100% specificity and sensitivity. If there is *any* deformity of the carotid upstroke, *valvular aortic stenosis is present.* This is true every time. It (valvular aortic stenosis) is the only condition that will cause this slurred upstroke. The only exception involves people over 80 (Figure 9.1).

Make palpation of the carotid the first part of your cardiac examination. (Most cardiologists don't, and they thereby miss some critical diagnoses.) Second, palpate the precordium and forget a fairy tale you learned in medical school. This tale concerns the point of maximum impulse on the precordium. In fact, it doesn't exist. In a normal adult, with normal body habitus, lying supine, you don't feel *anything* when you palpate the precordium. Try it, and you'll see.

If you feel a forceful, sustained, or complex lift over any part of the precordium, you're dealing with a diseased ventricle. Always stand on the patient's right side when you examine the heart. Palpate for a right ventricular lift with the heel of your right hand in the left parasternal region, approximately from the second to the fifth interspaces. If you feel a forceful or sustained lift here, there's increased right ventricular pressure, usually associated with pulmonary hypertension. Palpate for a left ventricular lift or heave anywhere from the midclavicular line to the midaxillary line in the fourth, fifth, and sixth interspaces. A forceful, sustained, or complex lift indicates a diseased left ventricle with almost 100% accuracy (Figure 9.2). If you feel a lift at about the midclavicular line relatively high in the precordium, in about the third or fourth

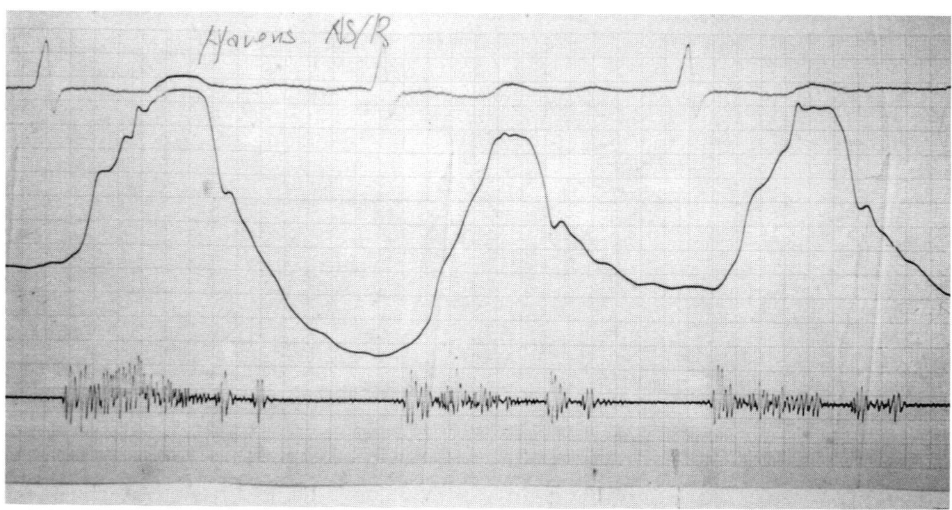

Figure 9.1 Typical delayed slurred upstroke of a carotid artery in the presence of aortic valvular stenosis. This type of slow, "shuddering" rise of the arterial pulse is easily detectable and is absolutely diagnostic of aortic valvular stenosis. Nothing else will cause it. The typical ejection murmur is recorded in the phonocardiogram below.

interspace, you're almost certainly dealing with a ventricular aneurysm. If you feel a forceful, sustained, or complex ventricular lift anywhere in the precordium, you're dealing with heart disease. Pursue the diagnosis!

Now listen to the heart. First, identify the first heart sound; palpate the carotid. Now listen carefully to the interval before the first heart sound for a soft, thumping noise. It sounds like "duh-lub-dub." The "duh" is the presystolic sound that comes with atrial systole. It's called an *S4* or *fourth heart sound gallop.* It comes before the first heart sound and hence before the carotid upstroke. (Keep your finger on that carotid!) (Figure 9.3). An S4 gallop is *always* abnormal in children and young adults. It may be normal in middle-aged and older patients but even then, if it's loud, it indicates heart disease. Always perform further tests.

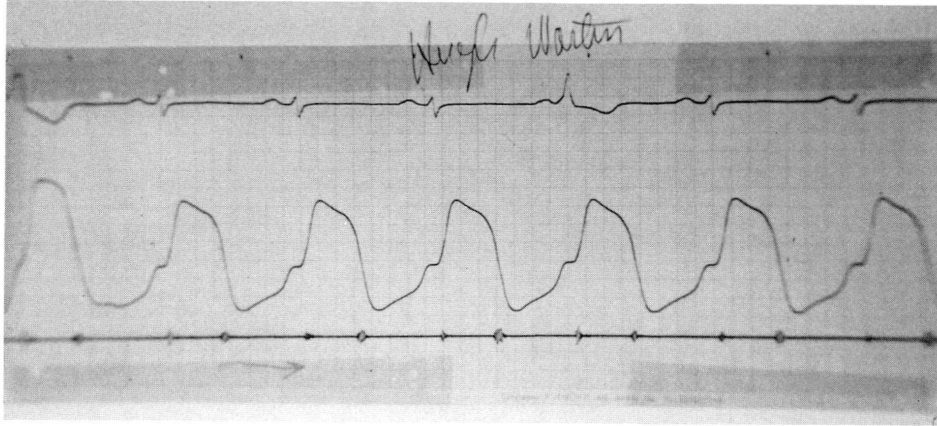

Figure 9.2 Left ventricular heave, or sustained rise, recorded over the mid-precordium. Note the initial rise directly below the P wave of the ECG; this is the atrial impulse or "a" wave. A palpable "a" wave and a sustained lift, as here, always indicate abnormal ventricular function.

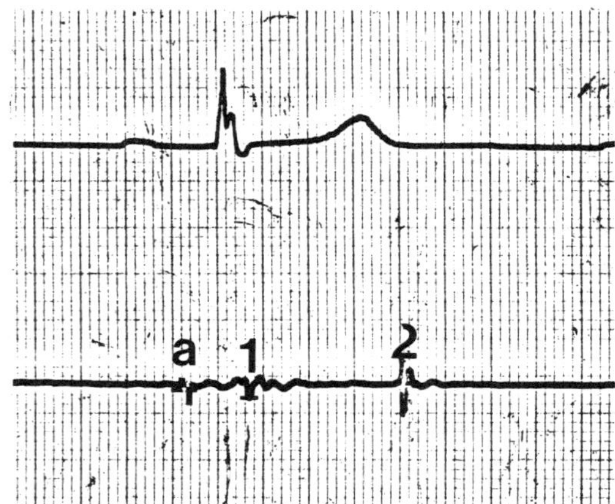

Figure 9.3 Atrial gallop or fourth heart sound "a." This is a presystolic sound caused by atrial contraction against an unyielding or overloaded left ventricle. Listen in the interval before S1 to hear it.

Now listen to the space after the second heart sound for another soft thumping sound that sounds like "lub-dub-duh." If you hear one here, it's an S3—a third heart sound gallop (Figure 9.4). An S3 is a ventricular gallop; it occurs just after the end of rapid diastolic filling. In the adult (over age 25), an S3 gallop is always a very bad sign. It means one of two things. Either the ventricle is seriously overloaded with an excess volume of blood or it's weakened so that it can't handle a normal volume. The excess volume almost always comes from a leaking valve, either aortic or mitral. The heart muscle can be weakened by ischemia, myocarditis, degenerative myocardiopathy, or, most commonly, by the excess load of pumping against an abnormally high blood pressure. In any case, the S3 gallop means imminent danger. Always call for help—at once.

A note on technique: every time you listen to a heart, search for gallops. Tell yourself that there's an S4 gallop before every first heart sound and listen for it. Tell yourself there's an S3 gallop after every second heart sound and listen for it. Focus your hearing!

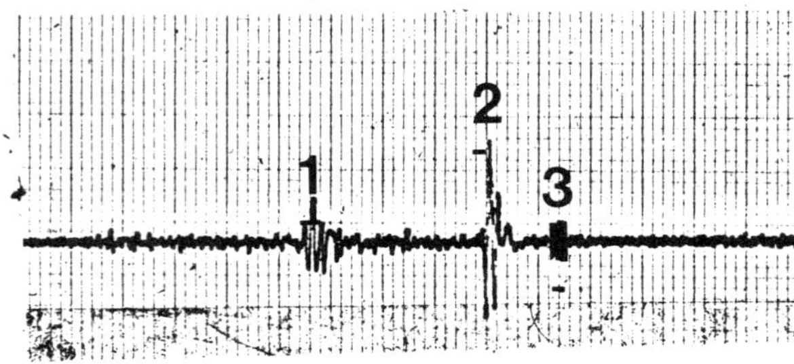

Figure 9.4 Ventricular gallop or third heart sound. This comes at the stage of rapid diastolic filling, and in the adult it always implies severe ventricular dysfunction. In the setting of a myocardial infarction it is a particularly bad prognostic sign.

An S4 gallop is always abnormal in children or young adults. If it's loud, it's abnormal in any patient. An S3 gallop is common and normal in children and young adults. If you hear it in anyone 25 years of age or older, it's a very bad sign. Summon cardiologic help at once.

Special note: gallops are very-low-frequency sounds. To hear them, use the bell of your stethescope and touch it as lightly as possible to the skin—just enough to screen out the air.

MURMURS

You still have your finger on the carotid, so you're ready to distinguish systole from diastole. Now divide murmurs into two main classes—systolic and diastolic.

There are two kinds of systolic murmurs—ejection and pansystolic. Learning to differentiate these murmurs is one of the most important skills any clinician can acquire. The pansystolic or holosystolic murmur starts with the first heart sound and goes all the way to the second heart sound. The murmur actually "runs into" the second heart sound like a person running into a door. You may have learned that you can't hear the second heart sound with a pansystolic murmur. Nonsense—of course you can. If there's pulmonary hypertension with a loud pulmonic valve closure, the second heart sound will be very loud and snapping. In any case, the second heart sound is clearly audible at the end of a pansystolic murmur (Figure 9.5).

This is the time to mention an important trick of auscultation. Psychologists who study sensation state that you can focus on hearing one item at a time so that you don't hear anything around it. Use this phenomenon when you listen to the heart. When you listen to the first heart sound, for instance, screen out everything else. Is there an S4 ahead of it? If there is a murmur, does it start precisely with the first heart sound or a little after it? When you're listening to a systolic murmur, focus on the *end* of the murmur. Ask yourself if the murmur runs into S2 with absolutely no gap or pause. If it does, there are only two diagnostic possibilities: mitral regurgitation or ventricular septal defect. That's an arresting differential diagnosis, and you made it by listening to the end of the murmur.

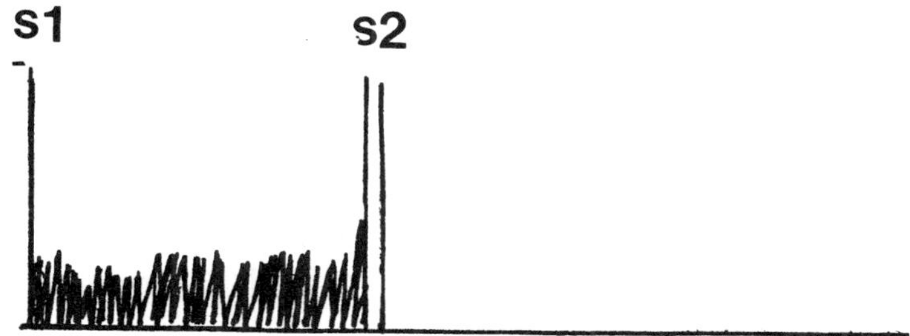

Figure 9.5 Pansystolic murmur. The murmur starts immediately with S1 and ends with S2. There is no interval between the end of the murmur and S2. A pansystolic murmur means one of two things—mitral insufficiency or a ventricular septal defect. A pansystolic murmur *always* indicates significant organic heart disease; it is never functional or innocent.

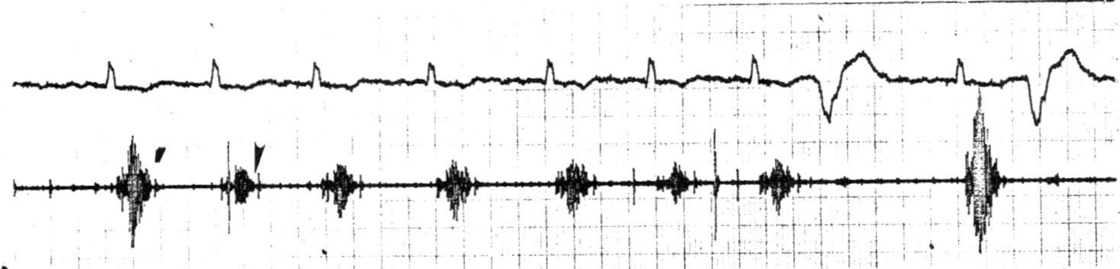

Figure 9.6 Systolic ejection murmur. There will always be a detectable pause before the second heart sound *(arrows)*. It is crucial to listen for this small interval since it indicates the distinction from pansystolic murmurs. Innocent and functional murmurs always have an ejection configuration; so do the murmurs of aortic or pulmonic stenosis, to name two causes.

Theoretically, tricuspid insufficiency should produce a pansystolic murmur, but in fact it doesn't. The murmur of tricuspid insufficiency is a short, midsystolic "whoosh." When you hear a real pansystolic murmur, it is *always* organic. It *always* means heart disease, and you're limited to the two diagnostic possibilities listed above.

The ejection systolic murmur is much more common. It starts after the first heart sound and it ends before the second heart sound (Figure 9.6).

The gap between the end of the murmur and the second heart sound is the essential factor in the diagnosis. Focus your hearing on the end of the murmur and listen for that short pause; it's the most important observation you can make. If you hear that pause, you're listening to an ejection murmur. There are many diagnostic possibilities—aortic stenosis, pulmonic stenosis, secundum atrial septal defect, aortic sclerosis (in older patients), functional murmurs, innocent murmurs. They all have an ejection configuration. They're never holosystolic.

Functional murmurs are caused by increased blood flow across a semilunar valve. Their causes include pregnancy, fever, anemia, hyperthyroidism, and atrioventricular (AV) shunts. They can also be caused by movement of blood in a high-pressure system; hypertension will often cause a murmur that disappears when the pressure falls to normal. Innocent murmurs are murmurs that appear even though the structure of the heart is normal and the hemodynamics of blood flow are normal. These murmurs are caused by eddies or whirlpools as the blood follows its tortuous course through the heart. *Remember that functional murmurs and innocent murmurs always have an ejection configuration. They are never pansystolic.*

Diastolic murmurs are always organic; they always connote heart disease. Let's repeat that: Diastolic murmurs are never functional and never innocent. When you hear a murmur in diastole, heart disease is present.

These days, in the Western world, the diastolic murmur you'll hear will practically always start immediately with the second heart sound and will fade away quickly—decrescendo. It will usually sound like a breath in your ear—soft and high-pitched (Figure 9.7). It's the murmur of aortic insufficiency. This is a really important diagnosis. Every time you listen to a heart, identify the second heart sound and listen carefully along the left sternal border for that breathy, soft, quickly fading murmur. Look for it! It's something you don't want to miss.

Fairy tale 2: In medical school, you were told to listen to the right side of the heart, off the sternum, for aortic murmurs and to the left side for pulmonic murmurs. This is

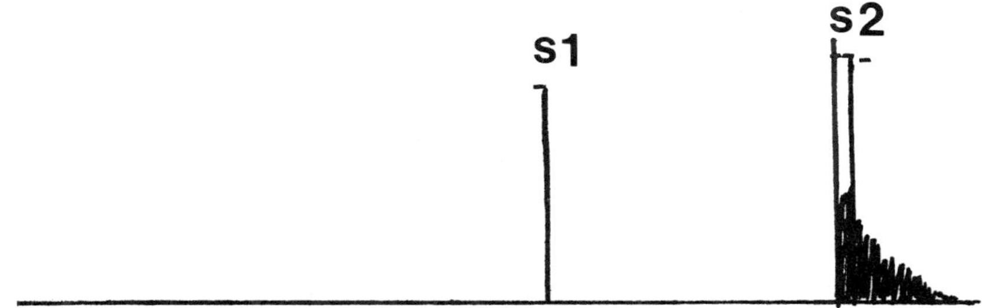

Figure 9.7 Early diastolic murmur. All diastolic murmurs indicate significant organic heart disease; they are never benign. The murmur of aortic insufficiency is by far the most common diastolic murmur; it starts immediately with the second heart sound and fades, diminuendo, as illustrated here. Sometimes it's so high-pitched that it sounds like a soft breath in your ear.

pernicious nonsense. The aortic and pulmonic valves lie directly over each other, with the aortic valve in front. You can hear both murmurs on the left side of the sternum. Organic pulmonic murmurs are very rare, so any early diastolic murmur left of the sternum means aortic insufficiency. The patient needs a definitive cardiologic workup.

ADVENTITIOUS SOUNDS

If you hear a sound in diastole after the second heart sound, it's either an S3 gallop or the opening snap of a stenotic mitral valve. A diastolic sound always means pathology: follow it up! If you hear a loud sound in systole well after the first heart sound, it may be the ejection click of a diseased aortic valve or the midsystolic click of mitral prolapse. In either case, expert cardiac consultation is essential. (Hint: try to find a cardiologist who knows how to use a stethescope; these days, that's not easy.)

THE ELECTROCARDIOGRAM

There are surprisingly few expert electrocardiographers even among cardiologists. On the other hand, any physician can make some simple observations that may well be lifesaving. In the dead of night, in an acute setting, there often won't be time to wait for expert consultation. If an acute cardiac emergency erupts in the middle of a delivery or during surgery, you must be ready to follow a few basic guidelines. *Most important, never rely on the computer interpretations of the ECG. They are riddled with mistakes, often lethal ones. No computer program performs with even marginal accuracy.* (Don't count on the anesthesiologist or anyone else in the operating room to tell you what those dancing lines on the oscilloscope mean. With the rarest exceptions, they won't have any idea.)

After these caveats, here are some easy principles any intelligent physician can apply:

1. What's driving the heart? Is a sinus rhythm present? First, always look for P waves. If you see P waves appearing at a normal rate and with a regular rhythm, the sinus node is firing normally.

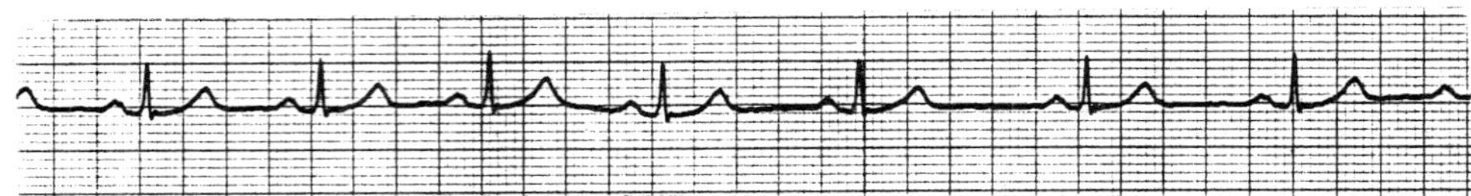

Figure 9.8 Normal sinus rhythm. Sinus P waves appear at regular intervals, followed at a normal distance by narrow (normal) ventricular complexes.

2. Is every P wave followed at the same normal interval by a ventricular response? If so, AV conduction is normal. There's no heart block. (Normal P-R interval = .12–.20 s or three to five small squares.)
3. Is the QRS complex narrow (.10 s or less.)? If so, conduction through the ventricles is normal (Figure 9.8). Diagnosis: normal sinus rhythm, normal AV and IV conduction.
4. Are there any early beats interrupting the sinus rhythm? If so, an ectopic focus is firing, producing extrasystoles. (Look for prematurity; think of the 5-month fetus.)
5. If there are premature beats, is the QRS complex narrow? If it is, the beats arise in the top half of the heart—in the atria or the AV node—and they're following the normal "fast track" down the bundle branches and through the ventricles. The ectopic beats are supraventricular (Figure 9.9).
6. Do the premature beats have a wide QRS complex (.12 s or greater)? If the premature beats have a wide QRS complex and if they're not preceded by a P wave, they are ventricular (Figure 9.10). If a premature beat arises in the atria, it will always be preceded by a P wave with a P-R interval of at least .12 s. A narrow premature beat (less than .12 sec) not preceded by a P wave can only come from the AV node or junction (Figure 9.11). (The practical distinction between atrial, junctional, and ventricular ectopic beats therefore is usually simple. It's based on three yes-or-no questions: QRS wide or narrow? P wave present? Distance of the P wave from the QRS complex?)

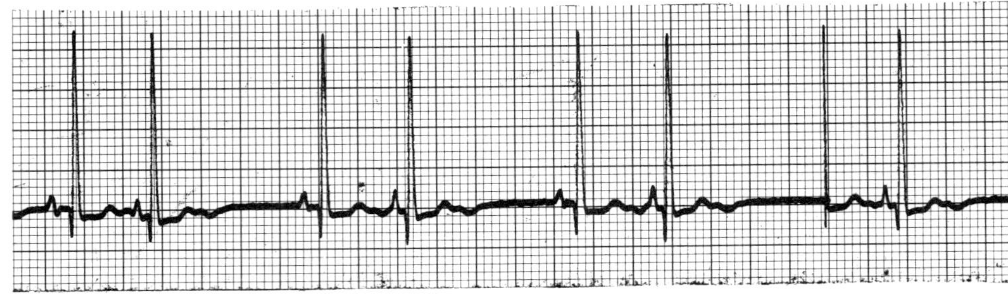

Figure 9.9 Premature atrial beats. After each sinus beat, there is an early beat forming a coupled or *bigeminal* rhythm. There is a P wave ahead of each early beat, so the beat arises in the atria. Note that the P wave of the atrial premature beat is different in shape from the sinus P wave. This is because it arises in a different place in the atria.

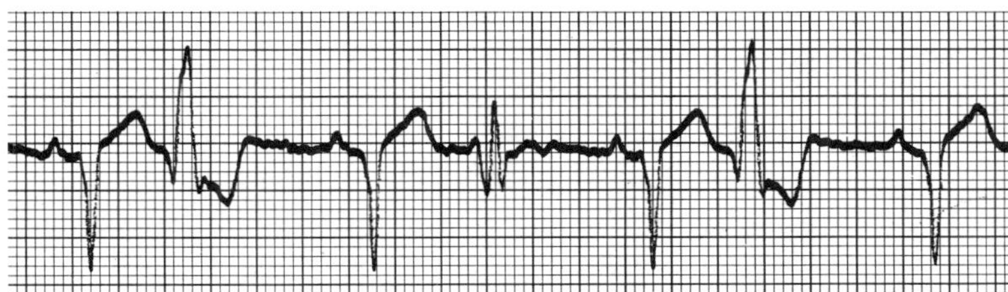

Figure 9.10 Ventricular premature beats. Every sinus beat is followed by a wide beat that is not preceded by a P wave. These are ventricular ectopic beats; they come in two different shapes, which means they arise in two different places in the ventricles.

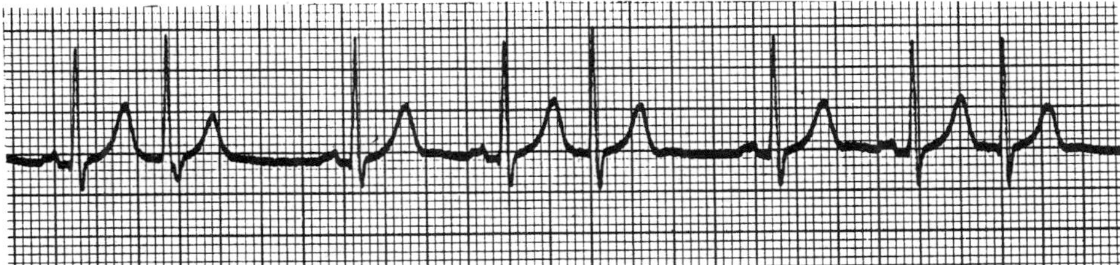

Figure 9.11 Premature junctional beats. A sinus rhythm is interrupted by early beats. These beats are narrow, so they can't be ventricular. There's no P wave ahead of them, so they can't be atrial. They can only arise in the AV node, also termed the *AV junction*.

Therapeutic Rule about Ectopic Beats: Don't Treat Them

Atrial and junctional premature beats are almost always benign. Everyone gets excited about ventricular ectopic beats because they look odd, but you still don't treat them. The only occasions for concern about ventricular ectopic beats occur (1) in the setting of an acute myocardial infarction; (2) if a patient is digitalis toxic with low serum potassium; or (3) if there's a congenital long Q-T syndrome (Romano-Ward). As you know, that eliminates about 99% of your patients. When those funny-looking beats appear on the oscilloscope during surgery, don't panic. They don't mean anything.

PAROXYSMAL TACHYCARDIA

Paroxysmal tachycardia is simply a rapid run of ectopic beats. The tachycardia starts and stops abruptly. The rhythm will be regular. There's only one question: where's the tachycardia coming from? It might be atrial, nodal, or ventricular. It's not important to distinguish atrial from nodal tachycardia acutely. There's really only one question: *Are the QRS complexes wide or narrow?* If they're wide and they're not preceded by P waves, you're looking at a rapid run of ventricular ectopic beats. *The diagnosis is ventricular tachycardia. This is always serious and may be life-threatening.* (Figure 9.12). If the QRS complexes are narrow, *the diagnosis is supraventricular tachycardia. This is never life-threatening and often appears in otherwise normal hearts* (Figure 9.13).

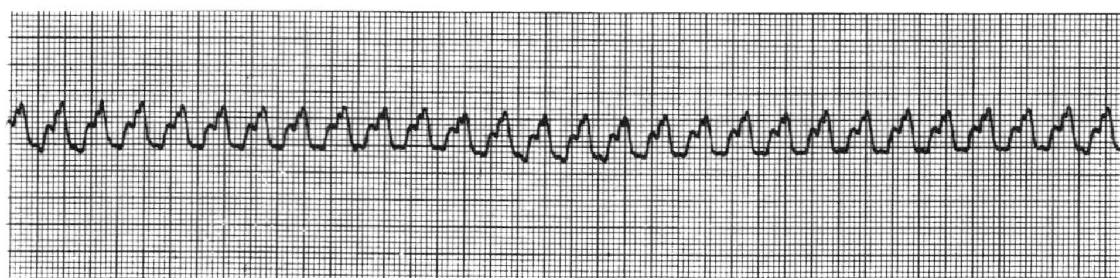

Figure 9.12 Paroxysmal ventricular tachycardia. This is simply a rapid succession of ventricular ectopic beats at a rate of 200 bpm. Wide beats with no P waves indicate ventricular tachycardia.

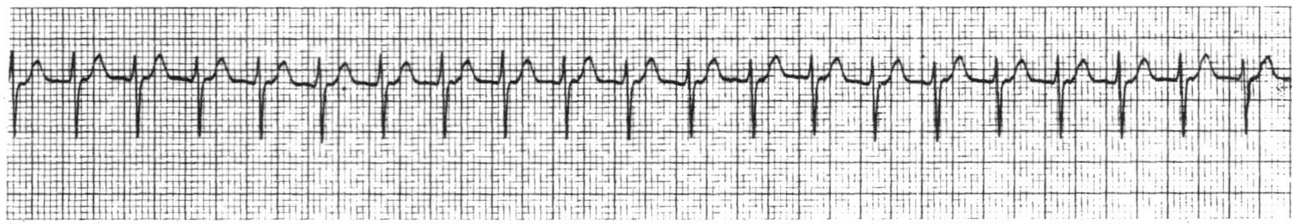

Figure 9.13 Paroxysmal supraventricular tachycardia. These are narrow beats and therefore suprventricular, either atrial or nodal; you can't be sure which. The distinction isn't important. What is important is that the narrow normal ventricular complexes indicate a benign supraventricular tachycardia.

Just answer the one overwhelming question: Are the QRS complexes wide or narrow?

Don't try anything fancy in the way of diagnosis when you see a wide-beat tachycardia. Always regard it as ventricular and treat it as such. It's the only safe approach.

ATRIAL FIBRILLATION AND THE DEADLY MIMIC

Atrial fibrillation is the most common sustained arrhythmia. The atria are twitching wildly, bombarding the AV over 400 times a minute with impulses; some come through, some don't. The ventricular rhythm will thus be totally irregular.

There are other arrhythmias that can produce the same kind of "irregular irregularity." This has led to the common shibboleth that an irregular irregularity means atrial fibrillation. That's a dangerous oversimplification. One could name at least 10 other disorders of rhythm that can produce an irregular irregularity. In one case at least, confusion with atrial fibrillation could be lethal. Look at Figures 9.14 and 9.15. The ventricular rhythm is rapid and completely irregular in both. Figure 9.14 illustrates typical atrial fibrillation—*there are no P waves.* The two conditions "no P waves" and "irregular ventricular rhythm" add up to atrial fibrillation with about 99.9% accuracy. In Figure 9.15, on the other hand, there are obvious P waves. These waves appear at a rapid rate, with a regular rhythm. This fact establishes the first half of the diagnosis—*atrial tachycardia.* Not all the P waves are reaching the ventricles. Some of them are

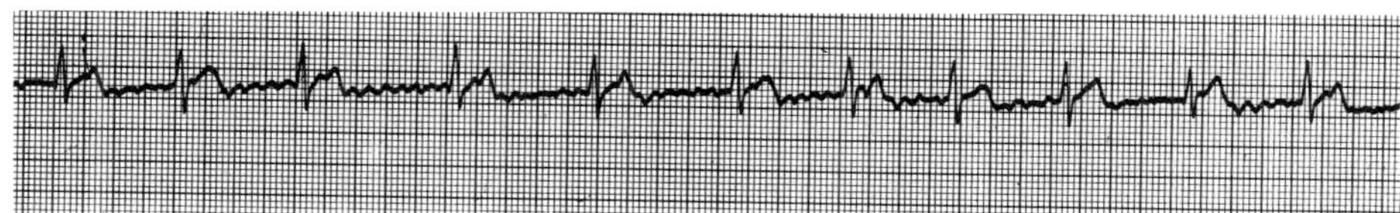

Figure 9.14 Atrial fibrillation. There are no P waves. There are rapid, fine atrial twitches in the baseline ("f" or fibrillary waves) and a totally irregular ventricular rhythm.

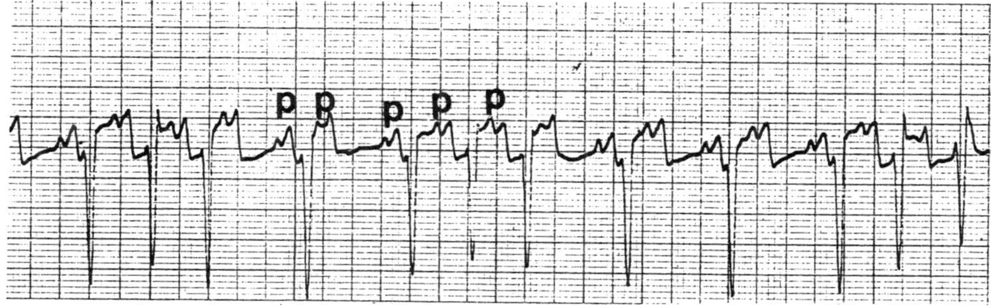

Figure 9.15 Paroxysmal atrial tachycardia with AV block. P waves are appearing with a regular rhythm and at a rapid rate (160 ppm). Some of the P waves are not followed by a ventricular response; they're blocked. This combination indicates paroxysmal atrial tachycardia with AV block, a potentially lethal arrhythmia almost always caused by digitalis toxicity.

blocked (arrows). Now you make the second half of the diagnosis—*AV block*. Total diagnosis—*paroxysmal atrial tachycardia (PAT) with AV block*. Because the degree of block changes from second to second, the ventricular rhythm is completely irregular, just like that in atrial fibrillation.

PAT *with block is a dangerous arryhthmia that is usually caused by digitalis toxicity in the setting of a low serum potassium level. The treatment is potassium. If more digitalis is given at this point, there's a 36% chance that the patient will die.*

Both atrial fibrillation and PAT with block can produce an irregular irregularity of the pulse. The proper treatment for one is lethal for the other.

Moral: When the pulse is rapid and irregular, get an ECG and find someone who knows how to read it. (This warning is tripled if the patient is taking digitalis of some kind.)

THE "SICK" SINUS NODE THAT REALLY ISN'T

In Figure 9.16 you see a sinus rhythm interrupted by two premature beats—junctional and atrial. Then the sinus rate slows dramatically to about 22 bpm. The patient was complaining of weakness and vertigo on minimal exertion. There were rumblings about a "sick sinus syndrome" and a possible pacemaker.

In Figure 9.17 you see a run of supraventricular tachycardia with a rate of 160 on the left-hand side of the strip. There are two ventricular premature beats ("V"), a late

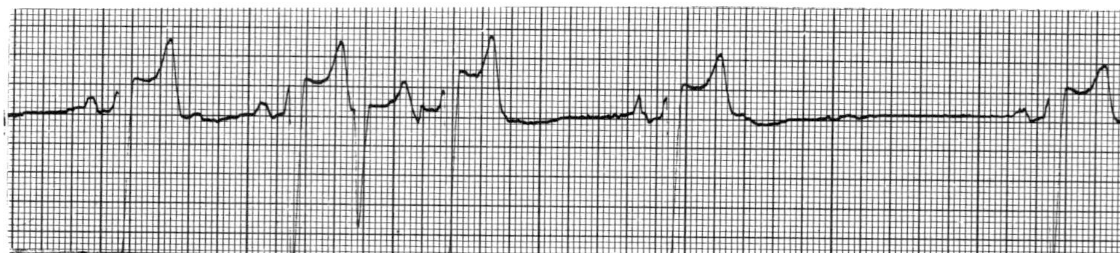

Figure 9.16 Sick sinus. Two sinus beats are followed by a premature atrial beat. Then the sinus rate slows dramatically to 18 bpm. The patient complained of faintness and dizziness. This depressed sinus node activity was the result of the antihypertensive drug clonidine. Most cases of sinus node depression are the result of drug effect.

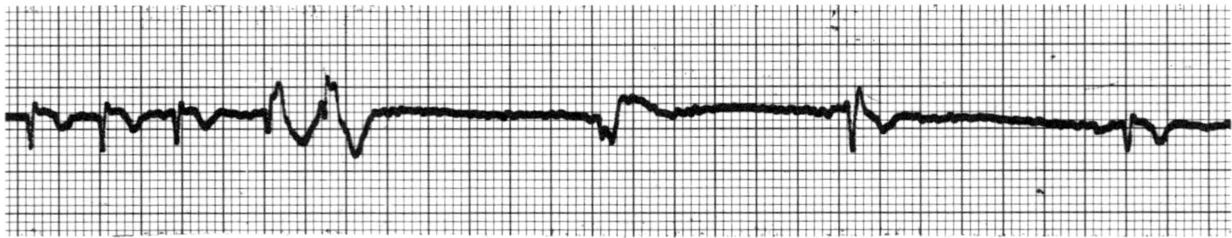

Figure 9.17 A run of paroxysmal supraventricular tachycardia (rate, 170 ppm) ends abruptly with the ventricular ectopic beats. There is no sinus node activity for some time. Two ventricular ectopic beats fire in their normal mode as "escape" or demand pacemakers before the sinus node resumes. This is true sick sinus behavior of the tachycardia-bradycardia type, in which rapid, abnormal rhythms alternate with periods of severe sinus bradycardia.

ventricular ectopic beat, and then a normal sinus rhythm with a rate of 53 bpm. Note that the third ventricular ectopic beat isn't premature—it's late. This is an example of an ectopic focus functioning the way it's supposed to; it discharges like a demand pacemaker when the normal system fails. That's why these ectopic potential pacemakers exist in the heart—they're potentially lifesaving.

Sick sinus again? Pacemaker? No in one case, yes in the other. The abnormally slow sinus in Figure 9.16 was the result of a drug. The patient was taking clonidine for hypertension; clonidine is one of the worst offenders in suppressing the sinus node. The rhythm illustrated in Figure 9.17 is the bradycardia-tachycardia type of sick sinus syndrome, occurring when runs of rapid, abnormal beating alternate with a slow sinus rate. This was a true sick sinus syndrome, not one caused by any medication.

Special note: When you see an abnormally slow sinus rhythm, always check the patient's medications. Ninety-nine times out of 100 you'll find the cause. Beta blockers, calcium blockers, digitalis, quinidine, procainamide, and many psychotropic drugs can all cause symptomatic and even dangerous slowing of the sinus rate.

True sick sinus syndrome is very rare. In our busy county hospital, I see fewer than one case every 2 years.

HEART BLOCK

Nobody expects you to be an expert on heart block, but here are two simple rules that anyone can apply:

1. If you see any sinus P wave that's not followed by a QRS complex, some kind of block is present.
2. If nonconducted P waves are present, look at the width of the QRS complex in the beats that are conducted. If the QRS is narrow, the block is in the AV node (Figure 9.18). If the QRS is wide—that is, if bundle branch block is present—the block may be down in the bundle branch system. The block may occur because one bundle branch is permanently blocked while the other fails intermittently—Mobitz II block. A wide QRS block is much more dangerous than a narrow QRS block (Figure 9.19). Any kind of AV block calls for immediate expert consultation.

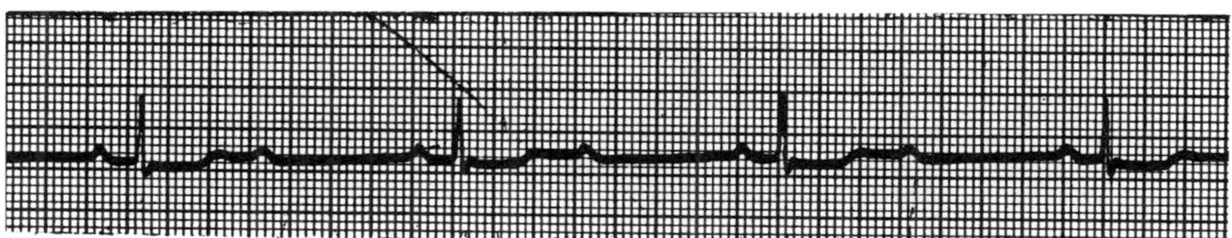

Figure 9.18 2:1 AV block. Every other P wave is blocked. The narrow ventricular complexes show that the bundle branch system is performing normally, so the block must be in the AV node.

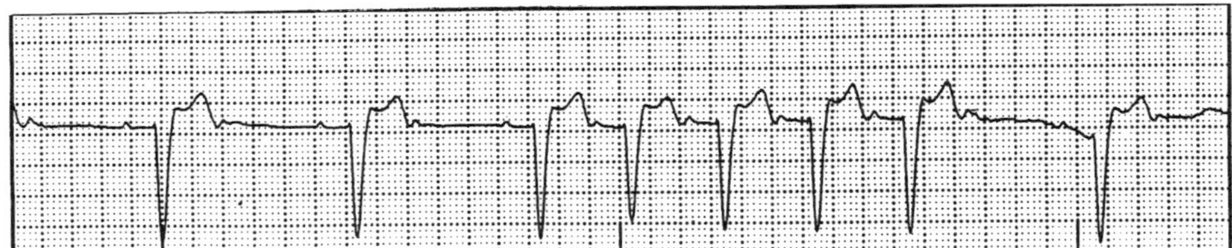

Figure 9.19 Mobitz II block. The wide QRS complexes show that one bundle branch is blocked. The strip starts with 2:1 block; then there are five conducted beats followed by a blocked P wave. This is a very dangerous type of block, and the wide QRS complex is the hallmark.

WHAT TO LOOK FOR IN THE PREOPERATIVE ECG

1. *Bundle branch block, or back to the wide QRS complex.* If you can count to 3 and distinguish up from down, you can diagnose bundle branch block. If the QRS of beats conducted down from the atria across the ventricles is .12 s wide, one bundle branch must be blocked. Look at lead V_1 to see which one is affected. If lead V_1 consists of a wide terminal upstroke or an R wave, right bundle branch block is present (Figure 9.20). If lead V_1 consists of a wide downstroke or an S wave, left bundle branch block is present. (Figure 9.21). Right bundle branch block can be benign, but left bundle branch block usually indicates heart disease. In either case, you should get a cardiac evaluation before surgery.
2. *Pathologic Q waves.* If the first detection of the QRS is down, with no upstroke ahead of it, it's a Q wave. Narrow, small Q waves are normal; they're produced by activation of the septum (Figure 9.22). By contrast, if a Q wave is wide—.04 s or more—it's pathologic. It usually means that there's dead myocardium, almost always the result of an infarct. *Pathologic Q waves can be a normal variant in leads III and V_1. In any other lead, they indicate pathology.* A cardiac consultation *is necessary* (Figure 9.23).

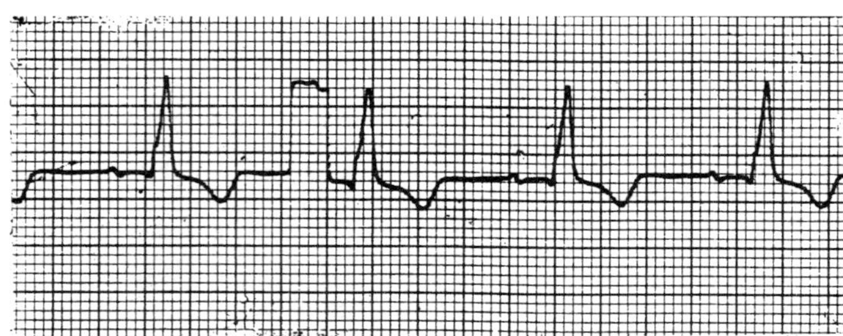

Figure 9.20 Lead V_1. The QRS complexes are .12 s wide, and the ventricular complex consists of a wide upward deflection or R wave. This demonstrates right bundle branch block.

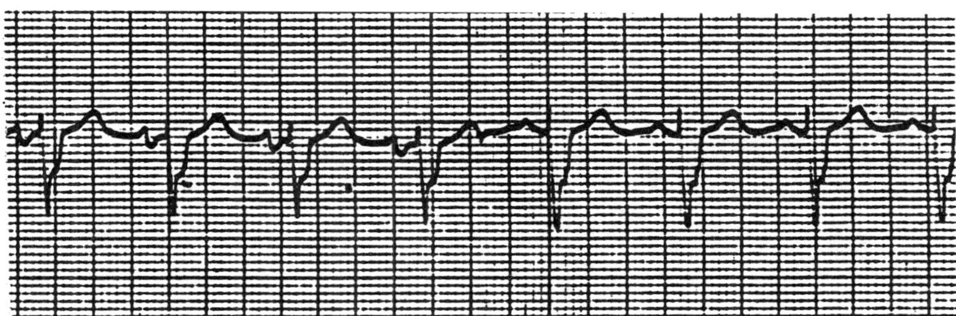

Figure 9.21 Lead V_1. The QRS complexes are .12 s wide, and the ventricular complex consists of a wide downward deflection, or S wave. This demonstrates left bundle branch block.

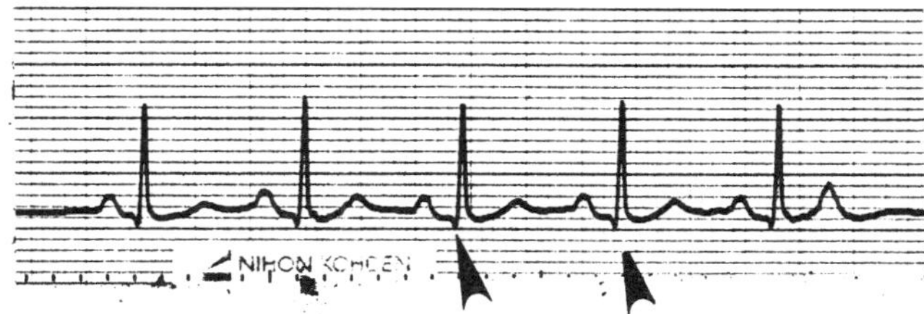

Figure 9.22 Normal physiologic septal Q waves *(arrows)*. These Q waves are narrow—about .01–.02 wide; this is the diagnostic feature.

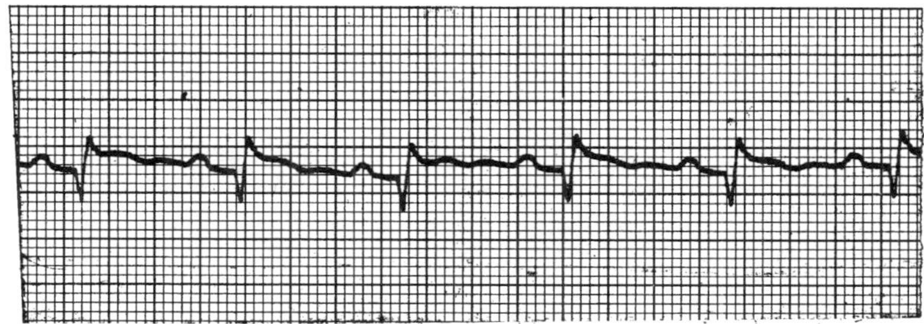

Figure 9.23 Pathologic Q waves. These Q waves are wide—at least .04 s wide. They always indicate myocardial pathology, usually a myocardial infarct.

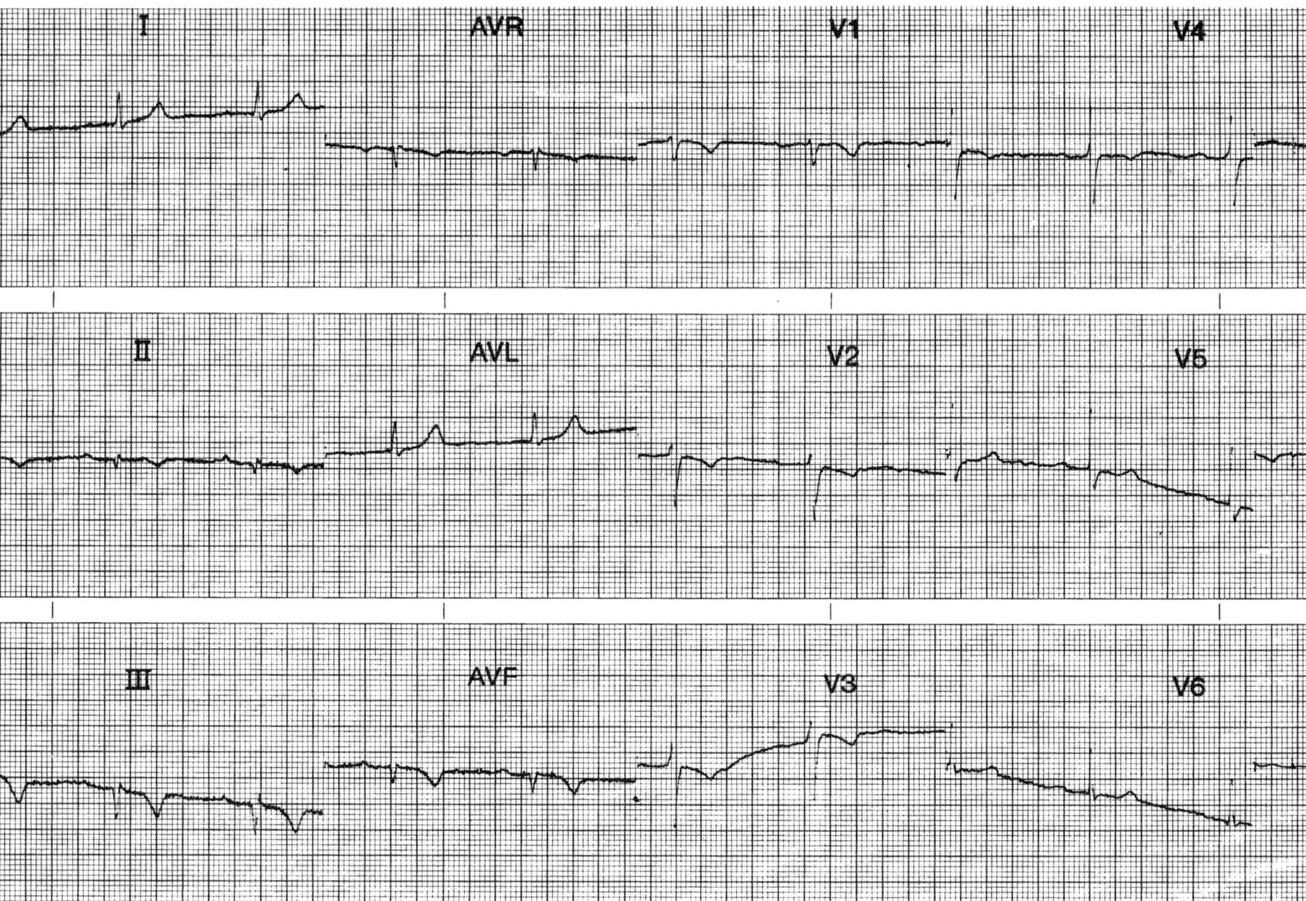

Figure 9.24 Nonspecific T-wave deformity. Inverted T waves occur in leads II, III, aV_F, and V_1 to V_4. This is always abnormal. When it appears in a preoperative tracing, halt the proceedings and obtain a cardiologic consultation. This kind of T-wave abnormality is a totally nonspecific finding.

3. *Invert T waves*. Simple rule: The T waves should be upright in all leads except III, aV_R and V_1. If they're inverted in any other leads, pathology is present (Figure 9.24).
4. *Current of injury*. Always inspect the ST segment. Acute ischemic insult to the myocardium will always register on this part of the ECG. The ST segment should be isoelectric—right at the baseline (Figure 9.25). If it's elevated or depressed, some kind of cardiac pathology, drug effect, or electrolyte abnormality is present. Figure 9.26 illustrates the early S-T segment elevation and depression of acute myocardial infarction, and Figure 9.27 is an example of ST segment depression caused by digitalis. Ventricular hypertrophy can also cause segment elevation or depression (Figure 9.28).

The moral for the noncardiologist in the preoperative holding area is simple: If the ST segments aren't right on the baseline, hold everything and call for help!

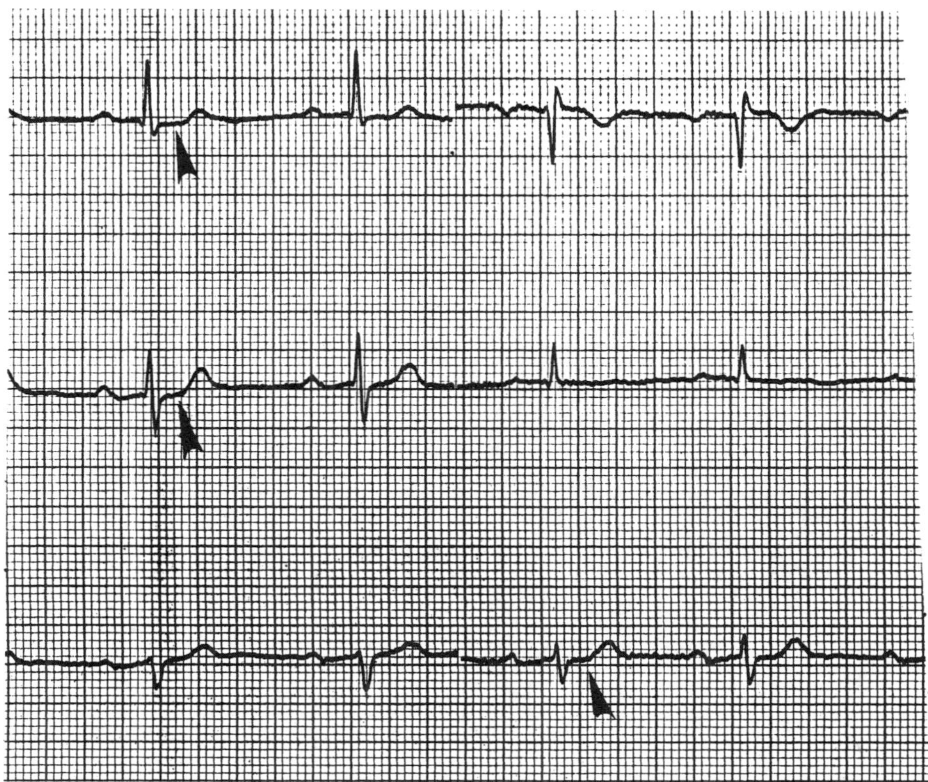

Figure 9.25 Normal, isoelectric ST segments *(arrows)*. The ST segment should be exactly on the baseline.

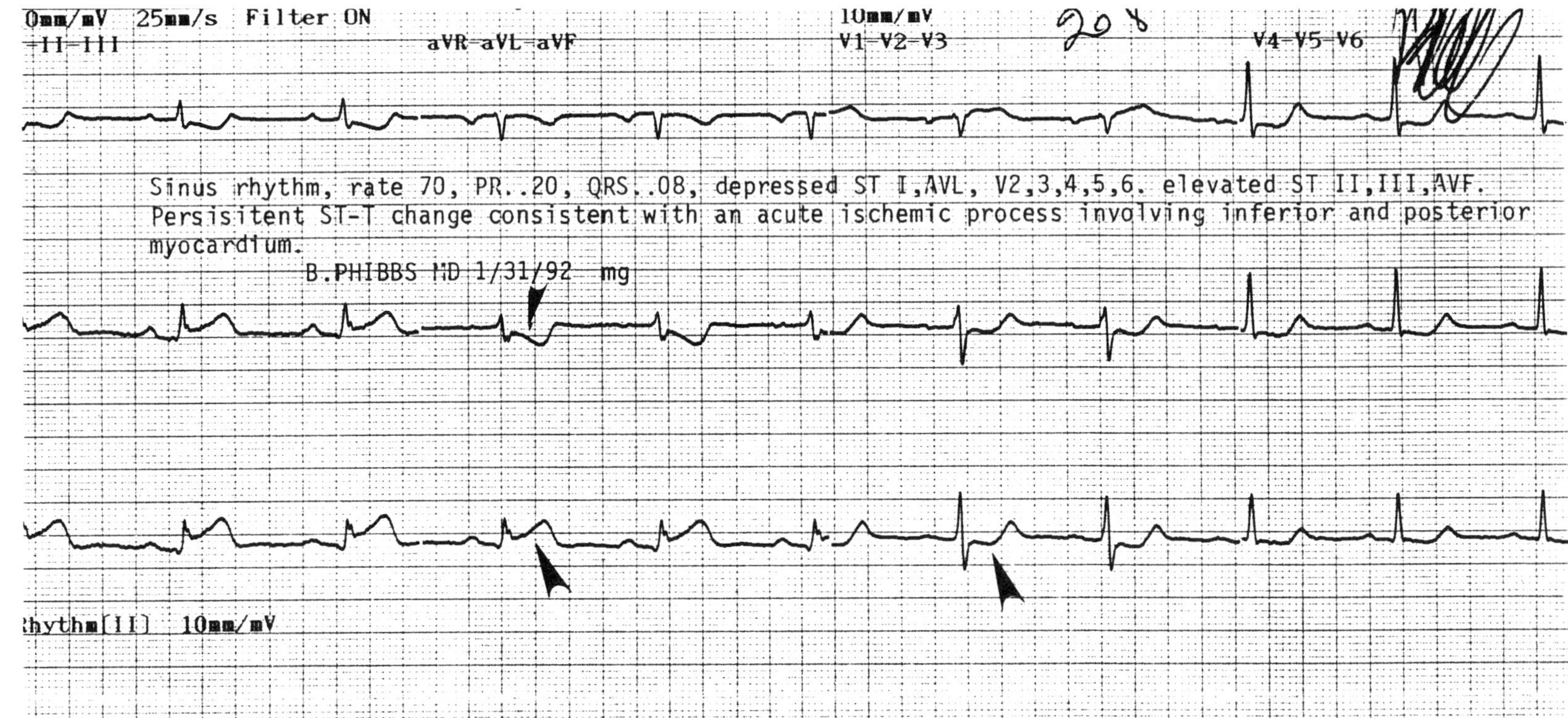

Figure 9.26 Elevation and depression of ST segments *(arrows)*. In this case, the ST segment deviation indicates an inferior-posterior myocardial infarct.

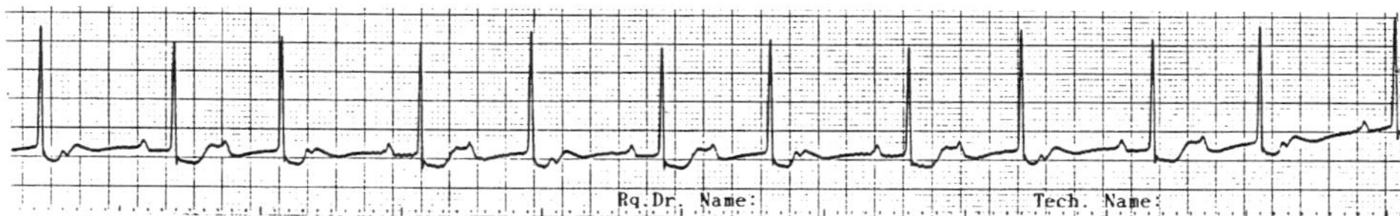

Figure 9.27 ST segment depression caused by the effect of digitalis. There is also a Wenckebach AV nodal block. Note that every third P wave is not conducted to the ventricles. This kind of block is a common manifestation of digitalis toxicity. The ST segment depression, on the other hand, merely indicates the digitalis *effect*, not toxicity.

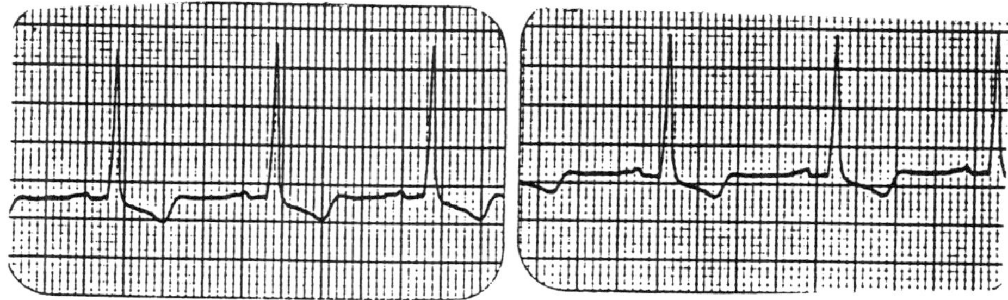

Figure 9.28 Typical S-T-T deformity produced by ventricular hypertrophy. The S-T segment is depressed with a long downslope and a quick return to baseline-a "hockeystick" configuration. The T wave is asymmetrically inverted, in comparison to the symmetrical T wave inversion of coronary disease. This is often called a "strain" pattern, even though there's no such thing as "strain" of heart muscle. It really means hypertrophy.

SUMMARY AND CONCLUSIONS

The diagnosis of heart disease is often a matter of a few simple observations that any competent physician can make right in the office or the emergency room. Life-and-death diagnoses are possible without elaborate machines or techniques. A careful history and physical examination will provide at least 95% of the information needed for any cardiac diagnosis. Don't be afraid to use them!

Chapter 10

Thyroid Disease

James R. Hurley

INTRODUCTION

Thyroid diseases can be divided into functional disorders, in which the thyroid produces too much or too little thyroid hormone, and anatomic disorders, in which the thyroid is enlarged or nodular. Most functional thyroid disease is caused by a disorder of the immune system. In Graves' disease, the most common cause of hyperthyroidism, an autoantibody binds to and stimulates thyroid-stimulating hormone (TSH) receptors, leading to overproduction of thyroid hormones. In Hashimoto's thyroiditis, the most common cause of hypothyroidism, the thyroid is infiltrated by lymphocytes, some of which produce antithyroid antibodies, while others release substances which damage thyroid cells. Both conditions are familial and may be associated with each other and with other organ-specific autoimmune diseases (Table 10.1). Both are significantly more common in women, with a 4:1 female:male ratio. It has been estimated that 5.5% of women over age 15 have functional thyroid disease severe enough to require treatment. Subclinical hypothyroidism (defined as an elevated TSH in the absence of symptoms) is present in 10% of women by age 50 and in 16.9% by age 60, while postpartum thyroid dysfunction occurs after 5–10% of deliveries.

Thyroid enlargement, or goiter, is often present in patients with Graves' disease and Hashimoto's thyroiditis but may also occur in patients with normal thyroid function. The most common cause worldwide is iodine deficiency, which is rare in the United States. In predisposed populations, thyroid enlargement is often first noted during or following pregnancy, which places additional stress on the gland. Thyroid nodules are discrete areas of differing consistency within the thyroid gland. They are common in patients with thyroid enlargement, and in this instance are usually multiple and benign. Solitary thyroid nodules in otherwise normal thyroid glands are often neoplasms. About 20% of thyroid neoplasms are malignant. Four percent of the population have palpable thyroid nodules, the majority occurring in women; thyroid cancer causes about 1.6% of all cancers in women.

TABLE 10.1 Organ-Specific Autoimmune Diseases

Hashimoto's thyroiditis
Graves' disease
Diabetes mellitus, type I
Addison's disease, idiopathic
Premature ovarian failure
Hypoparathyroidism, idiopathic
Pernicious anemia
Vitiligo
Alopecia areata
Myasthenia gravis
Idiopathic throbomcytopenic purpura

THYROID FUNCTION TESTING

Thyroid function testing can be either complex or simple, depending on one's approach. The complexity arises from the following factors:

1. The thyroid produces two hormones: thyroxine (T_4) which contains four iodine atoms, and triiodothyronine (T_3), which contains three. Under normal circumstances, about 95% of the hormone secreted is T_4. The circulating thyroid hormones are tightly bound to carrier proteins, so that only 0.03% of T_4 and 0.3% of T_3 are free to diffuse into the cells. The large amount of bound T_4 acts as a reservoir which stabilizes the level of free T_4. The standard tests for T_4 and T_3 measure the total hormone levels, which correlate with free hormone levels only if thyroid hormone binding is normal.
2. There are many situations in which thyroid hormone binding is not normal (Tables 10.2 and 10.3). Normal patients with high thyroid-binding capacity often have serum T_4 and T_3 levels which are above normal, while those with low binding capacity often have T_4 and T_3 levels which are below normal.
3. Free T_4 and T_3 can be accurately measured by direct dialysis or equilibrium dialysis, but these assays are time-consuming and expensive. For many years, free T_4 has been estimated by calculating a free T_4 index (FT_4I) from the total T_4 and an estimate of T_4 binding capacity such as the T_3 uptake test. In most instances, the FT_4I correlates very well with directly measured free T_4. However, the index is often inaccurate when T_4 binding is very abnormal. More recently, new assays for free T_4 have been introduced which use immunoassay techniques. Despite the name, these are also indirect measurements of free T_4, and many have significant technical problems. For routine evaluation, they are more expensive and less accurate than the old FT_4I.
4. The normal ranges for T_4, T_3, and the free hormone indices are population based and include 95% of the normal population. However, a result within the normal range is not necessarily normal for an individual patient.

In conclusion, abnormal levels of T_4 and T_3 do not necessarily indicate abnormal thyroid function, nor do normal levels eliminate the possibility of hyper- of hypothyroidism. The simplest and most accurate initial thyroid function test is the measurement of TSH (Figure 10.1). With currently available high-sensitivity assays, a TSH

TABLE 10.2 Causes of Increased Thyroid-Binding Capacity

High estrogen levels
- Pregnancy, postpartum and neonatal period
- Oral contraceptives
- Replacement estrogen
- Estrogen-secreting tumors (adrenal, ovary)

Drugs
- Heroin and methadone
- 5-Fluorouracil
- Clofibrate
- Perphenazine

Disease
- Hepatitis
- Chronic biliary cirrhosis
- Acute intermittent porphyria

Inherited abnormalities of thyroid-binding proteins
- Increased thyroid-binding globulin (TBG)
- Familial dysalbuminemic hyperthyroxinemia

within the normal range rules out hyperthyroidism of any cause and hypothyroidism due to thyroid gland failure, which is the cause of 95% of all hypothyroidism.

A TSH below the limit of detectability is consistent with hyperthyroidism. The diagnosis is confirmed if the estimated free T_4 (FT_4E) by any technique is elevated. If the FT_4E is normal, an FT_3E should be obtained since an occasional patient with hyperthyroidism may have elevation of T_3 alone (T_3 toxicosis). Patients with suppressed TSH and normal FT_4E and FT_3E may have very mild hyperthyroidism, TSH suppression due to medication use, the "sick euthyroid syndrome," or pituitary and/or hypothalamic disease (Table 10.4).

A TSH above the upper limit of normal is consistent with hypothyroidism due to thyroid gland failure. A low FT_4E confirms the diagnosis. Since hypothyroidism often develops slowly, it is common for the FT_4E to remain within the normal range and for patients to remain asymptomatic for prolonged periods after TSH becomes elevated.

TABLE 10.3 Causes of Decreased Thyroid-Binding Capacity

Drugs
- Androgens or anabolic steroids
- Glucocorticoids

Disease
- Major systemic illness
- Protein/calorie malnutrition
- Nephrotic syndrome
- Advanced cirrhosis

Inherited abnormalities
- Decreased thyroid-binding globulin

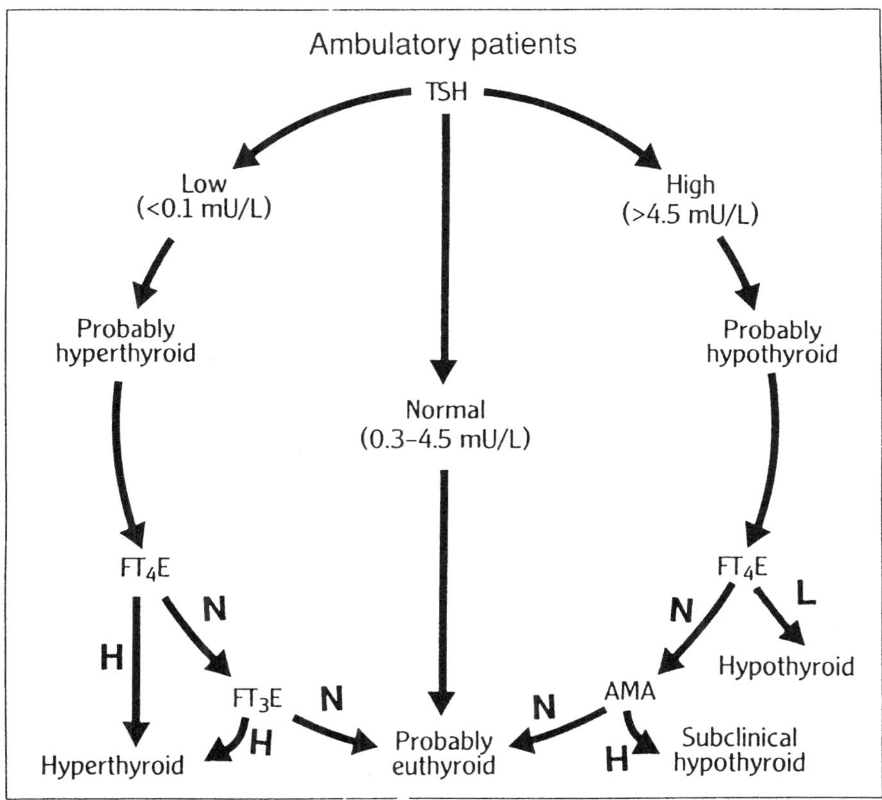

Figure 10.1 Diagnostic scheme for using the sensitive TSH assay as the initial thyroid function test in ambulatory patients. FT_4E = estimated free T_4; FT_3E = estimated free T_3; AMA = antimicrosomal antibodies (same as anti-TPO antibodies); L = low value; H = high value; N = value within the normal range. (Reprinted from *Clinical Chemistry News* 1989;15(12) with permission.)

TABLE 10.4 Causes of Suppressed TSH with Normal or Low T_4 and T_3

With Normal T_4 and T_3
- Subclinical hyperthyroidism
  - Graves' disease (mild or early)
  - Toxic nodule or toxic nodular goiter
  - High hCG in early pregnancy
  - Excessive T_4 replacement
  - Following an iodine load (transient)
- Drug-induced TSH suppression
  - Glucocorticoids
  - Dopamine

With Low T_4 and T_3
- Failure to secrete TSH (central hypothyroidism)
- Severe systemic illness (sick euthyroid syndrome)

This state is known as *subclinical hypothyroidism*. For patients with an elevated TSH and normal FT_4E, determination of antimicrosomal antibodies (AMA)—also known as *antibodies to thyroid peroxidase (TPO)*—may be helpful, since their presence indicates Hashimoto's thyroiditis, the major cause of thyroid gland failure.

Thyroid Function Testing During Pregnancy

The physiologic changes of pregnancy affect thyroid function tests in two ways:

1. Increased estrogen levels lead to increased production of thyroid-binding globulin (TBG) by the liver, which causes an increase in protein-bound thyroid hormones. T_4 and T_3 are often elevated during pregnancy, but the free hormone levels and free hormone indices remain within normal limits.
2. Human chorionic gonadotropin (hCG) has a weak stimulatory effect on the TSH receptors. Pregnant women with high levels of hCG may become hyperthyroid, with low and occasionally undetectable TSH during the first trimester.

HYPERTHYROIDISM

Clinical Presentation

Once hyperthyroidism is suspected, confirmation by laboratory testing is rapid and reliable. Since few patients present with a textbook list of symptoms, the physician's challenge is to suspect the diagnosis on the basis of a few clues which may be related to virtually any organ system. Hyperthyroidism causes a speeding up of body processes. The heart beats faster, causing palpitations; more oxygen is required, causing shortness of breath; intestinal motility is increased, causing frequent bowel movements; and thought processes are speeded up, causing decreased concentration, poor memory, irritability, and insomnia. Metabolism becomes inefficient, with less useful energy extracted for each calorie burned. Since hyperthyroidism is an excellent appetite stimulant, healthy individuals may gain weight in the early stages. Older individuals and those with more severe hyperthyroidism tend to lose weight and may become anorexic. Unused energy is released as heat. Previously cold-intolerant individuals may become normal, and normal individuals may become heat intolerant. Increased perspiration is common.

Thyroid hormone also sensitizes the body to adrenalin, which results in a rapid, strong heartbeat, increased irritability, and increased anxiety. Patients overreact to normal stress with emotional lability (mood swings), frequent tearful episodes, and depression. Other symptoms include decreased physical strength and stamina, increased fatigue, shorter and lighter menstrual periods, and infertility. Younger individuals tend to manifest the "activated" form, dominated by anxiety, palpitations, and tremors, while older individuals tend to manifest the "apathetic" form, with decreased appetite, significant weight loss, and profound muscular weakness. The latter are often suspected of having a malignancy. Hyperthyroid patients may also consult their physician for a lump in the neck due to an enlarged thyroid or eye symptoms, including bulging, pain, itching, redness, tearing, and double vision.

On physical examination, typical signs of hyperthyroidism include restlessness, tremor, prominent eyes, thyroid enlargement, warm moist skin, rapid pulse, wide pulse pressure, and a rapid return of the ankle reflex. Nonspecific laboratory abnormalities may include a low-normal white blood cell count with a relative lymphocytosis and a low cholesterol level. Elevated calcium, alkaline phosphatase, and liver enzymes may occur in severe or long-standing disease. If hyperthyroidism is suspected, the best confirmatory symptoms are heat intolerance and an increased appetite coupled with either stable or declining weight. All patients presenting with palpitations, unexplained weight loss, anxiety, mood swings, depression, and infertility should be evaluated for hyperthyroidism.

Thyroid storm is an extremely rare, life-threatening complication of hyperthyroidism. It usually occurs in patients with uncontrolled or inadequately controlled hyperthyroidism when they are subjected to additional metabolic stress such as surgery or a serious infection. The cardinal manifestation is mental obtundation, which is often associated with high fever and rapid tachycardia. Heart, liver, and kidney failure may develop. Most patients are severely dehydrated. Prompt recognition, diagnosis, and treatment are necessary to avoid a fatal outcome.

Varieties of Hyperthyroidism

There are two major types of hyperthyroidism: *active* hyperthyroidism, in which the thyroid is stimulated to synthesize and secrete thyroid hormones, and *destructive* hyperthyroidism, in which thyroid damage causes release of stored thyroid hormone but no new hormone is synthesized. Active hyperthyroidism requires specific treatment, while destructive hyperthyroidism resolves spontaneously when the supply of stored hormone in the gland is exhausted. This usually requires 2 to 3 months and is often followed by a transient episode of hypothyroidism before full recovery. Hyperthyroidism can also be caused by ingestion of excessive thyroid hormone. Active hyperthyroidism is characterized by elevated or occasionally normal radioiodine uptake despite a suppressed TSH, while radioiodine uptake in the other two types is very low.

Active Hyperthyroid States

Graves' Disease Graves' disease is the most common type of hyperthyroidism. It is caused by antibodies which bind to and stimulate TSH receptors (TSAb). The thyroid is usually diffusely enlarged but is occasionally normal in size or asymmetric. Radioiodine uptake is elevated or occasionally normal, and the scan shows a uniform distribution of radioiodine. If incidental thyroid nodules are present, they usually do not collect radioiodine. From 10% to 20% of patients with Graves' disease also have or develop a specific eye condition known as *ophthalmopathy,* in which the extraocular muscles and orbital fat are attacked by the immune system. About 1% have thickening of the skin in the anterior tibial region known as *pretibial myxedema* or *infiltrative dermopathy,* which also appears to be autoimmune.

Autonomously Functioning Thyroid Nodules (Toxic Nodules) These are benign neoplasms which produce thyroid hormone in the absence of TSH. There is usually a single palpable thyroid nodule. Radioiodine uptake is elevated or normal, and on the scan virtually all of the radioiodine is concentrated in the palpable nodule. The normal thyroid tissue is not visualized because TSH is suppressed.

Toxic Multinodular Goiter Many large goiters develop the ability to produce thyroid hormone in the absence of TSH (autonomy), which may cause hyperthyroidism in older patients or in young patients with very large glands. The hyperthyroidism is usually milder than that seen in Graves' disease. Radioiodine uptake is often within normal limits. The scan usually shows an irregular distribution of radioiodine, with palpable nodules either hot or cold.

Unusual Causes of Active Hyperthyroidism hCG has a weak stimulatory effect on TSH receptors. High levels can cause transient hyperthyroidism in the early stages of pregnancy. This condition is more common in women with multiple fetuses. Very high levels in molar pregnancy or choriocarcinoma can cause acute severe hyperthyroidism. Very rarely, inappropriate TSH secretion occurs due to malfunction of the hypothalamus or a pituitary tumor. In patients with hyperthyroidism due to either hCG or inappropriate TSH secretion, the uptake and scan findings are similar to those seen in Graves' disease.

Destructive Hyperthyroidism (Thyroiditis)

Subacute Thyroiditis Subacute thyroiditis is thought to be due to a viral inflammation of the gland. Pathologically, the gland shows giant cells and granulomas. There is significant thyroid pain, usually aggravated by swallowing and often radiating to the ears, associated with prominent systemic symptoms of fever, fatigue, and malaise, which often dominate the clinical picture. On palpation the thyroid is very firm and exquisitely tender. Only one lobe may be involved initially. T_4 and T_3 may be within normal limits, but TSH is invariably suppressed and the radioiodine uptake is zero. The sedimentation rate is markedly elevated. In mild cases the pain can be relieved by nonsteroidal anti-inflammatory drugs. For more severe cases, a short course of prednisone, initial dose 30 mg/day, will result in complete resolution of all symptoms within 24 h.

Silent Thyroiditis Silent thyroiditis has an autoimmune etiology. Pathologically, the gland is infiltrated with lymphocytes. There are no systemic symptoms, and hyperthyroid symptoms are often minimal. The thyroid may be only slightly enlarged and is not tender. T_4 and T_3 are often normal. Radioiodine uptake is zero, and the sedimentation rate is normal. Antibodies to TG and TPO are usually detectable. Patients with silent thyroiditis are rarely symptomatic enough to require treatment. Since this is an autoimmune thyroid disease, there is an increased risk of repeat episodes and of developing Graves' disease or Hashimoto's thyroiditis.

Postpartum Thyroiditis Postpartum thyroiditis occurs after 5–10% of deliveries. It is an autoimmune disorder with a clinical course and pathologic findings similar to those of silent thyroiditis. However, only 26% of patients have the classic pattern of hyperthyroidism followed by hypothyroidism. Further, 37% manifest only the hyperthyroid phase and 36% only the hypothyroid phase. The hyperthyroid phase usually occurs within 6 months of delivery and the hypothyroid phase within 1 year. Depression is common during the hypothyroid phase. In women with anti-TPO antibodies detectable in the early stages of pregnancy, 33% will develop postpartum thyroiditis, and women with type 1 diabetes have a threefold increased risk. There is an increased risk of recurrence with subsequent pregnancies. There is also an increased risk of developing Graves' disease or Hashimoto's thyroiditis, often after a subsequent pregnancy.

Hyperthyroidism Due to Medications

Thyroid Hormones The most common cause of TSH suppression in patients with normal thyroid hormone levels is the use of excessive thyroid hormone. Except for some patients with thyroid cancer, individuals receiving thyroid hormone should have the dose adjusted to maintain TSH within the normal range. An occasional patient will secretly take large amounts of thyroid hormone, usually in the hope that this will result in weight loss. If hyperthyroid symptoms result, the condition is known as *thyrotoxicosis factitia.* Radioiodine uptake in these patients is usually low. In patients who are abusing T_3 (Cytomel), serum T_4 may be low or undectable.

Iodine Patients with enlarged, partially autonomous thyroid glands or subclinical Graves' disease may have an acute increase in thyroid hormone levels and develop hyperthyroid symptoms after exposure to large amounts of iodine in radiographic contrast, food supplements containing kelp, Japanese food containing large amounts of seaweed, or amiodarone, an antiarrhythmic agent containing large amounts of iodine. Radioiodine uptake is usually low, and the hyperthyroidism is usually transient.

Treatment of Hyperthyroidism

Available treatments for active hyperthyroidism include antithyroid drugs, surgery, radioiodine, and beta-blocking drugs.

Antithyroid Drugs (ATDs) Treatment with ATDs can control hyperthyroidism in all patients with active disease, but it produces a permanent cure (remission) in only about 25% of those with Graves' disease. Unfortunately, it is not possible to identify the responders in advance. The available ATDs in the United States are propylthiouracil (PTU) and methimazole (MMI, Tapazole). Their mode of action and side effects are similar. Both inhibit the synthesis of new thyroid hormone but not the release of stored thyroid hormone. Blood levels of T_4 and T_3 fall slowly, usually reaching normal after 6 to 8 weeks, at which point the dose of ATD is decreased to maintenance. If one is attempting to obtain a permanent cure, the duration of treatment is usually 6 to 24 months. Reactions to ATDs are common, most often a drug rash. Serious side effects including agranulocytosis, hepatitis, and migratory polyarthralgias occur in 0.2–0.5% of patients. Hypothyroidism eventually develops in about 20% of patients who have a remission due to the late development of Hashimoto's thyroiditis.

Surgery Although it is very effective, thyroidectomy is little used currently in the treatment of hyperthyroidism due to a general desire to avoid surgery and the availability of acceptable alternative treatments. The major current indications for surgery are very large thyroid glands which are often difficult to control with radioactive iodine and recurrent hyperthyroidism after treatment with ATDs in patients who choose not to be treated with radioiodine. The incidence of recurrent hyperthyroidism and permanent hypothyroidism varies with the amount of thyroid tissue remaining. The risks of permanent hypoparathyroidism and recurrent laryngeal nerve paralysis vary with the experience and skill of the surgeon.

Radioiodine Approximately 90% of hyperthyroid patients in the United States are treated with radioiodine. Radioiodine is popular because it is simple, effective, and allows the patient to avoid surgery. The only known side effect is permanent hypothyroidism, which is rare in patients with toxic nodules and toxic nodular goiter but common in patients with Graves' disease. The risks of early hypothyroidism (within 1 year of treatment) and persistent hyperthyroidism are related to the amount of radioiodine administered. The full effect is usually apparent within 3 months. During this period, TSH often remains completely suppressed and T_4 is a better indicator or early hypothyroidism. Patients with normal thyroid function 1 year after treatment develop late hypothyroidism at a rate of 2.5% per year and should be followed with annual TSH determinations.

Radioiodine has been used to treat hyperthyroidism since 1942 and extensively since the 1950s. Because the thyroid is the only part of the body which retains radioiodine, it is possible to deliver a large radiation dose to the thyroid with a very small dose to the rest of the body. The radiation dose to the ovaries for an average hyperthyroid patient is approximately 1 to 2 rad, equivalent to the radiation dose from a diagnostic x-ray procedure such as a barium enema or GI series. Initial concerns that radioiodine might cause thyroid or other malignancies or result in congenital malformations or genetic defects have not been substantiated.

Treatment Decisions In reaching a decision regarding treatment, patients should be informed about the available methods, as well as the risks and benefits. Radioiodine is generally recommended for most patients. Pregnancy should be delayed for 6 months after radioiodine treatment. Women in their late 30s or early 40s who wish to become pregnant in the near future should seriously consider thyroidectomy if a skilled surgeon is available since this is the most rapid way to eliminate hyperthyroidism. Radioiodine is the second choice. For women who do not wish to become pregnant within 2 to 3 years, either ATD or radioiodine treatment is acceptable. Those who relapse after a course of ATD should be encouraged to accept radioiodine or thyroidectomy since the chance of achieving a permanent cure after a second course of ATD is only about 10%.

Ancillary Treatment Patients with palpitations, tremors, and anxiety often benefit from treatment with beta blockers which do not interfere with diagnostic evaluation or treatment. These drugs can be discontinued once blood thyroid hormone levels have normalized from specific treatment. In patients with a history of asthma or other lung disease, beta blockers must be used with extreme caution. Very agitated patients may benefit from mild tranquilizers and depressed patients from antidepressive agents. Hyperthyroid patients metabolize all drugs more rapidly than normal, and higher doses may be required. However, it is important to reduce the dose as they become euthyroid.

Hyperthyroidism During Pregnancy

Hyperthyroidism should be suspected if a pregnant woman fails to gain weight normally or develops hyperemesis. Many typical symptoms of hyperthyroidism can be present during normal pregnancy, including fatigue, heat intolerance, increased perspiration, palpitations, shortness of breath, poor stamina, and irritability. However, if these conditions are exaggerated or persistent, an evaluation is warranted.

Mild hyperthyroidism during pregnancy does not require specific treatment. If it is due to high levels of hCG, it will resolve as the hCG level falls. If it is due to Graves' disease, it often improves without specific treatment since levels of TSAb commonly decrease as pregnancy progresses. However, severe hyperthyroidism can result in congestive heart failure or thyroid storm associated with the stress of delivery or severe intercurrent infection. If there are significant symptoms and/or marked elevation of the free hormone indices, treatment with an ATD is indicated. PTU is preferred because of reports of aplasia cutis in children of women treated with MMI during pregnancy. ATDs cross the placenta and can cause in utero hypothyroidism. Therefore, the lowest possible dose should be used, aiming to maintain the free hormone indices just above the upper limit of normal. TSH should remain within the lower limits of normal. Thyroid hormones do not cross the placenta and should not be used in the management of hyperthyroidism during pregnancy. In women with hyperthyroidism due to high levels of hCG, ATDs can usually be discontinued during the second trimester; in those with Graves' disease, they can often be discontinued during the third trimester. If hyperthyroidism is severe and cannot be controlled with ATD, thyroidectomy can be performed during the second trimester. Radioiodine is always contraindicated during pregnancy.

Women with Graves' disease and very high levels of TSAb may transfer enough TSAb across the placenta to affect the fetal thyroid. If the mother requires treatment with ATD during pregnancy, the medication will also cross the placenta and prevent fetal hyperthyroidism. However, because TSAb may persist for months, children born to women with high levels of TSAb may develop neonatal hyperthyroidism manifested by failure to thrive, weight loss, tachycardia, and congestive heart failure. If the mother was treated in the past with radioiodine or surgery and is not taking ATD during pregnancy, in utero hyperthyroidism may develop during the third trimester, with tachycardia and failure of growth. Ultrasound may show a goiter. In utero hyperthyroidism can be treated by giving ATD to the mother. These infants are also at risk for neonatal hyperthyroidism.

HYPOTHYROIDISM

Clinical Presentation

Hypothyroidism causes a general slowing of body processes and usually develops gradually over a period of years. In the early stages there are few or no symptoms. When they do develop, the most common symptom is fatigue. There is an increased need for sleep, and patients may fall asleep at inappropriate times. Fewer calories are burned and less heat is produced, resulting in increased sensitivity to cold and a preference for warm environments. The intestines work more slowly than normal, often leading to constipation. Thought processes are also slower, which may cause frustration and increased irritability. Depression is common, and social activity is often restricted. Menstrual periods tend to be heavier and longer than normal, and fertility is diminished. In the late stages, an increase in mucopolysaccharides causes salt and water retention, as well as nonpitting swelling of the face, hands and feet known as *myxedema*. If untreated, hypothyroidism can proceed to coma, usually precipitated by a stressful event such as an acute infection and often associated with hypothermia, carbon dioxide retention, and a low blood sugar level.

A history of prior treatment with radioiodine or surgery should trigger a search for signs and symptoms of hypothyroidism. If hypothyroidism is suspected, the presence of new cold intolerance or new constipation are helpful confirmatory symptoms. On physical examination a goiter suggests Hashimoto's thyroiditis, the most common cause of hypothyroidism. A neck scar may indicate prior thyroid surgery. In patients with mild hypothyroidism, the physical examination may be otherwise normal. In severe hypothyroidism, the pulse and respiration are often slow due to the decreased demand for oxygen. The pulse pressure is narrow. Hair tends to be dry and brittle; the skin is dry and may be rough around the knuckles and elbows. It may also have a yellowish color due to retained carotene. Nonspecific laboratory abnormalities in severe hypothyroidism include mild normocytic anemia, elevated cholesterol, and elevated creatine phosphokinase. Some patients develop inappropriate antidiuretic hormone secretion, resulting in a low serum sodium level.

Causes of Hypothyroidism

Primary Hypothyroidism (Thyroid Gland Failure) Ninety-five percent of hypothyroidism is due to thyroid gland failure. The most common cause is Hashimoto's thyroiditis. Primary hypothyroidism can also be caused by radioiodine treatment or thyroid surgery. Patients with subclinical Hashimoto's thyroiditis and those who remain normal after treatment for Graves' disease with radioiodine or surgery may develop hypothyroidism after exposure to a number of drugs including iodine, lithium, and amiodarone.

Central Hypothyroidism About 5% of hypothyroidism is caused by inability of the pituitary to secrete TSH (secondary hypothyroidism) or failure of the hypothalamus to secrete thyrotropin-releasing hormone (tertiary hypothyroidism). Most patients with central hypothyroidism have other signs and symptoms of hypothalamic and/or pituitary dysfunction such as amenorrhea. The laboratory diagnosis of central hypothyroidism is difficult. It should be suspected when both FT_4I and TSH are low, although similar findings occur in the "sick euthyroid syndrome" and in patients taking T_3 (Cytomel).

Treatment of Hypothyroidism

Patients with a TSH over 10 μU/mL should be treated with enough thyroid hormone to normalize the TSH. The preparation of choice is T_4 (Synthroid, Levoxyl, Levothroid; generic name: levothyroxine). Due to differences in bioavailability, it is preferable to keep patients on the same branded preparation and to recheck thyroid function tests if a change is made. The average full replacement dose for an individual with no thyroid function is 100–150 μg (0.1–0.15 mg) daily. It tends to be higher in patients with larger lean body mass and decreases gradually with increasing age.

Because T_4 binds tightly to plasma proteins, it has a prolonged duration of action and can be given once a day. Administration of T_3 or preparations containing T_3, such as desiccated thyroid, results in widely fluctuating T_3 levels which are often above normal, resulting in transient hyperthyroidism.

The usual starting dose of T_4 in a patient with mild hypothyroidism and detectable serum T_4 is one-half of the anticipated full replacement dose, or 50–75 μg (0.5–0.075 mg) daily. After 4 weeks this can be doubled to the estimated full replacement dose. Because T_4 is metabolized slowly, the final adjustment should be made after an equilibration period of at least 2 months. In patients with significant symptoms and unmeasurable T_4 and in those with significant cardiac disease, the usual starting dose is 25 μg (0.025 mg) daily, with the dose slowly increased at 4-week intervals until the TSH is normalized. In patients with stable treated hypothyroidism, it is usually sufficient to check the TSH on an annual basis.

Patients with normal serum T_4 and a TSH between the upper limit of normal and 10 μU/mL are usually asymptomatic. The majority have Hashimoto's thyroiditis and eventually develop symptomatic hypothyroidism, while a few represent the tail of the normal distribution curve for TSH and remain euthyroid. These two groups can be separated by determining their levels of anti-TPO antibodies. Those with detectable antibodies have Hashimoto's thyroiditis and are much more likely to develop symptomatic hypothyroidism than those with slightly elevated TSH alone. Patients with slight TSH elevation and symptoms compatible with hypothyroidism should be placed on T_4. However, controversy exists regarding the treatment of asymptomatic patients with TSH between 5 and 10 μU/mL. Some thyroid specialists advocate treating all such patients, while others adopt a more flexible approach. Patients who are not treated should have their TSH determined on an annual basis.

Hypothyroidism and Pregnancy

Hypothyroidism should be suspected in a pregnant woman with a goiter or a history of treatment for hypo- or hyperthyroidism. Typical symptoms of hypothyroidism, such as fatigue and weight gain, occur in almost all pregnant women, but cold intolerance is suspicious for hypothyroidism. Pregnant women with any degree of TSH elevation should be treated with sufficient T_4 to normalize the TSH.

Due to the increased demand for thyroid hormone during pregnancy, most women on thyroid hormone replacement need an increase in their dose. TSH should be checked at 8 weeks of gestation and then every 2 months until delivery. Decisions should be based solely on the TSH level since total T_4 is often elevated above the non-pregnant normal range due to estrogen-induced elevation of thyroid-binding globulin.

Goiter and Nodules

An enlarged thyroid gland or thyroid nodule is most easily detected by watching the patient swallow with the neck slightly hyperextended. A thyroid sonogram is the best test to confirm the presence of a nodule or an enlarged thyroid.

Goiter Patients with diffuse thyroid enlargement may have Graves' disease or Hashimoto's thyroiditis and should have their TSH and antibodies to TPO determined. Those with normal TSH levels and no detectable antibodies most likely have simple goiter. As long as the goiter remains small and asymptomatic, no treatment is required. If the gland enlarges, suppression of TSH into the low normal range by administration of T_4 may prevent further enlargement.

Thyroid Nodules The challenge with thyroid nodules is to detect the minority which are malignant and to avoid surgery for the majority which are benign. Unfortunately, there is no single test or combination of tests which can reliably make this distinction. The best currently available method is cytologic examination of cells from the nodule obtained by fine needle aspiration (FNA). This is 95% accurate in papillary cancer, the most common form of thyroid cancer, and 99% accurate in benign nodules due to nodular goiter. However, 20% of nodules show a microfollicular pattern. About 20% of these are follicular cancers, while 80% are benign follicular adenomas.

The history and physical examination can serve as a rough guide in selecting patients for FNA (Tables 10.5 and 10.6). In the course of this evaluation, it is important to keep in mind that thyroid cancer can coexist with benign thyroid disease. An abnormal TSH level usually indicates a benign etiology. An elevated TSH level is compatible with Hashimoto's thyroiditis, in which firm swelling of the lower thyroid lobes may be appreciated as a nodule. A suppressed TSH level is compatible with an autonomously functioning nodule, and these are always benign.

Thyroid sonography can help to evaluate the risk of malignancy and can also serve as a guide for FNA of very small or partially cystic nodules. Solid nodules which have increased flow on Doppler ultrasound are usually neoplasms. Pure cysts are usually benign, but complex (partially cystic and partially solid) nodules are solid nodules which have undergone hemorrhagic degeneration and have an intermediate risk. Sono-

TABLE 10.5 Factors Suggestive of an Increased Risk of Malignancy

History
Previous radiation treatment to the head/neck region
Family history of thyroid cancer
Symptoms
Rapid recent increase in size of thyroid
Recent onset of hoarseness
Physical exam
Solitary nodule (rest of thyroid normal)
Hard, irregular nodule
Nodule fixed to underlying structures
Enlargement of adjacent cervical lymph nodes
Sonography
Solitary vascular nodule (rest of gland normal)
Fine, stippled calcification in nodule
Scanning
Nonfunctioning nodule (cold nodule)

TABLE 10.6 Factors Suggestive of a Decreased Risk of Malignancy

History
Family history of benign thyroid disease
Long duration of nodule
Early childhood spent in an iodine-deficient region
Physical exam
Enlarged thyroid
Multiple nodules
Nodule smooth, soft, and mobile
Lab
Suppressed or elevated TSH
High titers of antithyroid antibodies
Sonography
Enlarged thyroid
Diffusely abnormal echotexture
Multiple nodules with low vascularity
Purely cystic nodule
Scan
Nodule contains all the radioiodine (hot nodule)

graphic findings suggestive of benign nodular goiter include an enlarged thyroid gland, diffusely abnormal echotexture, and multiple nodules with low or no flow.

If an FNA suggests papillary thyroid cancer, surgery is indicated. If it is compatible with nodular goiter, the nodule can be observed or the patient can be placed on T_4 to suppress TSH in an attempt to prevent further enlargement. As long as the nodule does not enlarge, surgery can be avoided. Nodules with a microfollicular pattern should be further evaluated by radioiodine scanning. Those which collect more radioiodine than the remaining thyroid (hot nodules) are almost always benign. Patients with microfollicular nodules which are nonfunctional (cold) on scan can be placed on T_4 to suppress TSH, and the size of the nodule can be followed by ultrasound. If the nodules do not decrease significantly within 6 months, they should be surgically removed.

Goiter and Nodules During Pregnancy Thyroid enlargement occurring during pregnancy may be physiologic due to an increased demand for thyroid hormone or secondary to Hashimoto's thyroiditis or Graves' disease. If thyroid function tests reveal hyper- or hypothyroidism, appropriate treatment should be given. If they are normal, the gland can be observed. If there is progressive enlargement, T_4 can be cautiously administered to suppress TSH into the low normal range.

Thyroid nodules occurring during pregnancy can be investigated with thyroid function tests and thyroid sonography. Radioiodine scanning should not be used during pregnancy. Nodules suspicious for malignancy can be evaluated by FNA, with surgery performed in the second trimester if thyroid cancer is detected. Alternatively, T_4 can be administered cautiously to suppress TSH into the low normal range and the size of the nodule followed. Further evaluation can be delayed until after delivery as long as the nodule remains stable.

BIBLIOGRAPHY

Becker DV: Choice of therapy for Graves' hyperthyroidism. *N Engl J Med* 311:464–466, 1984.

Becks GP, Burrow GN: Thyroid disease and pregnancy. *Med Clin North Am* 75:121–150, 1991.

Borst GC, Eil C, Burman KD: Euthyroid hyperthyroxinemia. *Ann Intern Med* 98:366–378, 1983.

Burch HB, Wartofsky L: Life-threatening thyrotoxicosis: Thyroid storm. *Endocrinol Metab Clin North Am* 22:263–277, 1993.

Cavalieri RR: The effects of nonthyroid disease and drugs on thyroid function tests. *Med Clin North Am* 75:27–39, 1991.

Cooper DS: Antithyroid drugs. *N Engl J Med* 311:1353–1362, 1984.

Cooper DS, Ridgway EC: Clinical management of patients with hyperthyroidism. *Med Clin North Am* 69:953–971, 1985.

Fisher DA: Neonatal thyroid disease in the offspring of women with autoimmune thyroid disease. *Thyroid Today* 9(4):1–7, 1986.

Glinoer D, De Nayer P, Bourdoux P, et al: Regulation of maternal thyroid during pregnancy. *J Clin Endocrinol Metab* 71:276–287, 1990.

Glinoer D, Riahi M, Grun JP, et al: Risk of subclinical hypothyroidism in pregnant women with asymptomatic autoimmune thyroid disorders. *J Clin Endocrinol Metab* 79:197–204, 1994.

Glinoer D: The thyroid in pregnancy: A European perspective. *Thyroid Today* 18(2):1–11, 1995.

Greenspan FS: The problem of the nodular goiter. *Med Clin North Am* 75:195–209, 1991.

Mandel SJ, Larsen PR, Seely EW, et al: Increased need for thyroxine during pregnancy in women with primary hypothyroidism. *N Engl J Med* 323:91–96, 1990.

Mazzaferri EL: Management of a solitary thyroid nodule. *N Engl J Med* 328:553–559, 1993.

McDougall IR: Graves' disease: Current concepts. *Med Clin North Am* 75:79–95, 1991.

Nicoloff JT, LoPresti JS: Myxedema coma: A form of decompensated hypothyroidism. *Endocrinol Metab Clin North Am* 22:279–291, 1993.

Oppenheimer JH, Braverman LE, Toft A, et al: A therapeutic controversy. Thyroid hormone treatment: When and what? *J Clin Endocrinol Metab* 80:2873–2883, 1995.

Peterson CM: Thyroid disease and fertility. *Immunol Allergy Clin North Am* 14:725–738, 1994.

Robertson JS, Gorman CA: Gonadal radiation dose and its genetic significance in radioiodine therapy of hyperthyroidism. *J Nucl Med* 17:826–835, 1976.

Roti E, Minelli R, Gardini E, et al: The use and misuse of thyroid hormone. *Endocrinol Rev* 14:401–423, 1993.

Sawin CT: Hypothyroidism. *Med Clin North Am* 69:989–1004, 1985.

Singer PA: Thyroiditis: Acute, subacute, and chronic. *Med Clin North Am* 75:61–77, 1991.

Spencer CA, Nicoloff JT: Serum TSH measurement: A 1990 status report. *Thyroid Today* 13(4):1–12, 1990.

Stagnaro-Green A: Postpartum thyroiditis: Prevalence, etiology and clinical implications. *Thyroid Today* 16(4):1–11, 1993.

Studer H: Pathogenesis of goiter: A unifying hypothesis. *Thyroid Today* 7(4):1–7, 1984.

Surks MI, Chopra IJ, Mariash CN, et al: American Thyroid Association guidelines for use of laboratory tests in thyroid disorders. *JAMA* 263:1529–1532, 1990.

Chapter 11

Common Neurologic Disorders

Nancy Nealon

MIGRAINE HEADACHE

Migraine headaches are the most frequent neurologic problem seen in an outpatient obstetric-gynecologic practice. A recent prevalence study reported that 25% of women and 8% of men had a lifetime history of migraine. For women the frequency of headache is highest during the reproductive years, between the ages of 25 and 45. There is a definite genetic predisposition, with an increased incidence in family members. Women are affected five times as frequently as men in the childbearing years.

Migraine is a syndrome that consists most frequently of a unilateral headache, often associated with nausea. There are both classic and common migraines. In classic migraine, the patient has a focal neurologic symptom that precedes the onset of the headache. The most common symptoms are visual and the most common visual ones are hemianopsias or scintillating scotomas, shimmering lights in a geometric pattern that move across the visual field in 20 to 30 min and are characteristic of migraine.

The focal deficit, however, may be any neurologic symptom. It could be aphasia, weakness, or numbness.

The focal deficit usually lasts for 30–40 min and is followed by the headache. In classic migraine the headache itself may not be as intense as it is in common migraine.

In common migraine the patient develops a gradually worsening headache that is usually unilateral and makes it difficult to concentrate and function. In both types of migraine, individual patients describe an aura, or prodrome, that warns them of the incipient headache. They may develop yawning, poor sleep patterns, or difficulty concentrating prior to the headache.

The headache itself usually lasts for 4 to 72 h.

Migraine was long been considered a vascular headache because the focal deficits resembled those of a stroke in a young person. Blood flow studies now show that there is diffuse vascular reactivity in both classic and common migraine. There is evidence to support dysfunction of the trigeminal neurovascular brainstem connections. The neurotransmitter involved in this system is serotonin. The best support for the serotonin hypothesis of migraine has been sumatriptan or Imitrex.

Since 67% of patients with migraine respond to sumatriptan in 20 min after a subcutaneous injection, serotonin must have something to do with the etiology or continuation of migraine, since sumatriptan contains only an agonist for the second receptor for serotonin; it contains no other analgesic.

For many women, the frequency of migraine fluctuates with hormonal changes. The headaches tend to begin at menarche and occur more frequently during estrogen and progesterone fluctuations. They therefore tend to occur around the time of menstrual periods. In women with hormonally related migraine, they tend to decrease during the second and third trimesters of pregnancy when the hormonal levels are high and constant. If these women breast-feed, the migraines may not return until they stop and again recycle.

Some women first experience migraine around the time of menopause, when the hormonal levels are again changing. For some of these women, hormone replacement therapy may decrease their migraines. Estrogen must, however, be given daily and progesterone added or also given daily.

Some women with migraine cannot take oral contraceptives because these seem to increase the frequency and intensity of their migraines.

Migraine is not, however, an absolute contraindication to hormonal manipulation. Very few young women have strokes. Those who do have an increased frequency of migraine, smoking, and use of oral contraceptives. Every case should be judged individually. If the woman has rare common migraine and does not smoke, it is probably safe for her to use oral contraceptives. If she smokes, has hypertension, has a positive anticardiolipin antibody or a strong family history of stroke in young women, she should not take oral contraceptives.

In menopause a woman's greatest risk factor for stroke is not migraine but routine cardiovascular disease. If she has a high cholesterol level or a family history of arteriosclerotic cardiovascular disease, she should probably consider hormone replacement therapy. Estrogen may improve the woman's cardiovascular profile and decrease the risk of cerebral vascular events over time.

Patients with migraines have a normal neurologic exam and computed tomography scans. They may have some nonspecific areas of demyelination on a magnetic resonance image scan which are presumably due to small vessel ischemia. Patients with migraine are either treated prophylactically to decrease the frequency and intensity of their headaches or are treated at the time of the acute attack. Inderol and other beta blockers, the tricyclic antidepressants in lower doses than their antidepressant doses, and the calcium channel blockers are used prophylactically. Sumatriptan or Imitrex is the only specific drug used for the acute attack. Ergots, barbiturates, caffeine, nonsteroidal anti-inflammatories, and aspirin are often helpful. Some of the more commonly used medications include Fiorinal, (butabital, ASA & caffeine) Esgic, Midrin, and Caffergot. Codeine demeral and other nonspecific narcotic analgesics are used for more severe pain. Antiemetics help to control the nausea.

PARKINSON'S DISEASE

Parkinson's disease is a progressive neurodegenerative disorder that usually presents in the fourth to fifth decade. It is caused by a loss of neurons in the substantia nigra and a decrease in striatal dopamine. The three classic features of Parkinson's disease are rigidity, tremor, and bradykinesia, which may vary in severity in the individual patient. In the early stages, patients may present with just a change in facial features or some stiffness or clumsiness of one or both arms, which makes it harder to perform fine motor acts. The gait may change, so that they become stiffer, slower, and stooped. They may suddenly look older. They have a harder time initiating movement.

The other cardinal feature, which may be the predominant one, is tremor. It may be unilateral or bilateral. It is present at rest and is described as pin rolling. The tremor in the dependant hand may be very noticeable as the patient walks. The patient will often try to conceal the tremor by holding the hand, carrying the purse or bag in the arm, or putting it in a pocket. Since the introduction of levodopa therapy, patients are markedly improved. At first, the medication may eliminate all their symptoms. However, over time (usually in 3 to 5 years), most patients require increased doses of medications and do not respond as well. They develop fluctuations in their responses, as well as dyskinesias and dystonias that interfere with the activities of daily living. Dopamine agonists and surgical procedures including nigral transplant, pallidotomy, and subthalamic stimulation have been tried in attempts to improve patient function.

ALZHEIMER'S DISEASE

Alzheimer's disease is another neurologic degenerative disease of unknown etiology. Patients present with a decrease in short-term memory but actually have a global decrease in higher integrative functions. They can become relatively withdrawn, appearing to be quieter and less interactive. They may ask fewer questions on a routine gynecological exam. Their appearance is well preserved at first, as are social graces, and they have no focal neurologic findings.

The etiology of Alzheimer's disease is not known. There are rare familial clusterings in which the gene focus has been identified, but the more common late-onset disease, representing more than 98% of cases, has not been shown to have a specific gene locus.

There is an association, however, with apolipoprotein E (*APOE*, gene; apoeE, protein). *APOE 4* is a susceptibility gene that increases the risk of Alzheimer's disease and lowers the age of onset. *APOE 2*, a more uncommon allele, lowers the risk of Alzheimer's disease and raises the age of onset. The most commonly inherited allele, *APOE 3*, falls between *APOE 4* and *APOE 2*. Each person inherits one *APOE* gene from each parent. The difference between inheriting *APOE 4* and *APOE 2* causes a two-decade difference in the age of onset of Alzheimer's disease but implies that it is universal by the age of 140. The metabolic interaction of the *APOE* gene and amyoloid, neurofibrillary tangles, and neuritic plaques is currently under investigation.

There is currently no known treatment for Alzheimer's disease. One drug, Cognex, or tacrine has been approved for use in these patients. It provides minimal slowing of the disease process in some patients, but careful monitoring of liver function is required.

EPILEPSY

Women with epilepsy are frequently seen in a routine gynecologic practice. Epilepsy affects about 10% of the population; 2.8 million persons in the United States have epilepsy, and 1.1 million women of childbearing age have a seizure disorder. There are many types of seizure disorders. There are childhood-onset epilepsy syndromes, which have a genetic predisposition. Petit mal is a brief lapse in awareness that occurs with a characteristic electroencephalographic abnormality consisting of three spikes and waves per second. Petit mal seizures are controlled relatively easily by zarontin or depakote. Most children outgrow true petit mal by adolescence. They may become seizure free or develop atypical petit mal or partial complex seizures. Grand mal seizures involve loss of consciousness and often uncontrolled tonic-clonic movements. They are treated with various anticonvulsants. Depakote controls both petit and grand mal seizures. The other drugs are not effective in petit mal. They include phenytoin (Dilantin), carpenazepine, phenobarbital, felbamate gabapentin, lamotrigine, and vigabratin. Dilantin, carpenazepine, phenobarbital, and valproate are considered first-line drugs.

Estrogen increases neuronal excitability and progesterone decreases it. Hormones therefore may play a role in seizure control. Some women describe an increased frequency of auras around the time of their periods. Thirty percent of patients with seizures have catamenial seizures, that is, seizures that occur at the time of menses. Different approaches have been tried to decrease the frequency of these events, including increasing the doses of anticonvulsants around the time of menstrual flow and some attempts to increase progesterone. However, the dose of progesterone needed to prevent seizures is one that often produces anovulatory cycles, making it an inappropriate long-term solution. There is a recent report, however, by Herzog of using natural progesterone therapy in women with inadequate luteal phase cycles. Twenty-five women were given progesterone lozenges, 200 mg tid for 3 months, and experienced a 72% decrease in daily seizure frequency. Women with temporal lobe seizures have an increases frequency of anovulatory cycles.

There is no contraindication to oral contraceptive use in women with seizures. Oral contraceptives, however, have a higher failure rate (6–10%) in women taking antiepileptic drugs that increase liver enzyme levels. These women need to receive higher-dose estrogen preparations (>50 mEq estrogen) to achieve the normal protective effect. Carpenazepine, dilatin, and phenobarbital increase liver enzymes, while valproate and felbamate inhibit them. The newer second-line drugs—gabapentin, lamotrigine, and vigabratin—cause no change.

The increased failure rate in these patients is due to the faster metabolism of estrogen.

All women of childbearing age who have a seizure disorder should take oral folate supplementation to prevent neural tube defects in the fetus. If an unplanned pregnancy occurs, the folate needs to be present on days 1–25 of gestation to protect against neural tube defects. Therefore, it should be given routinely to any woman who may become pregnant and should be maintained throughout the pregnancy.

During pregnancy 25% of women with epilepsy have an increased frequency of seizures. This is felt to be due to a combination of changes in antiepileptic drug metabolism, compliance, and sleep deprivation. Many women try to decrease their medication during pregnancy because of the fear of fetal malformations. The same percentage of malformations occurs, however, due to exposure and not to the absolute dose. Most malformations occur in the first trimester. Women should therefore be encouraged to continue their medications and even increase their dose, if needed in pregnancy, to prevent seizures.

If a woman has a single seizure in pregnancy, miscarriage is rare, but the probability increases if the patient goes into status epilepticus or has many frequent seizures. One of the most common reasons for a woman to go into status is sudden discontinuation of her antiepileptic drug.

The risk of fetal malformations in the general population is 2–3%. Maternal epilepsy, with a single drug in the therapeutic range, increases the risk to 4–6%. The most common malformations are orofacial clefts (30%), followed by midline heart defects. Maternal but not paternal epilepsy increases the risk of epilepsy in the child. If maternal epilepsy began before the age of 18, it is twice as likely that the child will have epilepsy. Seizures in pregnancy increase the seizure risk in the offspring by a factor of 2. Fetal malformations are more common in women with seizures in the first trimester (12.3%) than with seizures that occur in the last two trimesters (4%). Seizures cause a decrease in fetal heart rate that lasts for 20 min postseizure. Tonic-clonic seizures occur during labor or delivery in less than 2% of women with a seizure disorder, but 1–2% of epileptic women have a seizure in the 24 h postpartum.

There is an increased risk of neonatal bleeding in the first 24 h in babies born to women taking antiepileptic drugs due to vitamin K deficiency. The antiepileptic drugs compete with vitamin K to cross the placenta. Therefore, the bleeding can be prevented by giving large doses of vitamin K to the mother prior to delivery. Phenobarbital withdrawal in the neonate occurs about 7 days postpartum, and results in restlessness and tremulousness. No intervention is usually needed.

Seizure disorders therefore increase the risk of obstetric complications, fetal malformations, and neonatal problems, but many of them can be prevented with adequate patient education and careful obstetric monitoring. The overall risk of obstetric problems has decreased by 70% in the last few years, including patients with underlying medical problems.

CONCLUSION

Women often consider their gynecologists their primary health care provider, and look to them for advice and medical referral. Patients with seizure disorders, migraine, and degenerative neurologic disorders add another dimension to routine obstetric and gynecologic care, but these patients are frequently seen and can be appreciative and intelligent patients.

BIBLIOGRAPHY

Davidoff RA: *Migraine: Manifestations, Pathogenesis and Management.* Philadelphia, FA Davis, 1995.

Devinsky O, Feldmann, E. Hainline, B. (eds): *Neurological Complications of Pregnancy.* New York, Raven Press, 1994.

Herzog, AG: Progesterone therapy in women with complex partial and secondary generalized seizures. *Neurology* 45:1660–1662, 1995.

Roses AD: Apolipoprotein E and Alzheimer's disease. *Sci Med* 2:16–25, 1995.

Chapter 12

Anemia and Blood Disorders

Jeanne A. Smith

INTRODUCTION

Hematologic disorders are not uncommonly seen in the office practice of obstetricians and gynecologists. These disorders may present either as a manifestation of the woman's underlying gynecologic condition (e.g., iron deficiency secondary to excessive gynecologic or obstetric blood loss) or as a manifestation of unrelated disorders as variable as pernicious anemia, Von Willebrand's disease, or leukemia. This chapter will focus on assisting the clinician to identify the presence of a hematologic disorder. Some of these conditions can and should be worked up and managed by the primary clinician (these will be indicated), while many others will require consultation with and/or management by a hematologist or oncologist. For ease of reference, the chapter is divided into four sections: History and Physical Findings, Anemia, White Blood Cell Disorders and Lymphomas, and Platelet and Coagulation Disorders.

HISTORY AND PHYSICAL FINDINGS

At initial visits, as well as when a hematologic disorder is suspected, a history should be taken which includes information on the woman's previous history of hematologic disorders, as well as her family's. Specific questions should be asked concerning gynecologic (menstrual) and obstetric blood loss, as well as gastrointestinal blood loss and the use of iron or other hematinics. The presence of hemoglobinopathy disease (sickle cell anemia, thalassemia, etc.) or trait in the woman or her family, and the presence of coagulation disorders should be discussed. Easy bruisability and any history of an abnormal hematologic response to drugs or foods should be ascertained. The human immunodeficiency virus (HIV) status may also be important for hematologic assessment.

The routine physical examination should include documentation of the presence or absence of mucosal pallor, jaundice, adenopathy, and hepatosplenomegaly. The skin and mucous membranes should be examined for the presence of petechiae or ecchymoses.

ANEMIA

Signs and Symptoms

The signs and symptoms of anemia can be very nonspecific. Patients may report increased fatigue, headache, or dyspnea on effort, all of which can also have other causes. Jaundice, associated with the above symptoms may suggest a hemolytic anemia, and intermittent episodes of pain may suggest sickle cell disease. Neurologic complaints such as paresthesia may suggest vitamin B_{12} deficiency.

Physical findings likewise may not be helpful in establishing the presence of anemia. Other than pallor, jaundice, and splenomegaly, the smooth tongue and the loss of position and vibratory sense in vitamin B_{12} deficiency are the most helpful signs.

Office Diagnostic Workup and Management

Interpretation of the CBC Report Today, most complete blood counts (CBCs) are performed by automated technology. They provide several tests which are useful in establishing the presence of anemia and suggesting its possible etiology. The most useful of these tests are the hemoglobin or hematocrit (either one can be used to establish the presence of anemia) and the mean corpuscular volume (MCV) (also known as the *packed cell volume*). The latter can be helpful in suggesting possible diagnoses. The normal, or reference, values for these tests are printed on the laboratory slip next to the patient's report.

Hemoglobin or hematocrit values more than 10% below the reference range suggest anemia. If the value is borderline and there is no obvious explanation, the test should be repeated before an extensive workup is performed. *Note: occasional patients with values 10–15% or more above the normal range may also be seen. If the finding is confirmed on repeat testing, a hematology consultation should be requested to evaluate the possibility of polycythemia, either primary (vera) or secondary (due to smoking, chronic lung disease, uterine fibroid, etc.)*

The MCV can be most easily interpreted if it is lower or higher than the normal range (Table 12.1) since in these situations only a few conditions need to be considered. Normal MCV anemias occur in a wide variety of conditions, most of which will require extensive evaluation.

TABLE 12.1 Interpretation of the MCV

MCV Value		Most Likely Diagnostic Possibilities
Low:	<80	Iron deficiency Presence of one or more alpha or beta thalassemia genes Anemia of chronic disease
Normal:	80–100	Multiple causes
High:	>100	Megaloblastic anemia High reticulocyte count Liver disease Certain chemotherapeutic agents

Low Mean Corpuscular Volume (MCV) Anemias

Iron Deficiency The most common low MCV anemia is iron deficiency. Iron deficiency anemia is almost invariably the result of blood loss. In men, the blood loss is usually from the gastrointestinal tract and may be the result of neoplastic disease. In women, gynecologic disease is common. Blood loss can be due to menometorragia, endometriosis, or associated with pregnancy and delivery. Except for women under the age of 30–35, the possibility of gastrointestinal blood loss should be considered and investigated. Iron deficiency can be confirmed by obtaining a serum ferritin level, which, if low, is diagnostic. Alternatively, bone marrow can be obtained to ascertain the presence or absence of iron stores, but this is usually not necessary. Replacement therapy should be given orally (ferrous sulfate 325 mg tid with meals) and should be continued for 6 months to ensure replacement of stores as well as correction of anemia. *Note: Over-the-counter preparations contain much lower doses of iron and may not provide adequate replacement. The other prescription formulations have not been consistently shown to improve gastrointestinal absorption or reduce gastrointestinal toxicity and are more expensive.*

Thalassemia Syndromes The thalassemia syndromes result from the inheritance of genes which are defective in their ability to produce the normal alpha- or beta-globin chains of hemoglobin. Defects can be found in either alpha- or beta-globin genes. Homozygous beta thalassemia produces the most severe anemia, usually requiring a chronic transfusion program, but this is not always true. On occasion the heterozygous state (thalassemia trait) may be associated with mild to moderate anemia, although most commonly there is only a low MCV with no anemia. It is also possible to inherit a beta thalassemia gene from one parent and a sickle gene from the other. This syndrome, known as *sickle beta thalassemia,* is one of the forms of sickle cell disease discussed later in this chapter.

Since there is no abnormal protein in thalassemia, the diagnosis cannot be made by routine tests for hemoglobinopathies such as cellulose acetate electrophoresis. For beta thalassemia trait, the diagnosis is usually established by the presence of a low MCV in the absence of iron deficiency and by the presence of an elevated level of one of the minor hemoglobins, hemoglobin A2. The diagnosis of alpha thalassemia trait may require DNA analysis. While individuals with the trait *do not* require medical management, all women should receive genetic counseling and be encouraged to have their partners tested to determine if the couple is at risk of having a child with homozygous or doubly heterozygous disease.

It is now clear that the thalassemia syndromes occur in many, if not all, racial and ethnic groups. The health care provider therefore should not allow race or ethnicity to govern his or her decision to order appropriate testing.

Anemia of Chronic Disease There are several chronic conditions which may lead to a moderate degree of anemia associated with either a low or, more commonly, normal MCV. Rheumatoid arthritis, diabetes, hypertensive cardiovascular disease, and chronic infection (bronchiectasis, osteomyelitis) are examples of such conditions. It has been shown that the underlying disease results in defective storage of iron, making it unavailable for incorporation into hemoglobin. Most commonly, this type of anemia occurs in older individuals. Iron deficiency must be ruled out in all such cases. The anemia usually does not improve unless the underlying condition improves.

Normal MCV Anemias As discussed above, the list of normal MCV anemias is long and includes such conditions as sickle cell disease, as well as other hemolytic anemias such as lupus and hereditary spherocytosis, the anemia of chronic disease, cancer-related anemia, HIV-related anemia, aplastic anemia, and the anemia of chronic renal failure. Such patients almost invariably require hematologic or other special consultation and collaborative management.

Sickle Hemoglobinopathies As with the thalassemias, the health care provider must be aware that sickle hemoglobin has been found in many ethnic and racial groups and that the disease can occur in the homozygous state, hemoglobin SS, or in one of several doubly heterozygous combinations such as hemoglobin SC, SD, SO arab, the S beta thalassemias, and others. Thus testing of women and their partners, and the provision of appropriate genetic counseling, is important for reproductive planning.

When ordering a test for a hemoglobinopathy, the provider should be aware that tests such as the sickle cell prep (metabisulfite) and solubility (dithionate) will only identify sickle hemoglobin and thus have a high false-negative rate. It is recommended that all testing be done by hemoglobin electrophoresis, isoelectric focusing, or column chromatography. It is also important to recognize that, by convention, laboratories report sickle cell trait as hemoglobin AS and sickle beta thalassemia disease as hemoglobin SA, thus putting the hemoglobin present in the largest percentage first.

On occasion, a report may be received of hemoglobin AF. F represents the hereditary persistence of fetal hemoglobin (HPFH). HPFH, when inherited together with hemoglobin S, does not usually produce clinical disease. On occasion, reports are received of individuals with hemoglobin CC, C thalassemia, CD, and so on. These individuals *do not* have sickle cell disease but usually have a mild hemolytic anemia.

Anemia in Pregnancy A mild normal MCV anemia is not uncommon during pregnancy. It is believed to be due to an increase in plasma volume which is disproportionately greater than the concomitant increase in red cell mass and is therefore described as a "dilutional anemia." The diagnosis is established by excluding known causes of anemia such as iron or folate deficiency and hemolytic disease in an otherwise healthy pregnant woman. No intervention is indicated.

Of more concern are the anemia, thrombocytopenia, and disseminated intravascular coagulation which can develop as a result of preeclampsia and eclampsia or the HELLP syndrome (*he*molysis, *l*iver dysfunction, *l*ow *p*latelets). The management of this condition requires multidisciplinary expertise and is beyond the scope of this chapter.

High MCV Anemias The megaloblastic anemias, which are probably the most common high MCV anemias, are due to a deficiency of one of two vitamins—folic acid or vitamin B_{12}—which are both involved in DNA synthesis. Both are characterized by high MCV anemia with peripheral smear findings of ovalomacrocytes and hypersegmented neutrophils. Bone marrow aspiration will show morphologic changes in both red cell and white cell precursors, but it does not distinguish between the two disorders. This distinction is important because the treatment of vitamin B_{12} deficiency with folic acid may correct the anemia but can result in the development or worsening of the neurologic complications of this deficiency.

Folic Acid Deficiency This disorder, most frequently caused in pregnancy by inadequate dietary intake and an increased requirement due to fetal needs, has been largely eliminated by the inclusion of folic acid in prenatal vitamins. However, in recent years, an association has been established between neural tube defects and folate deficiency in early pregnancy even in the absence of maternal megaloblastic anemia. Excessive alcohol consumption (probably through dietary inadequacy) and diphenylhydantoin, used in the treatment of epilepsy, can also result in folate deficiency. The increased requirements of patients with hemolytic anemia, such as those with sickle cell disease, hereditary spherocytosis, and others, have also been implicated. The 1-mg daily dose contained in prenatal vitamins appears to be adequate to correct all of these conditions. However, in patients with excessive alcohol consumption, compliance with a regimen of daily vitamin ingestion may be unlikely.

Vitamin B_{12} Deficiency Pernicious anemia, the classic form of vitamin B_{12} deficiency, results from a loss of intrinsic factor, a cofactor produced by the gastric mucosa required to enable transport of vitamin B_{12} across the epithelium of the terminal ileum. The disorder is unusual in women of childbearing age, except for a rare congenital form, but it can occur. Other causes of vitamin B_{12} deficiency are subtotal gastrectomy, tropical or nontropical sprue, blind loop syndrome, gastric or intestinal lymphoma, other diseases of the terminal ileum, and a strict vegetarian diet (no animal protein). The last condition may be devastating to the fetus without producing significant anemia in the mother. For this reason, a careful dietary history is important.

As discussed earlier, a serum vitamin B_{12} level will establish the presence of vitamin B_{12} deficiency, and replacement therapy with 1000 μg of vitamin B_{12} intramuscularly for 5 days can be instituted. At the same time, the patient should be referred for evaluation to determine the cause, as several of the conditions listed can be corrected and will not require lifelong vitamin B_{12} replacement.

High Reticulocyte Count as a Cause of High MCV Anemia Reticulocytes are larger than more mature red cells. Since the MCV is an average of all red cells, a high reticulocyte count can result in a high MCV. This can be seen when there is a brisk marrow response to hemolysis. No intervention is indicated.

Chemotherapeutic Agents as a Cause of a High MCV The agent most consistently known to produce this picture is hydroxyurea. This agent is used in the treatment of polycythemia vera, essential thrombocytosis, chronic myelocytic leukemia, and, most recently, sickle cell disease.

WHITE BLOOD CELL DISORDERS AND LYMPHOMAS

Signs and Symptoms

With the exception of the leukemias and lymphomas, white blood cell disorders rarely present with characteristic or diagnostic physical findings or symptoms. Fever, night sweats, weight loss, and generalized malaise, while also characteristic of chronic infections such as tuberculosis, are frequently seen in lymphomas, and sometimes also in both acute and chronic leukemia.

Physical examination may reveal lymphadenopathy, either localized to one region or diffuse, and hepatosplenomegaly. Acute leukemia may present with petechiae, ecchymoses, gingival bleeding, and conjunctival and retinal hemorrhages.

Interpretation of the White Blood Cell Count

In order to interpret the white blood cell (WBC) count, a few principles must be observed. First, the WBC test measures all nucleated cells found in the blood. Thus, if nucleated red blood cells are present, the count must be corrected. The "corrected WBC" is the true WBC count. Second, the differential reports the percentage of the different types of WBCs found in the specimen of blood analyzed. Therefore, it can only be interpreted in conjunction with the WBC count. Some examples of correct interpretation are given in Table 12.2. The absolute neutrophil (or lymphocyte) count can be calculated as follows:

$$\text{WBC count} \times \%\ \text{neutrophils} = \text{absolute neutrophil count}$$

Each cell line has a normal range; the most important of these are neutrophils (and bands) 2000 to 8000 and lymphocytes 2000 to 5000. In the third example in Table 12.2, what might appear to be a lymphocytosis if only the percentages are considered is actually a neutropenia. Neutropenias are not uncommonly seen by primary care practitioners, and while thorough hematologic evaluation is usually required, the practitioner should be aware that many drugs are capable of producing neutropenia. Some of

TABLE 12.2 Interpretation of the WBC Count and Differential

Total WBC Count	% of Polys	Absolute No. of Polys	% of Lymphs	Absolute No. of Lymphs	Interpretation
10,000	35%	3,500	55%	5,500	Normal neutrophil count, borderline lymphocyte count
7,500	35%	2,625	55%	4,125	Normal neutrophil count, normal lymphocyte count
3,750	35%	1,313	55%	2,063	*Neutropenia*, normal lymphocyte count

Note: A complete differential in each case would also include a total of 10% monocytes, eosinophils, and basophils.

TABLE 12.3 Drugs Often Associated with Neutropenia*

Antiarrhythmics
- Procainamide HCL (Pronestyl) (with or without lupus syndrome)
- Quinidine

Antibiotics
- Semisynthetic penicillins
- Cephalosporins
- Sulfonamides
- Trimethoprim-Sulfamethoxazole (especially in AIDS and bone marrow transplant patients)

Anticonvulsants
- Phenytoin (Dilantin)
- Trimethadione (Tridione)

Antihypertensives
- Methyldopa (Aldomet)
- Captopril (Capoten)

Anti-inflammatory agents
- Gold compounds
- Penicillamine (Cuprimine, Depen)
- Phenylbutazone (Azolid, Butazolidin)
- Aminopyrine
- Indomethacin (Indocin, Indo-Lemmon)

Antineoplastic and immunosuppressive agents

Antithyroid agents
- Propylthiouracil
- Methimazole (Tapazole)

Psychotropic agents
- Tricyclic antidepressants
- Phenothiazines

Miscellaneous
- Cimetidine (Tagamet)
- Alcohol
- Thiazides

Source: Russin SJ, Fillipo BH, Adler AG: Neutropenia in adults—What is its clinical significance? *Postgrad Med* 88(2):209–215, 1990. Used with permission of McGraw-Hill, Inc.

*Many of these drugs can also cause Thrombocytopenia.

the most common drugs are listed in Table 12.3. It is good clinical practice to discontinue the use of possibly offending agents while the patient is being evaluated. Elevation of the absolute number of a cell line may indicate infection or leukemia and will require further evaluation.

Specific WBC Disorders

Neutropenia Neutropenia, particularly when the absolute neutrophil count is under 500 per cu mm, places the patient at severe risk of overwhelming bacterial infection and sepsis. Management of these patients requires special consultations. The condition is common in patients with HIV infection.

Leukemias and Lymphomas Leukemias are classified as either acute or chronic, depending on whether the abnormal cells involved are mature or immature (blasts). Both types of leukemia can involve any of the cell lines. Bleeding, frequently gingival and sometimes gynecologic, due to thrombocytopenia, is often the first manifestation of an acute leukemia. The CBC report will usually show the presence of immature cells. This should prompt further evaluation. Patients with chronic lymphocytic or chronic myelocytic leukemia have a more indolent course and may survive for 5 or more years; patients with lymphomas may be cured. The diagnosis and management of these disorders are beyond the scope of this chapter, but the primary care practitioner is reminded that routine preventive gynecologic care should be provided to these patients.

Bone marrow transplantation is becoming an important therapeutic option in attempting to cure all of the above disorders, as well as others such as aplastic anemia and sickle cell anemia. Some of the children transplanted several years ago have now reached adulthood and are fertile. In addition to routine gynecologic management, the potential for pregnancy exists. The teratogenic risk is unknown at this time.

PLATELET AND COAGULATION DISORDERS

Signs and Symptoms

Bleeding is the most common manifestation of platelet and coagulation disorders. Patients may present with complaints of bleeding from one or more sites, such as the conjunctiva, gingiva, skin, gastrointestinal or urogenital tract, or joints. Patients should be questioned carefully concerning a personal or family history of a bleeding disorder, any medications taken, and a history of recent viral infection, as well as the possibility of trauma. Less commonly, thrombotic disorders or vasculitis may result from platelet or coagulation disorders such as essential thrombocytosis, protein S deficiency, or Weber-Osler-Rendu disease.

The most frequent physical findings in bleeding disorders are petechiae and/or ecchymoses, hemarthroses, and blood in a body cavity. These findings may also be seen in patients with a vasculitis. The thrombotic disorders may result in signs consistent with either central nervous system (CNS) thrombosis or peripheral venous thrombosis or, at times, both.

Interpreting the Platelet Count

In most laboratories the normal range for platelet counts is 150,000–400,000/mm^3. The range for a particular laboratory is usually printed on the report slip. Platelet counts 15–20% higher or lower than this range should be retested before any other action is taken to account for diurnal variation, laboratory error, and the possibility of menstrual or other bleeding. Many laboratories also describe the appearance of the platelets on the peripheral smear, reporting that their level appears to be "low," "normal," or "high" or that they are clumped. The last description is particularly helpful with borderline low counts, as it suggests that the specimen was inadequately mixed.

It should be noted that bleeding manifestations usually do not occur if the platelet count is 50,000/mm^3 or above.

Thrombocytopenia

Idiopathic Thrombocytopenic Purpura This disorder is not infrequent in women of childbearing age. Its etiology is unknown, but viral infections are a suspected cause. The disorder is believed to be due to the development of an antiplatelet antibody which results in destruction of platelets by the spleen. Purpura and mucosal bleeding are the most common manifestations. CNS bleeding is rare. Bone marrow examination in these patients shows normal to high numbers of megakaryocytes. To date, there are no specific laboratory tests; thus, the diagnosis is made by excluding the causes of thrombocytopenia discussed below. The platelet count may be moderately to severely reduced.

The degree of thrombocytopenia and the bleeding manifestations form the basis of decisions on whether to treat and what type of therapy is indicated. Some patients will experience a permanent remission, while others may remain thrombocytopenic for many years. Successful pregnancy has occurred in many patients who were only mildly thrombocytopenic; however, it should be noted that transient thrombocytopenia may occur in the neonate, who will therefore need close monitoring. Patients receiving therapy with steroids or chemotherapy should probably be advised against conception.

Thrombocytopenia indistinguishable from idiopathic thrombocytopenic purpura is a not infrequent manifestation of early HIV infection. Many clinicians now recommend HIV testing of patients suspected of having the disorder.

Drug-Related Thrombocytopenia Many drugs and alcohol can cause thrombocytopenia (see Table 12.3). As with neutropenia, withdrawal of any possibly offending agents is a wise first step in managing the patient. Chemotherapeutic agents may also be responsible.

Thrombocytopenia of Pregnancy Mild thrombocytopenia has been reported to occur during the third trimester of pregnancy. Its etiology is unknown. There are usually no bleeding manifestations, and the condition corrects itself after delivery.

The HELLP Syndrome and Thrombotic Thrombocytopenic Purpura The pathogenesis of both of these conditions involves a vasculitis, with resultant platelet and red blood cell destruction through adherence to the abnormal vascular endothelium. Many clinicians believe that the two disorders have a similar etiology (unknown) and differ only in that the HELLP syndrome is associated with preeclampsia and eclampsia, whereas thrombotic thrombocytopenic purpura occurs in the nonpregnant state. Both syndromes are characterized by hemolytic anemia, renal and/or hepatic dysfunction, and CNS manifestations, as well as thrombocytopenia. These syndromes represent medical emergencies and require urgent special consultation.

Thrombocytopenia in the Setting of Other Disorders Thrombocytopenia is a common finding in patients with vitamin B_{12} or folate deficiency. It is seen in the acute leukemias and late in the course of the chronic leukemias. In addition, it may occur as the result of bone marrow invasion by neoplastic cells and in patients with cirrhosis or other causes of hypersplenism such as lupus.

Thrombocytosis As noted earlier, elevation of the platelet count may occur in patients with significant bleeding from any site. The platelet count will return to normal within 5–10 days after bleeding ceases. Mild elevation of the platelet count (up to 700,000 –800,000/mm^3) are common in hemolytic anemias. Platelet counts of over 1,000,000/mm^3 are seen in polycythemia vera, essential thrombocytosis, and chronic myelocytic leukemia. These latter situations invariably require intervention, as either thrombosis or bleeding is likely to occur.

COAGULATION DISORDERS

Most disorders of coagulation factors, whether they produce bleeding or thrombosis, are inherited. The personal or family history of such a disorder should therefore prompt the primary care practitioner to confirm the correct diagnosis and discuss with the patient the advisability of genetic counseling for her and her partner if childbearing is planned. Coagulation disorders, primarily factor deficiencies or antibodies to coagulation factors, can also occur in the setting of other disorders such as liver disease, neoplastic disease, and severe infection. Full discussion of these disorders, all of which require expert intervention, is beyond the scope of this chapter.

BIBLIOGRAPHY

Brown RG: Determining the cause of anemia. General approach, with emphasis on microcytic hypochromic anemias. *Postgrad Med* 89(6):161–164, 167–170, 1991 May.

Cruikshank DP: Cardiovascular, pulmonary and hematologic diseases in pregnancy. In Scott JR, DiSaia PJ, Hammond CB, et al (eds): *Danforth's Obstetrics and Gynecology*. Philadelphia, JB Lipincott, 1994, pp 367–392.

Goebel RA: Thrombocytopenia. *Emergency Med Clin North Am* 11(2):445–461, 1993.

Russin SJ, Filipo BH, Adler AG: Neutropenia in adults. What is its clinical significance? *Postgrad Med* 88(2):209–216, 1990.

Weaver DW: Differential diagnosis and management of unexplained bleeding. *Surg Clin North Am* 73(2):353–361, 1993.

Chapter 13

Hypertension

Velvie Pogue

INTRODUCTION

Cardiovascular disease is the leading cause of death in the United States, causing nearly 1 million deaths in 1989. Approximately 1.5 million people suffer myocardial infarctions per year, and about one-third of these die. Stroke is the third leading cause of death in the United States after myocardial infarction and all forms of cancer. Approximately 500,000 strokes occur per year in the United States. Hypertension is one of the most important contributing risk factors for coronary heart disease and the predominant risk factor for stroke. Hypertension contributes to 498,000 coronary deaths, 147,000 stroke deaths, and 35,000 cases of heart failure. More than 50 million Americans suffer from hypertension if one uses a definition of systolic blood pressure (SBP) >140 mmHg and/or diastolic blood pressure (DBP) >90 mmHg. The prevalence of hypertension increases with age, is greater in blacks than in whites, and in both races is greater in less educated than in more educated persons. Nonfatal and fatal cardiovascular disease, as well as renal disease and all-cause mortality, increase progressively with higher levels of both SBP and DBP.

Steady improvement in blood pressure control in the U.S. population has followed a successful series of randomized, controlled clinical trials of hypertension treatment, the development of potent antihypertensive agents, and the dissemination of information through the National High Blood Pressure Education Program. Despite these gains, however, poorly controlled hypertension remains a health problem of major proportions, particularly among minority populations, the poor, those with lower levels of education, and those with limited access to medical care. Obstetricians/gynecologists, as the only primary care physicians for many women, can play an important role in the diagnosis and treatment of hypertension. In this chapter we will discuss criteria for the diagnosis of hypertension, diagnostic evaluation, and choice of antihypertensive therapy.

DIAGNOSIS AND EVALUATION

The initial step in the management of hypertension is a careful assessment of the level of blood pressure. Ambulatory blood pressure monitoring has demonstrated that blood pressure varies greatly during awake hours in association with physical and emotional stresses. The diagnosis of hypertension should not be made until several readings have been done over several weeks unless the blood pressure is very high (SBP >210 mmHg, DBP >120 mmHg) or there is evidence of hypertensive target organ damage. The blood pressure should be measured in such a manner that the values obtained are representative of patients' usual levels. At least two readings should be done at each visit; if they differ by more than 5 mmHg, additional readings should be obtained. The patient should be seated for at least 5 min, with the arm unconstricted and supported at the level of the heart on a platform or table.

An average DBP level of ≥90 mmHg and/or an average SBP level of 140 mmHg is required for the diagnosis. Once the average pressure is obtained, both SBP and DBP are used to classify subjects into one of the four stages using the criteria of the Fifth Report of the Joint National Committee on the Evaluation, Detection, and Treatment of High Blood Pressure (JNC V). The JNC V stages of hypertension are stage 1 (SBP 140–159 mmHg, DBP 90–99 mmHg), stage 2 (SBP 160–179 mmHg, DBP 100–109 mmHg), stage 3 (SBP 180–209 mmHg, DBP 110–119 mmHg), and stage 4 (SBP ≥210 mmHg; DBP > 120 mmHG (Table 13.1). If the SBP and DBP yield different stages of severity, the higher stage is used to classify the subject.

The major goals of evaluation of the hypertensive subject are (1) to exclude secondary causes, (2) to assess target organ damage (Table 13.2), and (3) to determine the overall cardiovascular risk. The evaluation of all patients should include a complete medical history, physical examination, hematocrit, urinalysis, serum creatinine, fasting glucose, serum electrolytes, total and high density lipoprotein cholesterol, and electrocardiogram.

Although not recommended for the routine evaluation of hypertensive subjects, 24-h ambulatory blood pressure monitoring may provide more information and may be a better predictor of the cardiovascular and renal disease risks (Table 13.3). Ambulatory blood pressure monitoring may be particularly useful in the diagnosis of white coat hypertension and in the assessment of the efficacy and duration of antihypertensive therapy in clinical trials.

TABLE 13.1 JNC V Classification of Hypertension for Adults Aged 18 and older

Category	Systolic (mmHg)	Diastolic (mmHg)
Normal	<130	<85
High Normal	130–139	85–90
Hypertension		
Stage 1 (mild)	140–159	90–99
Stage 2 (moderate)	160–179	100–109
Stage 3 (severe)	180–209	110–119
Stage 4 (very severe)	≥210	≥120

TABLE 13.2 Manifestations of Target-Organ Damage

Organ System	Manifestations
Cardiac	Clinical, electrocardiographic, or radiologic evidence of coronary artery disease Left ventricular hypertrophy or strain by electrocardiography or left ventricular hypertrophy by echocardiography Left ventricular dysfunction or cardiac failure
Cerebrovascular	Transient ischemic attack or stroke
Peripheral vascular	Absence of 1 or more major pulses in extremities (except for dorsalis pedis) with or without intermittent claudication; aneurysm
Renal	Serum creatinine ≥ 1.5 mg/dL; proteinuria (1+ or greater); microalbuminuria
Retinopathy	Hemorrhages or exudates, with or without papilledema

TABLE 13.3 Situations in Which Automated Noninvasive Ambulatory Blood Pressure Monitoring Devices May Be Useful

"Office" or "white-coat" hypertension; blood pressure repeatedly elevated in office setting but normal out of office
Evaluation of drug resistance
Evaluation of nocturnal blood pressure changes
Episodic hypertension
Hypotensive symptoms associated with antihypertensive medications or autonomic dysfunction
Carotid sinus syncope and pacemaker syndromes*

If the results of the baseline evaluation suggest secondary causes of hypertension, additional tests may be necessary.

SECONDARY CAUSES OF HYPERTENSION

As many as 10% of patients with hypertension will have a secondary cause of hypertension. The possible causes include (1) renal parenchymal disease, (2) renal vascular hypertension, (3) diseases of the adrenal gland (pheochromocytoma, Cushing's disease, and primary aldosteronism), (4) thyroid disease, and (5) illicit drug use.

Renal Parenchymal Disease

The blood pressure tends to rise as renal function is lost, mainly from inability of the damaged kidneys to excrete sodium and water. As renal function deteriorates, hypertension becomes more prevalent; it is present in about 85% of those with end-stage renal disease (ESRD). It is sometimes difficult to determine whether hypertension in patients with renal disease is primary or secondary to intrinsic renal disease. All forms of progressive renal disease may lead to hypertension, including (1) polycystic disease, (2) analgesic nephropathy, (3) vasculitis, (4) pyelonephritis, (5) diabetic nephropathy, and (6) obstructive nephropathy.

Renal Vascular Hypertension

Renal vascular hypertension should be suspected in patients with any of the following clinical features: (1) the onset of hypertension before age 30 or after age 50, (2) rapid progression of hypertension, and (3) the presence of an abdominal bruit, (4) a poor response to most antihypertensive drugs, and (5) rapid progression of renal insufficiency after the use of an ACE inhibitor. The most common causes of renal vascular hypertension are medial fibroplasia in young patients, especially young women, and atherosclerotic plaques in older patients.

Adrenal Disease

Hypertension accompanies diseases of the adrenal medulla or cortex. Pheochromocytoma is frequently unilateral and benign in 80% of subjects. The hypertension may be episodic or sustained, but intermittent "spells" are almost always noted and include headache, tachycardia, sweating, and tremor. The excess catecholamines usually induce a hypermetabolic state with weight loss, hyperglycemia, and intense peripheral vasoconstriction with paleness. Pheochromocytoma should be suspected in patients with widely fluctuating blood pressure and repeated spells.

Hypertension is present in approximately 85% of patients with Cushing's syndrome, regardless of the cause. Cortisol excess is usually manifested by truncal obesity, thin skin with striae and ecchymoses, osteoporosis, and hyperglycemia.

Primary Aldosteronism The diagnosis of primary aldosteronism should be considered in patients with hypokalemia that is not provoked by diuretic use, renal tubular acidosis, or gastrointestinal fluid loss. Almost all patients will have hypertension, which is often severe, and hypokalemia, which may be intermittent. The excess mineralocorticoid in this syndrome may arise from a solitary benign adenoma or from bilateral hyperplasia.

Hypercalcemia Hypercalcemia from any cause may increase peripheral resistance and raise the blood pressure. Most patients with hyperparathyroidism are hypertensive, although the blood pressure becomes normal only in a minority after cure of the hyperparathyroidism.

Hypothyroidism

Patients with hypothyroidism may have an increase in DBP which results from an increase in peripheral vasoconstriction. The SBP is usually not increased since cardiac output is reduced.

Hyperthyroidism

Hyperthyroidism usually results in a high cardiac output, which causes an increase in the SBP. The DBP is usually reduced, presumably because of peripheral vasodilation in response to increased metabolic demands.

TREATMENT OF HYPERTENSION

Current recommendations concerning the treatment of hypertension do not differentiate between women and men. Patients with uncomplicated mild hypertension, defined as DBP between 90 and 100 mmHg, should not be started on antihypertensive drugs immediately. Although an immediate start of therapy has become common practice, a more conservative approach is recommended. Patients with mild hypertension are at little short-term risk and will not be endangered by postponement of drug therapy. A delay in the start of antihypertensive drug therapy will allow confirmation of the presence of sustained hypertension and will provide sufficient time to determine whether lifestyle modification will be adequate to return the blood pressure to normal.

Once hypertension is confirmed, treatment should be started with lifestyle modifications. In addition to controlling hypertension, lifestyle modifications improve the cardiovascular risk profile. In subjects whose blood pressure is not adequately controlled with lifestyle modification, such modification may reduce the number and doses of antihypertensive medication. Therefore, clinicians should encourage their patients to adopt lifestyle modification; this provides multiple benefits with minimal risks.

Lifestyle Modifications

Weight Reduction Excess body weight is correlated closely with increased blood pressure. Almost half of the hypertensive people are overweight. Weight reduction reduces blood pressure in a large proportion of hypertensive individuals who are more than 10% above ideal body weight. Weight reduction can lead to lowering of blood pressure even if ideal body weight is not attained. In addition, weight reduction of overweight subjects enhances the blood pressure–lowering effect of concurrent antihypertensive agents and can reduce the cardiovascular risk.

In overweight hypertensive subjects with stage 1 hypertension, weight reduction should be tried for 3–6 months prior to initiating pharmacologic therapy. Calories should be restricted in a manner appropriate to the individual patient. For most patients, a 1200-calorie low-fat diet will provide gradual weight loss without discomfort.

Sodium Restriction Epidemiologic studies and clinical trials show an association between dietary sodium intake and blood pressure. Multiple clinical trials document a reduction of blood pressure in response to reduced sodium intake. Restriction of dietary sodium to 2.4 grams per day (100 mmol or 6 g of NaCl) will lower the SBP by 5 to 10 mmHg in a significant number of sodium-sensitive hypertensives. This degree of restriction can be attained by avoiding highly salted foods (e.g., pickles, processed meats, canned tomato juice) and adding no salt at the table or in cooking. Awareness of the hidden sodium content of most processed foods, such as canned vegetables and many breakfast cereals, is necessary. Fresh or unprocessed frozen foods should be used whenever possible. More rigid sodium restriction may be needed for patients with renal failure or severe heart failure.

Potassium Supplementation A high dietary potassium intake may protect against the development of hypertension, and potassium deficiency may increase blood pressure. Correction of hypokalemia may lower the blood pressure. Although supplemental potassium chloride has been shown to lower the blood pressure in some normokalemic hypertensives, it is usually unnecessary to provide supplemental potassium if high-potassium foods are substituted for processed, high-sodium foods in the diet.

Isotonic Exercise A number of studies have shown that regular aerobic exercise is accompanied by a fall in blood pressure. Although some of the antihypertensive effects of exercise may reflect coincidental weight loss, hypertensive subjects should be encouraged to perform regular isotonic exercises. In addition, regular exercise may enhance the functional health status and reduce the risk of cardiovascular and all-cause mortality. To reach the "conditioned" state of cardiac performance, 20 to 30 min of sustained exercise at 70% of maximal capacity, usually determined from the rise in pulse rate, is required three times each week. The level of exercise that leads to the greatest fall in blood pressure has not been determined.

Relaxation and Biofeedback Therapy Almost all forms of relaxation therapy have been said to lower the blood pressure. However, most controlled studies have not shown a sustained effect beyond the duration of the relaxation procedure. Those patients who seem to benefit and are willing to continue the practice of some form of relaxation therapy should be encouraged to do so.

Moderate Use of Alcohol Besides adding calories, alcohol consumption may raise the blood pressure and cause resistance to antihypertensive therapy. Patients who drink alcoholic beverages should be advised to limit alcohol intake to 1 oz of ethanol per day. This amount is unlikely to raise the blood pressure, and it provides protection against coronary heart disease. However, in multiple population surveys, daily consumption of more than 1 oz of alcohol per day is associated with higher blood pressure, and more than 2 oz per day is often associated with overt hypertension.

Smoking Cessation Although cigarette smoking is not related to sustained hypertension, it is a major risk factor in cardiovascular disease. Avoidance of smoking is essential in the risk reduction of the hypertensive patient. Repetitive counseling, including referral to smoking cessation programs, should be provided to all patients who smoke. The rate of relapse in cigarette smokers is high, and the addition of nicotine therapy to counseling should be considered in heavily addicted smokers.

Pharmacologic Therapy

Although women were not included in some of the major clinical trials which demonstrated the efficacy of antihypertensive therapy in preventing the complications of hypertension, the available data have not clearly demonstrated gender differences in blood pressure response and outcomes. Therefore, the recommended approach to women with hypertension is the same as that to men. The goals of treatment are to prevent the morbidity and mortality associated with high blood pressure and to control high blood pressure by the least intrusive means possible. Patients with severe hypertension, target organ damage, other cardiovascular risk factors, or an inadequate response to lifestyle modification will require pharmacologic therapy. Many antihypertensive drugs are available, so that the patient's therapy can be tailored individually. The antihypertensive medications currently available include:

Diuretics Diuretics work by decreasing plasma and extracellular fluid volume and by reducing cardiac output. Total peripheral resistance is also reduced with normalization of cardiac output. Chronic effects include a slight decrease in extracellular fluid volume. These drugs may cause hypokalemia, hypomagnesemia, hyponatremia, hyperglycemia, and hyperlipidemia. Sexual dysfunction and weakness are also possible.

JNC V states that in blacks diuretics have been proven in controlled trials to reduce hypertensive morbidity and mortality. Thus, diuretics should be the agents of first choice in the absence of other conditions that prohibit their use.

When using diuretics, the following facts should be kept in mind: (1) cholestyramine and colestipol decrease the absorption of diuretics and may decrease the antihypertensive effect; (2) non-steroidal anti-inflammatory agents (NSAIA) may antagonize the effectiveness of diuretics; (3) diuretics may raise lithium levels and increase tonicity by enhancing proximal tubular reabsorption of lithium; and (4) diuretics may make it more difficult to control dyslipidemia and diabetes.

Adrenergic Inhibitors Adrenergic inhibitors decrease blood pressure by reducing output and increasing total peripheral resistance. Plasma renin activity may also be reduced. When using adrenergic inhibitors, the following interactions/side effects should be kept in mind:

1. Beta blockers and alpha-beta blockers should not be used in patients with asthma, chronic obstructive pulmonary disease, left ventricular failure secondary to systolic dysfunction, heart block of second degree or greater, or sick sinus syndrome.
2. Beta blockers should be used with caution in insulin-treated diabetics and in patients with peripheral vascular disease.
3. Adrenergic inhibitors should not be withdrawn abruptly in patients with ischemic heart disease.
4. Alpha$_1$-receptor blockers can cause orthostatic hypotension, syncope, weakness, palpitations, and headache and should be used cautiously in older patients.
5. NSAIA, rifampin, smoking, and phenobarbital may decrease the antihypertensive effect of beta blockers.
6. Cimetidine may increase serum levels of beta blockers that are metabolized primarily by the liver due to enzyme inhibition.
7. Beta blockers may have additive sinoatrial and atrioventricular node depressant effects when combined with diltiazem or verapamil. This combination may also promote negative inotropic effects on the failing myocardium.
8. The combination of beta blockers and reserpine may cause marked bradycardia and syncope. Nonselective beta blockers may prolong insulin-induced hypoglycemia and promote rebound hypertension due to unopposed alpha stimula-

tion. All beta blockers mask the adrenergically mediated symptoms of hypoglycemia and have the potential to aggravate diabetes.

ACE Inhibitors ACE inhibitors block the formation of angiotensin II, promoting vasodilation and decreased aldosterone. These agents also increase bradykinin and vasodilator prostaglandins.

Common side effects of ACE inhibitors include cough, rash, angioneurotic edema, hyperkalemia, and dysgeusia. Hyperkalemia is of particular concern in patients with renal insufficiency. Acute renal failure can occur in patients with bilateral renal arterial stenosis or unilateral stenosis in a solitary kidney, as well as in patients with cardiac failure and with volume depletion. Much less commonly, neutropenia or proteinuria can develop.

ACE inhibitors are absolutely contraindicated in the second and third trimesters of pregnancy.

The following drug interactions should also be considered:

1. NSAIA and antacids may lead to decreased antihypertensive effects of ACE inhibitors.
2. Diuretics may cause increased antihypertensive effects of ACE inhibitors due to hypovolemia.
3. ACE inhibitors, when combined with potassium supplements, potassium-sparing diuretics, or NSAIAs, may cause hyperkalemia.
4. ACE inhibitors may also increase serum lithium levels.

Calcium Antagonists Calcium antagonists block the inward movement of calcium ions across cell membranes and cause smooth muscle relaxation. These agents also block the slow channels in the heart, and may reduce the sinus rate and produce heart block. Calcium antagonists should be used with caution in patients with congestive heart failure; they may also aggravate angina and myocardial ischemia. Side effects are headache, dizziness, peripheral edema, tachycardia, and gingival hyperplasia.

When using these agents, the following interactions/side effects should be considered:

1. A decreased antihypertensive effect may occur when calcium antagonists are combined with rifampin, carbazepine, phenobarbital, or phenytoin.
2. Cimetidine may increase the pharmacologic effects of calcium antagonists due to inhibition of hepatic metabolizing enzymes, resulting in increased serum levels.
3. Calcium antagonists cause an increase in the serum levels of the following drugs: digoxin, carbamazepine, preseason, quinidine, theophylline, and cyclosporine.

Centrally Acting Alpha Agonists Centrally acting alpha$_2$-agonists stimulate central alpha$_2$-receptors that inhibit efferent sympathetic activity. These drugs cause rebound hypertension with abrupt discontinuance, particularly with prior administration of high doses. Common side effects include drowsiness, sedation, dry mouth, fatigue, and orthostatic dizziness. Transdermal clonidine patches are replaced once a week. These agents should be avoided in noncompliant patients because of the risk of rebound hypertension after abrupt drug withdrawal.

The severity of clonidine withdrawal may be increased by beta blockers.

Peripherally Acting Adrenergic Antagonists Peripherally acting adrenergic antagonists inhibit catecholamine release from neuronal storage sites. These drugs may cause serious orthostatic and exercise-induced hypotension. Side effects of guanethidine include diarrhea, as well as orthostatic and exercise hypotension. Side effects of reserpine include lethargy, nasal congestion, and depression. Reserpine is contraindicated in patients with a history of mental depression or with active peptic ulcer.

Direct Vasodilators Direct vasocilators act by direct smooth muscle vasodilation (primarily arteriolar). They should be used with a diuretic and a beta blocker to prevent fluid retention and reflex tachycardia. The following possible side effects should be noted:

1. Hydralazine may cause a positive antinuclear antibody test, and lupus syndrome may develop.
2. Minoxidil may cause or aggravate pleural and pericardial effusions.
3. Hypertrichosis is a common side effect of minoxidil.

All of these drugs may precipitate angina pectoris in patients with coronary artery disease.

Coexisting Cardiovascular Disease The presence of concomitant medical conditions should also be considered in the selection of antihypertensive therapy. The presence of hypertensive target organ damage is an indication for antihypertensive therapy. Conditions which should be considered are cerebrovascular disease, coronary artery disease, cardiac failure, left ventricular hypertrophy, and peripheral vascular disease.

BIBLIOGRAPHY

Cappuccio FP, MacGregor GA: Does potassium supplementation lower blood pressure? A meta-analysis of published trials. *J Hypertension* 9:465–473, 1991.

Cutler JA, Brittain E: Calcium and blood pressure. An epidemiologic prospective. *Am J Hypertens* 3:137S–146S, 1990.

Fodor JG, Chockalingam A: The Canadian Concensus Report on Non-Pharmacological Approaches to the Management of High Blood Pressure. *Clin Exper Hypertens* A12:729–743, 1990.

*Joint National Committee: The Fifth Report of the Joint National Committee on Detection, Evaluation, and Treatment of High Blood Pressure. *Arch Intern Med* 1993; 153:154–183.

Kaplan NM: Long-term effectiveness of nonpharmacological treatment of hypertension. *Hypertension* 18(Suppl 1):153–160, 1991.

Kelemen MH, Effron MB, Valenti SA, et al: Exercise training combined with antihypertensive drug therapy. *JAMA* 263:2766–2771, 1990.

Law MR, Frost CD, Wald JN: III—Analysis of data from trials of salt reduction. *Br Med J* 302:819–824, 1991.

Lind L, Jacobson S, Palmer M, et al: Cardiovascular risk factors in primary hyperparathyroidism: A 15-year follow-up of operated and unoperated cases. *J Intern Med* 230:29–35, 1991.

Martin JE, Dubbert PM, Cushman WC: Controlled trial of aerobic exercise in hypertension. *Circulation* 81:1560–1567, 1990.

Mueller FB, Sealey JE, Case DB, et al: The captopril test for identifying renovascular disease in hypertensive patients. *Am J Med* 80:633–644, 1986.

Nally JV Jr, Chen C, Fine E, et al: Diagnosic criteria of renovascular hypertension with captopril renography. A consensus statement. *Am J Hypertens* 4:749S–752S, 1991.

Pickering TG: The role of laboratory testing in the diagnosis of renovascular hypertension. *Clin Chem* 37:1831–1837, 1991.

Schotte DE, Stunkard AJ: The effects of weight reduction on blood pressure in 301 obese patients. *Arch Intern Med* 150:1701–1704, 1990.

Stamler R, Stamler J, Gosch FC, et al: Primary prevention of hypertension by nutritional-hygienic means. Final report of a randomized, controlled trial. *JAMA* 262:1801–1807, 1989.

Streeten DHP, Anderson GH Jr, Howland T, et al: Effects of thyroid function on blood pressure. Recognition of hypothyroid hypertension. *Hypertension* 11:78–83, 1988.

Swain JF, Rouse IL, Curley CB, et al: Comparison of the effects of oat bran and low-fiber wheat on serum lipoprotein levels and blood pressure. *N Engl J Med* 322:147–152, 1990.

**The Fifth Report of the Joint National Committee on Detection, Evaluation, and Treatment of High Blood Pressure.* National Institutes of Health/National Heart, Lung and Blood Institute, 1993.

The good news about hypertension. National High Blood Pressure Education Program, National Heart, Lung, and Blood Institute. *Stat Bull Metrop Insur Co* 70(2):29, 1989.

Trials of Hypertension Prevention Collaborative Research Group: The effects of 2 nonpharamacologic interventions on blood pressure of persons with high normal levels. Results of the Trials of Hypertension Prevention, Phase 1. *JAMA* 267:1213–1220, 1992.

Whelton PK, Klag MJ: Magnesium and blood pressure: Review of the epidemiologic and clinical trials experience. *Am J Cardiol* 63:26G–30G, 1989.

Working Group on Ambulatory Blood Pressure Monitoring, National High Blood Pressure Coordinating Committee: National High Blood Pressure Education Program working group report on ambulatory blood pressure monitoring. *Arch Intern Med* 150:2270–2280, 1990.

Working Group on Management of Patients with Hypertension and High Blood Cholesterol: National Education Programs Working Group report on the management of patients with hypertension and high blood cholesterol. *Ann Intern Med* 114:224–237, 1991.

*These references are the same. The recommendations are available as a monograph from the NIH, but were published in the Archives of Internal Medicine.

Chapter 14

Current Concepts in Diabetes Mellitus

Abbas E. Kitabchi
Connie J. Holladay

Diabetes mellitus, a chronic disease state, is characterized by a relative or absolute deficiency of pancreatic insulin production and/or function. This, in turn, creates abnormal metabolism of carbohydrates, proteins, and fats resulting in hyperglycemia. Multiple metabolic, microvascular, and macrovascular complications follow. Therefore, patients with uncontrolled diabetes have a decreased life expectancy and a poorer quality of life compared to those without diabetes. In the United States and Western Europe, persons with diabetes have 2 times the risk of heart disease and stroke, 5 times the risk of peripheral vascular disease, 17 times the risk of renal disease, and 25 times the risk of blindness compared to nondiabetics.[1,2] It is therefore imperative that the primary practitioner understand the pathophysiology of the disease, make an early diagnosis to prevent or delay the onset of complications, and treat aggressively to prevent or delay the progression of disease.

EPIDEMIOLOGY

There are an estimated 14 million diabetics in the United States.[2] Fully half of those are undiagnosed, which translates into a huge health care problem.[3] In excess of $90 billion were spent in 1992 on diabetes care and hospitalization.[4]

Approximately 90% of all diabetics are type II. The incidence of type II diabetes is 600,000 per year in the United States. This disease is ethnically related, with a prevalence in Pima Indians of 35%, native Americans of 17%, Hispanics 12%, African-Americans 5%, and the general population 2.5%.[5]

Type I diabetes constitutes about 10% of all diabetes and accounts for about 3% of newly diagnosed cases per year. The incidence is similar in males and females. The incidence is higher in whites than in African-Americans and is much more common than in Hispanics, Asian-Americans, and Native Americans.[2]

TABLE 14.1 Characteristics of Two Spontaneous Forms of Diabetes

Characteristic	Type I (IDDM)	Type II (NIDDM)
Proportion of diabetics	~10%	~90%
Symptom occurrence	Subacute or acute	Gradual
Risk of ketoacidosis	Common	Rare
Seasonal trend	Fall and winter	None
Usual age of onset	<20 years old	>40 years old
Association with obesity	Uncommon	Common
Plasma insulin concentration	Decreased	Variable
Beta cell number	Decreased	Variable
Islet cell inflammation	Initially present	Absent
Association with HLA	Present	Absent
Family history of diabetes	Uncommon	Common
Concordance in identical twins	25–50%	90–95%
Islet cell antibodies	Present	Absent
Insulin autoantibodies	Present	Absent
Glutamic acid decarboxylase (GAD) antibodies	Present	Absent
Treatment	Diet and insulin	Diet ± oral hypoglycemics ± insulin

Source: Adapted from Ref. 1.

CLASSIFICATION

There are two major types of diabetes.[6] Type I, or insulin-dependent diabetes (IDDM), was formerly called *juvenile-onset diabetes*. It constitutes about 10% of all diabetics. Type II, or non-insulin-dependent diabetes (NIDDM), was formerly referred to as *adult onset diabetes*. It is by far the most common form, affecting about 90% of all diabetics. Of the type II diabetics, nearly 85% are obese. Table 14.1 gives the major features of these two types of diabetes.[1]

Type I Diabetes Mellitus

The less common of the two major forms of diabetes, type I (IDDM), has an estimated incidence rate of 15 per 100,000 in people younger than 20 years of age, with the rate dropping to 5 per 100,000 in those older than 20. So, although previously called *juvenile onset,* it can in fact occur at any age. There is a propensity for the development of ketosis since the major defects are the destruction of pancreatic beta cells and the absence of insulin. This occurs when more than 90% of the islet cells are destroyed. There is then a failure of efficient glucose metabolism in muscle, liver, and fat cells, all of which are insulin-dependent tissues.[7] Excess counterregulatory hormonal interaction involving glucagon, catecholamines, and cortisol follows, causing breakdown of muscle (proteolysis), fat (lipolysis), and glycogen stores (glycogenolysis). Excess release of amino acids, free fatty acids, and glycerol provides substrates for gluconeogenesis (i.e., glucose production in the presence of precursors from noncarbohydrate sources in the presence of an increased glucagon:insulin ratio), thus worsening the hyperglycemia and promoting ketogenesis in the liver. The results are diabetic ketoacidosis, coma, and even death if the patient is not adequately treated with insulin.[8]

Type I diabetes is thought to be an autoimmune process which is activated either by viral or toxic exposure to some environmental component. The seasonal tendency to develop the disease may point to a viral etiology. There is a strong association with human leukocyte antigen (HLA), especially the DR3 and DR4 genes. The DQ locus (DQW32) has been identified as the susceptibility gene for type I diabetes. Islet cell autoantibodies have been found in up to 85% of type I diabetics when tested in the first few weeks after diagnosis. The newly discovered "64K" antibody has now been identified to be glutamic acid decarboxylase (GAD). The antibody is present about 75% of the time at the diagnosis of type I diabetes, and it may persist for years.[9] Up to 60% of younger IDDM patients may also have insulin antibodies prior to being treated with insulin.

Type II Diabetes

People with type II diabetes (NIDDM) continue to produce insulin, but there is a deficiency in secretion and/or action. This may occur due to reduced beta cell mass, loss of pulsatile secretion of insulin, beta cell unresponsiveness to insulin (hyperinsulinemia), or even glucose toxicity. Although these persons produce normal and even supranormal amounts of insulin, there is a cellular defect which causes inefficient glucose utilization, otherwise known as *insulin resistance.*[10] Since some insulin is produced, ketosis does not develop. Metabolic decompensation in NIDDM is accompanied by a hyperglycemic, hyperosmolar, nonketotic state. However, ketosis may eventually occur if the person with NIDDM has progressed to an insulinopenic stage and is subjected to severe stresses such as intercurrent infections, myocardial infarction and so on.

The period of hyperinsulinemia is variable, and there may be progression from impaired glucose tolerance (IGT) to NIDDM to IDDM. This occurs as pancreatic insulin production gradually fails. The rate of conversion of IGT to overt diabetes is 5–8% per year, depending on the ethnic composition of the population. Insulin resistance is the hallmark of the disease, and obesity is a major contributing factor; 85% of type II diabetics are obese. When obesity and insulin resistance (hyperinsulinemia) are accompanied by hypertension and dyslipidemia, the condition is referred to as *Syndrome X.*[11]

There is a subclass of maturity-onset diabetes in the young (MODY) which occurs in late childhood or early adulthood. Circulating islet cell antibodies are rare in this form of disease compared to type I diabetes. MODY is inherited as an autosomal dominant trait. Another recessively inherited form of diabetes, called *type II diabetes of early onset,* occurs between the ages of 25 and 40. It may be difficult initially to classify new diabetics, especially during the "honeymoon phase" that may occur in type I. This occurs in the early phase of autoimmune islet cell destruction, when some insulin is initially produced prior to absolute insulinopenia. Close follow-up of those patients who at first require insulin after an episode of ketosis and then appear to be in remission is essential.

TABLE 14.2 Oral Glucose Tolerance Test in the Diagnosis of Impaired Glucose Tolerance (IGT) and Diabetes Mellitus (DM)

		Criteria of the WHO		Criteria of NDDG	
	Normal	IGT	DM	IGT	DM
Fasting	<115 mg/dL	<140 mg/dL *And*	<140 mg/dL *Or*	≥140 mg/dL *And*	≥140 mg/dL *Or*
2-h OGTT	<140mg/dL	140–199 mg/dL	≥200 mg/dL	140–199 mg/dL	≥200 mg/dL
OGTT (samples at 30-, 60-, and 90-min hr intervals)	<200 mg/dL	(Not required for diagnosis)		≥200 mg/dL	≥200 mg/dL

OGTT = oral glucose tolerance test; WHO = World Health Organization; NDDG = National Diabetes Data Group.
Source: Adapted from Ref. 12.

Impaired Glucose Tolerance

Impaired glucose tolerance (IGT), previously called *chemical diabetes,* is especially important when considering the scope of diabetes. It is even more prevalent than NIDDM and often heralds the progression to frank diabetes. Improvement in diagnosis and treatment at this stage could hopefully prevent many of the complications associated with NIDDM. A large multicenter study of the Diabetes Prevention Program (DPP), supported by the National Institutes of Health (NIH), has now been initiated in an attempt to modify the progression of disease by various interventional strategies.

IGT is the state of glucose control between normal and frank diabetes, as per the World Health Organization criteria (Table 14.2).[12] IGT is a risk factor for NIDDM and macrovascular disease, although it has not been shown to increase the risk of retinal, renal, or neuropathic complications. Eleven percent of Americans aged 20–74 have IGT compared to 7% with NIDDM. IGT is often associated with hyperinsulinemia. The risk of IGT increases with age; it also increases and parallels the risk of NIDDM in minority populations.[13] For this reason, screening of at-risk populations may prove prudent.

Diabetes Secondary to Other Disease Processes

Although types I and II diabetes are by far the most common forms of diabetes, other conditions may predispose to or cause hyperglycemia. These entities include diseases of the pancreas, other endocrine disorders, insulin receptor abnormalities, as in acanthosis nigricans, and drug toxicities. These are mentioned briefly just as a caution to rule out potentially curable diabetes.

Pancreatic disease requires the loss of at least two-thirds of the pancreas for diabetes to occur. Loss of pancreatic function may be due to pancreatectomy or chronic pancreatitis, whether caused by alcoholism or other reasons. The loss of pancreatic islet cells results in diabetes. Concomitant loss of pancreatic exocrine function causes other abnormalities, such as digestive disturbances, or loss of countregulatory hormonal function, as with glucagon deficiency. In these patients there is a tendency toward a wide swing of hypoglycemia or hyperglycemia (brittle diabetes) when treated with insulin because of the loss of counterregulation.

Other endocrine disorders can cause a type II picture of diabetes. This is often due to impaired peripheral responsiveness to insulin. Examples include increased production of glucocorticoids in Cushing's disease, growth hormone in acromegaly, and catecholamines in pheochromocytoma. Glucagonomas and somatostinomas may also yield a diabetes-type picture. When these diseases are treated, normalization of blood glucose occurs. Diabetes secondary to hyperaldosteronism is due to hypokalemia, which inhibits insulin secretion.

Some drugs may impair the utilization of glucose, so it is important to do a complete drug history for each patient. Examples are thiazides and phenytoin, which interfere with pancreatic insulin release; glucocorticoids and oral contraceptives, which may lead to insulin resistance peripherally; and pentamidine, which can destroy the pancreatic beta cells.

Other, much rarer forms include diabetes associated with certain diseases. These include ataxia-telangiectasia, Prader-Willi syndrome, leprechaunism, and some forms of myotonic dystrophy.[14]

SCREENING

Two types of screening will be addressed. The first is community programs, which are not done in physicians' offices or under direct physician supervision. The goal here is to determine risk factors for diabetes; if they are present, medical referral is given. Second are screenings done under direct physician supervision, with the intention to treat if diagnosed.

Plasma glucose determinations should be used as screening procedures only for those at risk for diabetes and for all pregnant women, usually those between weeks 24 and 28 of gestation. A glucose sample should be obtained diagnostically for anyone with symptoms of diabetes or complications consistent with diabetes. Recommendations for screening programs have been made by the American Diabetes Association.[15] The purpose is to identify asymptomatic individuals who have a high probability of having diabetes in the hope that early diagnosis and good control can prevent or delay the onset of complications.

Recommendations for screening by type of diabetes will now be discussed.

Type I Diabetes (IDDM)

Type I diabetes usually occurs in younger persons, represents only about 10% of diabetics, and tends to occur with an acute, symptomatic onset. Due to its low incidence and abrupt presentation, screening is unlikely to yield significant information and is not recommended.

Type II Diabetes (NIDDM)

Type II diabetes usually occurs in older persons (>30), with a more gradual onset; these persons may already have underlying pathology due to the disease. About 90% of all diabetics have NIDDM. Therefore, because of the increased prevalence of this disease and the possibility of ameliorating the underlying complications, this is an ideal group to screen.

Impaired Glucose Tolerance

Abnormal blood glucose levels which do not meet the criteria for diagnosis of diabetes (see below) are classified as IGT. These subjects are at risk for macrovascular complications and progression to frank diabetes mellitus. Wide screening for IGT is not recommended unless one is screening for risk factors in that group of people who are likely to have or develop NIDDM (those with more than one risk factor).

Gestational Diabetes Mellitus (GDM)

About 3% of women develop diabetes during pregnancy. Although the symptoms are usually mild, there are increased fetal complications and an increased fetal death rate in those with the disease. Therefore, it is important to determine the glucose status in all pregnant women. Women with GDM are also at risk for developing diabetes later, although pure GDM resolves with delivery.

RISK FACTORS APPROPRIATE FOR SCREENING

People should be screened who have one or more of the following risk factors:[15,16]

1. Obesity (>20% over ideal body weight), especially with upper body or central adiposity.
2. Ethnic group membership, including Native Americans, African-Americans, and Hispanics.
3. History of diabetes in first-degree relatives.
4. Hypertension.
5. A previous history of impaired glucose tolerance.
6. A woman who has a history of GDM or who has delivered a baby weighing >9 lb.
7. A history of recurrent genital, urinary, or skin infections.
8. Age above 65 years.

DIAGNOSIS OF DIABETES

Any person who has screened positive for diabetes or has classic signs and symptoms needs evaluation. Definitive diagnosis[6] is made by the following criteria.

Diabetes Mellitus

1. Classic symptoms of polyuria, polyphagia, and polydipsia accompanied by weight loss and a random blood glucose >200 mg/dL

   or

2. Fasting blood glucose >140 mg/dL on at least two occasions

   or

TABLE 14.3 Standardization of the OGTT

1. This test should be done only on otherwise ambulatory, healthy patients who do not have a definite diagnosis of diabetes.
2. Three days of an unrestricted diet of >150 g of carbohydrate and normal activity should precede the test.
3. There should be a 10- to 14-h fast just before the start of testing, which should begin in the morning.
4. A glucose load is given in the following amounts:
   75 g for adults
   100 g for pregnant women
   1.5 g/kg body weight for children to a maximum of 75 g
5. The patient should remain seated, should use no caffeine, and should not smoke during the examination.
6. Blood is drawn at 30-min intervals for 2 h in nonpregnant patients and hourly for 3 h in pregnant patients.

Source: Adapted from Ref. 3.

3. Plasma glucose concentration >200 mg/dL in at least two time periods during an oral glucose tolerance test (OGTT), i.e., 30, 60, 90 or 120 min. See Table 14.3 for the standard OGTT.

(Remember, if diabetes is diagnosed in steps 1 or 2, a glucose tolerance test is **not** indicated and could be extremely harmful.)

Impaired Glucose Tolerance

(World Health Organization criteria, which are different from American Diabetes Association criteria)

1. Fasting glucose >115 mg/dL but <140 mg/dL

   and

2. Blood glucose between 140 and 199 mg/dL at 2 h.

Gestational Diabetes

Table 14.4[6,17] gives information for the screening and diagnosis of GDM. Do not do an oral glucose tolerance test in a pregnant woman with diabetes, as serious hyperglycemia may ensue.

Initial Visit

The single most important aspect of good patient care is a thorough history and physical examination.[17] This becomes the baseline for treatment strategies and complete follow-up. This is the time to present information, as well as build lasting rapport with the patient. A diagnosis of diabetes can be devastating in some cases, requiring a complete lifestyle change in a person who may be resistant or in denial. It is a time for good medical advice and treatment, but it should also be a time for empathy and understanding by the physician.

TABLE 14.4 Screening and Diagnosis of GDM

Screening Process

1. Give a 50-g oral glucose load to all pregnant women who are not known to be glucose intolerant or diabetic. This should be done during the 24th through the 28th week of pregnancy.
2. The glucose load may be given regardless of when the last meal was taken.
3. A venous blood sample is taken 1 h later.
4. A venous glucose level ≥140 mg/dL is an indication for a full OGTT.

Definitive Diagnosis of GDM

1. A 100-g glucose load is given after an overnight fast of 8–14 h. The woman should have been on an unrestricted diet and activity for the preceding 3 days.
2. Glucose levels are measured while fasting and hourly for the next 3 h, for a total of four samples. The patient should remain seated, have no caffeine, and not smoke during the testing period.
3. More than two values exceeding the following limits is the basis for definitive diagnosis:
   Fasting ≥105 mg/dL
   1 hour ≥190 mg/dL
   2 hour ≥165 mg/dL
   3 hour ≥145 mg/dL

Source: Adapted from Refs. 6 and 7.

The medical history may disclose symptoms pointing to the diagnosis of diabetes or confirm a previous history of the disease. The history should include the following:

1. Reason for the visit, including any symptoms, results of any previous exams or laboratory tests, and any history of previous diabetes, impaired glucose tolerance, or GDM.
2. Nutritional history, including eating patterns, recent weight loss or gain, and growth and development patterns in the young patient.
3. Previous treatments and level of understanding of the disease.
4. Results of glycosylated hemoglobin values, if known.
5. Current medications, diet plan, type and results of glucose monitoring.
6. Previous hospitalizations, especially if required for diabetic ketoacidosis or a hyperosmolar state.
7. Presence of other endocrine disorders.
8. History of eating disorders.
9. History of recurrent urinary, oral, foot, genital, or skin infections, especially candidiasis.
10. Exercise history.
11. Risk factors for atherosclerosis, including smoking, obesity, family history, hyperlipidemia, and hypertension.
12. Complete review of systems to determine whether complications have already occurred. This should include ocular (especially fluctuating acuity), oral (mouth pain and poor dentition), cardiovascular, gastrointestinal, renal, genitourinary (including sexual function), cerebrovascular, peripherovascular, and complete neurologic complaints.
13. Complete medication history, including prescribed and over-the-counter medications.
14. Family history of diabetes and other endocrine disorders.
15. Complete obstetric history, including miscarriages, toxemia, birth of a child weighing >9 lb, polyhydramnios, or any other complications.

16. A complete social history, including educational level, present lifestyle, living arrangements, means of transportation and communication, economic situation including occupation and avocation, and support systems.

The physical examination should be thorough and include the following:

1. General assessment of nutritional status and appearance.
2. Height and weight. It may be helpful to calculate the body mass index (BMI):

$$\text{BMI} = \frac{\text{Body wt (kg)}}{\text{height } (\text{M}^2)}$$

3. Blood pressure should include sitting and standing measurements to check for evidence of orthostasis.
4. Ophthalmologic examination, including visual acuity, extraocular muscle function, and retinal exam (with dilation if possible).
5. Oral examination with attention to dental and periodontal disease, and examination of the tongue and buccal mucosa.
6. Neck examination should include palpation of the thyroid.
7. Cardiac examination should note the presence of murmurs, rubs, gallops, hypertrophy on palpation of the chest wall, and other abnormalities.
8. Abdominal examination should include palpation for evidence masses, hepatosplenomegaly, and so on.
9. Palpation and auscultation of all pulses to evaluate for character of the pulse and presence of bruits.
10. Close examination of the hands and feet, with note of any infection.
11. Close examination of the skin, especially insulin injection sites, noting any areas of poor healing.
12. Thorough neurologic examination for any signs of loss of vibratory, positional, light touch, pain sensation, or motor strength, as well as deep tendon reflex abnormalities.
13. Breast examination.
14. Genitourinary evaluation, including Pap smear and bimanual examination, should be offered if not done recently.

Laboratory Examination

The ability to do blood glucose and urine ketone tests in the office is essential for treatment of the diabetic patient. After establishment of the diagnosis of diabetes, specific laboratory tests are ordered to evaluate glycemic control and test for the presence of other diseases associated with or resulting from the diabetes. These tests should include the following:

1. Fasting glucose level.
2. A random glucose level can be used for screening in an undiagnosed patient with symptoms that may be attributable to diabetes.
3. Glycohemoglobin A_{1c} (HbA_{1c}).
4. Renal function tests, including creatinine and blood urea nitrogen.
5. Urinalysis, including glucose, protein, nitrites, ketones, and sediment.
6. Urine culture if indicated by urinalysis.

7. Complete lipid profile, including total cholesterol, high and low density lipoprotein cholesterol, and triglyceride levels.
8. Thyroid studies (at least thyroid-stimulating hormone and free thyronine).
9. Electrocardiogram in adults.
10. Liver function tests (if therapy with oral agents is planned or if evidence of hepatic disease exists).

TREATMENT STRATEGIES

Diabetes is a chronic disease, and the patient will have to adapt to a lifetime of change. It is therefore recommended that he or she be under the care of a multidisciplinary team of health care providers. This should include the physician, a registered dietitian, a diabetes educator, and a mental health specialist. Sometimes the physician will need to assume several of these roles. He or she should be fully versed in total treatment or refer the patient to such a multidisciplinary program.

The Diabetes Control and Complications Trial (DCCT), a 10-year NIH-supported multicentered trial studied 1441 patients with IDDM with intensive vs. conventional therapy of insulin for a mean follow-up of 6-1/2 years in a prospective randomized fashion. There was conclusive evidence that intensive therapy decreased the onset and progression of diabetic complications in IDDM patients. Microvascular complications leading to development of nephropathy, retinopathy, neuropathy were significantly reduced by 54, 76, and 60%, respectively. Hyperglycemia was reduced, as evidenced by reduction of HbA_{1c} toward normal levels, with the goal being <7%, and blood glucose levels of 70–120 mg/dL preprandially and at bedtime, and <180 mg/dL 1.5–2 h postprandially in IDDM with the use of three or more insulin injections or insulin pump. Intensive therapy in these groups was associated with a threefold increase in the incidence of hypoglycemia and an increase in weight. The ability to check blood glucose levels frequently, follow nutritional advice, and solve problems is necessary for tight control.[18] Although NIDDM was not specifically addressed by the DCCT, it would seem appropriate to follow a similar course of normalizing glucoses and HbA_{1c} since micro- and macrovascular complications also occur in this type of diabetes. The therapeutic regimen may be different since insulin is not always a part of the treatment, and hyperinsulinemia and insulin resistance may predominate.[19]

Education is the key to good diabetic control. No matter how much good information is given, if the patient does not understand the disease, hyperglycemia will not be well controlled and complications are almost certain to develop.[16]

DIETARY GUIDELINES

The key to treatment of any type of diabetes is in dietary management. The goal is establishment and maintenance of ideal body weight (IBW) in both the nonpregnant and pregnant woman. IBW can be determined as follows:

For women, use 100 lb for the first 5 ft and add 5 lb for each additional inch.
For males, use 110 lb for the first 5 ft and add 6 lb for each inch thereafter.

Caloric requirements are then determined for each patient by multiplying IBW by 10 and adding 30–100% for daily activity. The patient with IDDM may be of normal

TABLE 14.5 Metabolic Goals in the Treatment of Diabetes Mellitus

	Normal	Goal	Consider Treatment
Blood glucose (mg/dL)			
Fasting			
Nonpregnant	70–115	70–120	<70 or >140
Pregnant	60–90	<100	<50 or >120
Postprandial			
Nonpregnant	<140	<180	>180
Pregnant	<120	≤120	>140
Glycosylated hemoglobin			
HbA_{1c} (%)	4.5–6	6–8	>8
Lipids (mg/dL)			
Triglycerides	<150	<150	≥200
Total cholesterol	<200	<200	≥200
LDL cholesterol	<130	<130	≥130
HDL cholesterol			
Females	>45	>45	≤45
Males	>35	>35	≤35

Source: Adapted from Ref. 16.

weight or even underweight. The patient with NIDDM is more likely to be obese. Once the calorie level has been established, the dietary components are divided as follows:

50–55% as carbohydrates, especially complex carbohydrates. Limitation of refined and simple sugars should be stressed.

15–20% as protein, with emphasis on poultry, fish, veal, and vegetable sources to decrease the level of saturated fats obtained with red meat.

30% as fat. There should be more intake of the monounsaturated fats, such as in olive oil and canola oil, less of the polyunsaturated fats, and least of the unsaturated fats.

30 g/day of dietary fiber. Insoluble fiber, such as that found in bran, increases intestinal transit time, which helps relieve constipation. Soluble fiber, as found in fruits and beans, decreases gastric and intestinal transit time, which helps stabilize blood glucose. For patients with a previous history of low fiber intake, it is prudent to advise them that they may have increased gas formation until they adjust to the diet.

The goals of dietary treatment are to return the person to a normal metabolic state. These goals are summarized in Table 14.5.[16] The bases of diet therapy are five: (1) achieve and maintain normal weight, (2) reduce hyperinsulinemia, (3) reduce and maintain lipids, (4) achieve and maintain normal blood pressure, and (5) provide essential vitamins and minerals. It goes without saying that the diet must incorporate the diabetic's food preferences. This can be most effectively accomplished on a one-to-one basis with an understanding nutritionist.

ORAL HYPOGLYCEMIA AGENTS

Table 14.6[12,20] lists the first- and second-generation oral hypoglycemia agents approved by the Food and Drug Administration for use in the United States. They are all sulfonylureas, with the exception of metformin, which has been recently released.

The proposed mechanism of action of the sulfonylureas includes the potentiation of insulin action at the target site and augmented release of insulin from the pancreas. Therefore, the patient must be able to produce some insulin for the drugs to have any effect, hence the warning that IDDM patients *cannot* be treated with these agents.

TABLE 14.6 Oral Hypoglycemic Agents

Generic Name	Trade Name	Daily Dosage	Duration of Action (h)	Comments
		First-Generation Sulfonylureas		
Chlorpropamide	Diabinese	100–500 mg, single dose	60	Causes hyponatremia, disulfiram effect, prolonged hypoglycemia
Tolbutamide	Orinase	1.5–3.0 g, divided doses	6–12	Hepatic metabolism to inactive product and short half-life better for the elderly
Tolazamide	Tolinase	100–1000 mg, single or divided	12–24	Slowly absorbed, hepatic and renal excretion
Acetohexamide	Dymelor	250–1500 mg, single or divided	12–24	Hepatic metabolism and renal excretion
		Second-Generation Sulfonylureas		
Glipizide	Glucotrol	2.5–20 mg, single or divided	3–8	Lower potency and short half-life better for the elderly
	Glucotrol XL	5–20 mg, single dose	24	Controlled release with sustained plasma levels
Glyburide	Diabeta, Micronase	1.25–20 mg, single or divided	16–24	Hepatic metabolism with hepatic and renal excretion
	Glynase	0.75–12 mg, single or divided	12–24	Small particle size causes rapid absorption
		Biguanides		
Metformin	Glucophage	1.5–2.5 g	Plasma $T_{1/2}$ ~5.5	Hepatic metabolism and renal excretion, may be used alone or in combination therapy

Source: Adapted from Refs. 12 and 20.

First-generation sulfonylureas include the long-acting drugs chlorpropamide, tolazamide, and acetohexamide and the shorter-acting tolbutamide (see Table 14.6). *Tolbutamide* has a shorter duration of action because it is completely oxidized by the liver and is therefore independent of renal function. For these reasons, it is probably the safest to use in the elderly when hypoglycemia would pose a serious risk. Skin rashes are the most common side effect; acute toxic reactions are rare. *Chlorpropamide* is slowly metabolized by the liver, with about 20–30% excreted unchanged by the kidney. Metabolites retain hypoglycemia effects and are almost completely excreted by the kidney; therefore, this drug is contraindicated in renal insufficiency. It is the most potent of the first-generation drugs, and with its long half-life, it is the most likely to cause prolonged hypoglycemia. The incidence of jaundice increases at doses >500 mg/day. Other side effects include hyponatremia and a disulfiram-like reaction in some patients who ingest alcohol. In less than 1% of patients, transient leukopenia and thrombocytopenia occur. *Tolazamide* is comparable to chlorpropamide in potency but does not have the disulfiram-like reaction or cause water retention. It is more slowly absorbed than other agents, and its long duration of action can cause prolonged hypoglycemia. *Acetohexamide* has an intermediate duration of action, has rapid hepatic metabolism, but does excrete active metabolites by the kidney. It does not have the water-retaining or disulfiram-like properties of chlorpropamide.

Second-generation medications include the more potent and shorter-acting glyburide and glipizide. Both are metabolized by the liver, with by-products that are renally excreted and so are contraindicated in persons with renal or hepatic impairment. *Glyburide* is the longer-acting of the two. The maximum dose is 20 mg/day. It does not cause water retention, and the most common side effect is its hypoglycemic potential. *Glipizide* is shorter-acting and equipotent to glyburide, and it provides a lower postprandial blood glucose level than glyburide. It must be taken on an empty stomach about 30 min before meals. The newer, long-acting forms of these oral hypoglycemic agents (Glynase and Glucotrol XL) can be given as one dose per day.

Metformin is a biguanide. This drug does not require intact pancreatic beta cell function in order to have an effect. The exact mechanism of action is not known, but it decreases fasting and postprandial blood glucose levels in type II diabetics and has no effect on a normal person's blood glucose. A benefit of therapy is the improvement of hypertriglyceridemia and hyperglycemia without the concomitant weight gain often seen with the oral hypoglycemic agents and insulin. The ability to correct hyperglycemia while sparing insulin makes it particularly helpful in treating patients with insulin resistance. It is contraindicated in patients with chronic renal (serum creatine ≥1.4 mg/dL) or hepatic disease and absolutely contraindicated in those with a propensity to develop acidosis, including those with cardiorespiratory insufficiency, advanced age, and alcoholism.[14]

INSULIN

Insulin is the mainstay of therapy for type I diabetics and for type II diabetics who require insulin. The types of commercially prepared insulins are noted in Table 14.7.[14,16] With the development of highly purified human insulin, many of the previous problems with immunogenicity have been circumvented. Immune insulin resistance, insulin allergies, and localized lipoatrophy have been greatly reduced.

TABLE 14.7 Summary of Bioavailability Characteristics of the Insulins

Type of Insulin	Trade Name	Onset	Peak Action	Duration
Short-acting	Regular Velosulin Semitard Semilente	15–30 min	1–3 h	5–7 h
Intermediate-acting	Lente, Lentard Monotard, NPH Insulatard Protaphane	30–60 min	4–6 h	12–16 h
Long-acting	Ultralente, PZI Ultratard	4–5 h	8–14 h	25–36 h

Source: Adapted from Refs. 14 and 16.

There are some newer insulin mixtures of intermediate NPH and short-acting regular insulin in a 50/50 or 70/30 combination. These may be very useful in patients with IDDM who are too young or unable to mix the insulins. Some type II diabetics may use them either alone or in combination with oral agents. There is some evidence that insulin in combination with oral agents may improve glucose control, but this has not been accepted by all diabetes experts.

Studies have estimated that basal insulin secretion is approximately 1 U/h, for a total of 24 U/day. Postprandial insulin secretion is about 25 U/day. It is secreted in response to meals through multiple mechanisms of gastric and cephalic phases. Therefore, the total estimated secretion in a 70-kg man is about 49 U, or about 0.7 U/kg. The IDDM treatment guidelines set forth in Table 14.8 reflect an attempt to reproduce this physiologic phenomenon. Other regimens include three injections per day (tid) insulin dosing, and multidose injections (MDI) preprandially and at bedtime, using sliding-scale regular insulin along with intermediate or long-acting insulin (Figure 14.1). Continuous subcutaneous insulin infusion (CSII) delivers a basal rate of insulin, with "bursts" of insulin given preprandially in accordance with a sliding scale based on blood glucose values. The MDI regimen or CSII use may require consultations with a diabetologist.

Present preparations of insulin should be given 30 min before a meal unless the preprandial blood glucose level is <60, in which case it should be given with the meal. With higher preprandial glucose levels, we recommend a longer waiting period after insulin injections before the meal is taken (e.g., if blood glucose is 200–250 mg/dL, wait 45 min; if it is 250–300 mg/dL, wait 60 min). There is one caveat regarding the use of ultralente (UL) insulin with regular insulin. When UL is mixed with regular insulin, it should be injected within a few minutes of mixing; otherwise, the effectiveness of the regular insulin will be nullified.

GENERAL GUIDELINES FOR MANAGEMENT OF TYPE I AND TYPE II DIABETES

Management differs when treating different types of diabetes and is the reason that classification is important. The treatment strategies are listed in Tables 14.8 and 14.9.[16]

TABLE 14.8 Management Guidelines for the Type I Diabetic (IDDM)

1. Establish the diagnosis by the WHO or NDDG criteria (listed in Table 14.3). Then classify as to type I.
2. Inform the patient of the diagnosis and refer to diabetes education classes, which should include counseling in nutrition, glucose monitoring, use of insulin, complications, etc.
3. Prescribe a diet based on ADA recommendations with 50% carbohydrates, 30% protein, and 20% fat. Caloric needs should be calculated and based on suitability for growth, development, and maintenance of IBW.
4. Do not give oral hypoglycemic agents for type I diabetes.
5. At least 3 meals a day with a bedtime snack are needed.
6. Give insulin based on actual body weight (0.5–0.8 U/kg), with 40–60% of the total as intermediate-acting and the rest as short-acting insulin.
7. BID insulin, given as short- and intermediate-acting insulin, must be given to all IDDM patients.
8. Therapeutic goals should be FBG 70–120 mg/dL, 2-h PPBG ≤180 mg/dL, and no blood glucose levels <50 mg/dL.
9. Divide the dosage of intermediate-acting insulin, with half given before breakfast and half before supper or bedtime.
10. Consider short-acting (regular) insulin injections before each meal and intermediate- or long-acting insulin at bedtime if bid dosing does not achieve the therapeutic goal.
11. Give short-acting (regular) insulin 30 min before each meal or snack. Adjust regular insulin dose based on preprandial blood glucose level and/or number of grams of carbohydrate intake.
12. Give a bedtime snack if short-acting (regular) insulin is given at bedtime and the blood glucose level is ≤200 mg/dL.
13. Initial patient follow-up visit is every 2 weeks until the glucose level is stabilized; then schedule a visit every 1–3 months to assess glycemic control and compliance with diet, and check for evidence of chronic complications.
14. Refer brittle diabetics (those with wide swings in their blood glucoses) to a diabetologist.

WHO = World Health Organization; NDDG = National Diabetes Data Group; ADA = American Diabetes Association; bid = twice a day; FBG = fasting blood glucose; PPBG = postprandial blood glucose.

Source: Adapted from Ref. 16.

The key difference in treatment to remember is that type I diabetes *always* needs insulin, whereas type II diabetes can usually be treated without it. An algorithm for management of type II diabetes is presented in Figure 14.2.

In both diseases, treatment is geared to the individual and must be tailored to his or her lifestyle. The assessment of glycemic control should be followed and records meticulously kept. The flow sheet used in our outpatient endocrine clinic is reproduced in Figure 14.3.

In the treatment of diabetes, the emphasis must be placed on the patient's understanding of the disease process and willingness to comply. This is one disease in which compliance is essential to prevent complications. A diabetes educator must discuss all aspects of the condition, with oral and especially written instructions that the patient can follow. It is not enough to state that the patient must follow an American Diabetes Association diet unless he or she has a copy of the diet and knows how to use it. The patient needs to be shown how to monitor blood glucoses, record results, what to do when the values are high or low, and how to monitor for signs of disease progression, such as good foot care, evidence of infection, and so on.

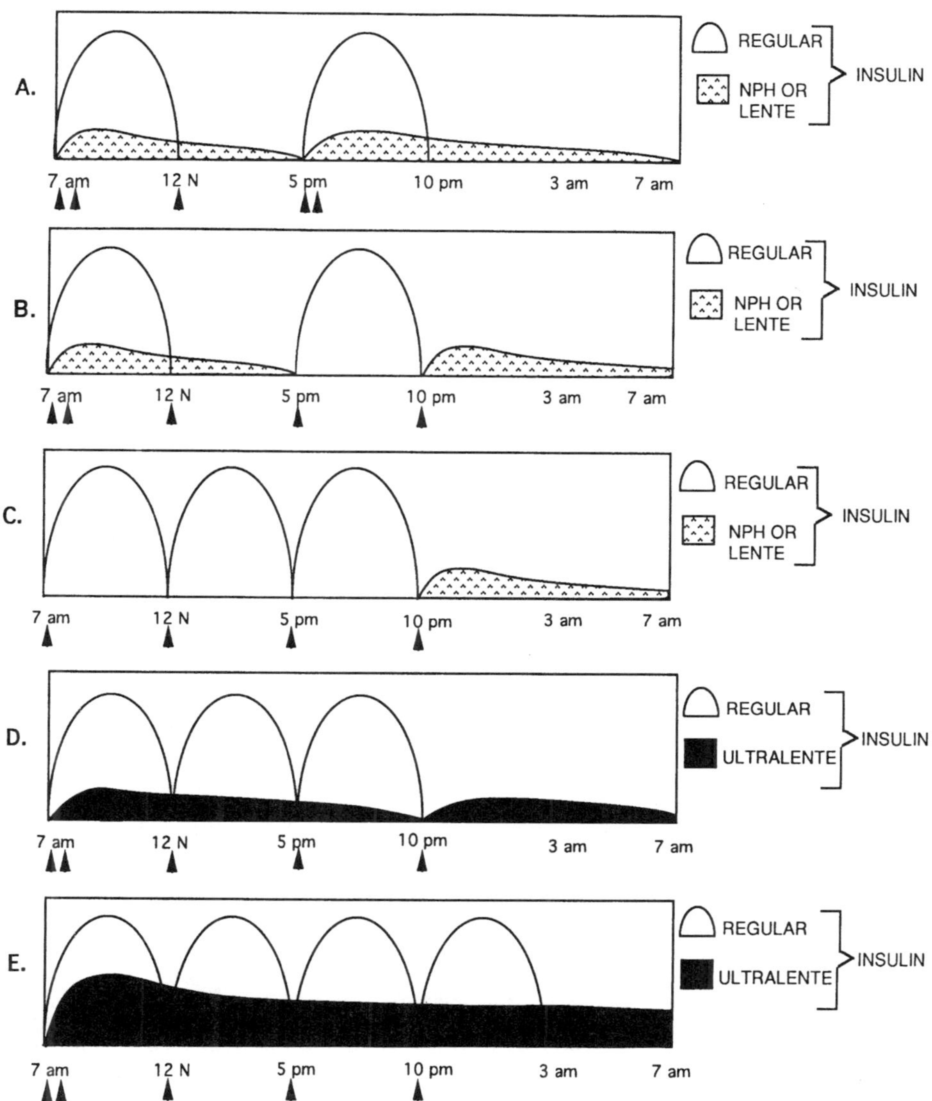

Figure 14.1 Proposed methods of insulin injection schedules in IDDM patients. (From Kitabchi AE, Diabetes mellitus. In Seltzer VL, Pearse WH [eds]. *Women's Primary Health Care: Office Practice and Procedures.* New York, McGraw-Hill, 1995, pp 541–553). Reproduced from Ref. 16 with permission.

TABLE 14.9 Management Guidelines for the Type II Diabetic (NIDDM)

1. Establish the diagnosis by the WHO or NDDG criteria (Table 14.3). Then classify as to type II.
2. Inform the patient of the diagnosis and refer to diabetes education classes. At this point, address risk factor interventions dealing with smoking, exercise, lipids, etc. Exercise should be prescribed of at least 100 kcal/day (about a 1-mile walk) with a total of 700 kcal/wk.
3. Place the patient on an ADA diet consisting of 50% carbohydrates, 30% protein, and 20% fat to achieve and maintain IBW. Three meals a day are recommended. In a majority of the cases, the patient will be obese and should be started on a weight reduction diet, with the goal of reducing weight by 7% in 6 months if >130% IBW.
4. While on the diet, check FBG by fingerstick every day for 2 months. The FBG will gradually decline during this period if diet and exercise are effective. If the FBG has not improved or worsens, consider oral hypoglycemic agents (OHA) if the patient
   Is not pregnant.
   Has had diabetes for <10 years.
   Has no history of severe renal or hepatic diseases.
   Has no allergy to sulfonylureas.
   Has no history of acidosis (in using metformin).
5. After adequate dietary restriction, the patient with an FBG ≥250 mg/day is not suitable for OHA.
6. Check the patient every 2 months while on OHA. FBG and 2 HPPBG are checked in the office at this time, and the patient should do daily monitoring of FBG and 2 HPPBG at home.
   If 2 HPPBG is <200 mg/dL, stop the OHA, place the patient on diet alone, and follow every 1–2 months.
   If FBG is consistently >20 mg/dL, begin insulin therapy.
7. Calculate the insulin dosage based on actual body weight at 0.5–1.0 U/kg weight.
8. For total insulin requirements 30 Units/day, may try to give the entire dose as NPH or Lente before a major meal and check control of hyperglycemia. The goals are FBG <140 mg/dL, 2 HPPBG <200 mg/dL, and no glucose <60 mg/dL.
9. If a single insulin dose cannot achieve the glycemic goals, insulin can be given as a mixture of regular: NPH (50:50) bid, 30 min before breakfast and 30 min before supper.
10. Very obese diabetics may be insulin resistant and require more insulin/per kilogram body weight and a greater percentage of the total insulin given as regular insulin than less obese or normal-weight diabetics.
11. If the above regimen fails to control the hyperglycemia, consider multiple regular insulin injections before each meal and NPH or Lente at bedtime.
12. Insulin-resistant diabetics who require >200 U insulin per day should be referred to a diabetologist.

WHO = World Health Organization; NDDG = National Diabetes Data Group; ADA = American Diabetes Association; IBW = Ideal Body Weight; bid = twice a day; FBG = Fasting blood glucose; 2 HPPBG = 2-h postprandial blood glucose; OHA = oral hypoglycemic agents; NPH = Neutral Protamine Hagedorn.

Source: Adapted from Ref. 16.

Continuing Care

The frequency of patient visits initially depends on the severity of the diabetes, the regimen implemented, and the presence of complications. Patients who are being treated with diet or oral agents should be contacted weekly until glycemic control is achieved. Those who are beginning insulin treatment or are having a major change in their therapy should be contacted daily until the diabetes is well controlled and the risk of hypoglycemia is reduced. There are times where hospitalization may be necessary for initiating or changing therapy.

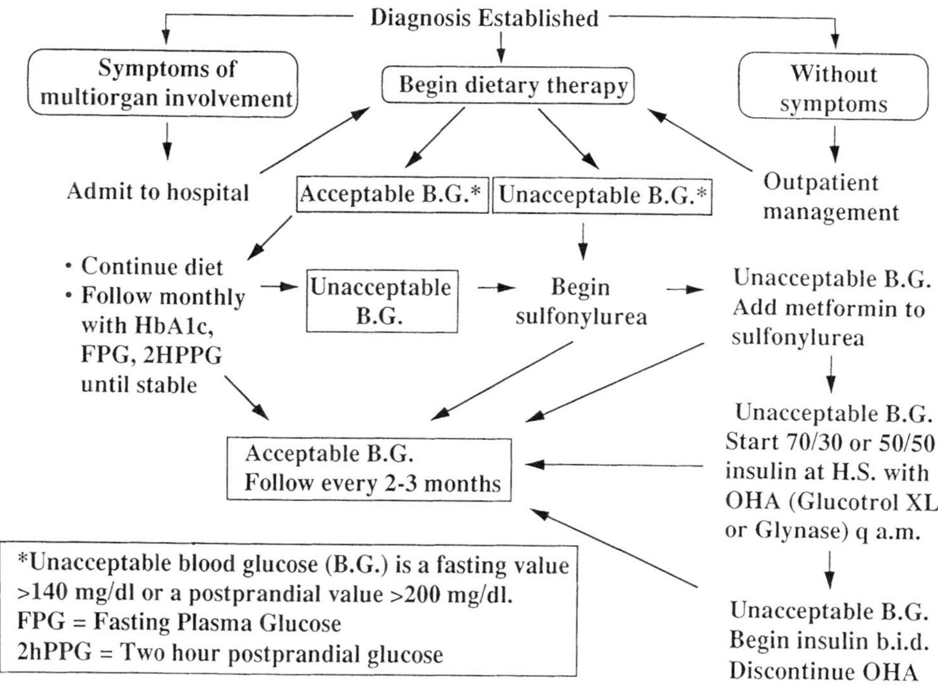

Figure 14.2 Medical management of NIDDM. NIDDM = non-insulin-dependent diabetes mellitus; BG = blood glucose; FBG = fasting blood glucose; 2 HPPBG = 2-h postprandial blood glucose; HbA_{1c} = hemoglobin A_{1c}, OHA = oral hypoglycemic agents. 70/30 and 50/50 insulins are premixed preparations of NPH and regular insulin in the proportions noted. Reproduced from Ref. 16 with permission.

After adequate control of the diabetes has been achieved, visits for patients on insulin should be scheduled every 2 to 3 months and for others every 3 to 6 months, depending on the patient. The interim history should include review of self-monitored glucose results, any episodes of hyper- or hypoglycemia and the surrounding circumstances, current medications, other illnesses, symptoms suggesting complications, and any change in the patient's social history. The physical examination needs to include height, weight, and blood pressure. A fundoscopic exam should be done regularly, and ophthalmologic consultation arranged at least annually for all patients 12 years of age and over with diabetes for more than 5 years, all patients over 30, and any patient with vision abnormalities. The feet need to be checked at each visit and the lower extremities evaluated for peripheral neuropathy or vascular insufficiency. An examination of any other area is done based on the current history. Laboratory tests should include quarterly glycosylated hemoglobins. We recommend a random blood glucose check at each visit, which may also be useful in comparing home monitored glucose levels. Abnormal lipid profiles need to be monitored annually unless the patient is taking lipid-lowering agents, which will increase the frequency of the determinations, as well as a liver function profile. Routine urinalysis should be done annually or if the patient is symptomatic. If albuminuria or proteinuria occurs, the creatinine and blood urea nitrogen values should be obtained.

NAME: ADDRESS:	PRIMARY DX: DATE: AGE:
PH: (H) (W) CONTACT: SSN: INS. DOB: RACE*: C B I H O	OTHER DX'S: DATE: REFER MD:

DATE						
HEIGHT / WEIGHT						
BMI / W/H						
WAIST / HIP						
BP / P						
GLUCOSE / C-PEP	F					
GLUCOSE / C-PEP	PP					
WBC / Hct						
HbA1c / UA						
CR / BUN						
CRCL / M'ALB						
GFR / OTHER PROC.						
CHOL / TG						
HDL / LDL						
FT4 / TSH						
T3 / Abn.SMAC						
EYES / NEURO.						
PAP Smr. / MAMMGR.						
RECTAL / FEET						
MEAL PLANS						
MEDICINES						
OTHER Rx OR CHANGES						
REFERRALS						
COMMENTS						

* RACE = C/Caucasian; B/Black; I/Indian; H/Hispanic; O/Other

Figure 14.3 UT Diabetes/Endocrine Outpatient Follow-Up Sheet

Indications for Hospitalization

Criteria have been established for determining the appropriateness of hospitalization.[15] These include the following:

1. Acute, life-threatening complications of diabetes.
   a. Diabetic ketoacidosis—blood glucose level >250 mg/dL; arterial pH <7.30; serum bicarbonate <15; and ketonuria or ketonemia.
   b. Hyperosmolar nonketotic state—glucose ≥6400 mg/dL; plasma osmolality ≥315 mOsm; and altered mental status.
   c. Hypoglycemia with neurologic symptoms.
      i. Glucose level <50 mg/dL, with no change in mental status after treatment.
      ii. Coma, seizures, behavioral changes due to hypoglycemia.
      iii. Sulfonylurea-induced hypoglycemia.
      iv. Instances of treated hypoglycemia where the patient would be without supervision for the next 12 h.
2. Poor metabolic control when necessary to determine the etiology and correct it.
3. New-onset diabetes in children and adolescents.
4. Newly diagnosed or uncontrolled diabetes in pregnancy.
5. Severe illness unrelated to diabetes but adversely affecting glycemic control or complications of diabetes and requiring intensive treatment.
6. Implementation of insulin pump therapy or other regimens of intensive insulin therapy.

Other Considerations

The DCCT has demonstrated that good glycemic control in the type I diabetic, as evidenced by a glycosylated HbA_{1c} level of 7%, reduced the risk of microvascular complications 40–60%. Achievement of this goal requires a team approach.[18] Some office settings are not able to provide this entire team, but the practitioner can work with a network of local health care professionals to provide the level of care the patient will need. A good reference point is the American Diabetes Association or the American Association of Diabetes Educators.

Patients should be referred to a diabetologist under certain circumstances. These include patients with brittle diabetes who have unpredictable and unacceptable variations in blood glucose levels. Other patients who need referral are diabetics on multidose regimens or insulin pumps, those who are pregnant or considering pregnancy, and those who are insulin resistant and require >200 U/day of insulin. Those diabetics with multisystem complications may also need referral to other subspecialists.

REFERENCES

1. Kitabchi AE, Fisher JN: Diabetes mellitus. In Conn R (ed): *Current Diagnosis*. Philadelphia, WB Saunders, 1991, pp 766–774.
2. Harris MI, Hadden WC, Knowler WC, et al: Prevalence of diabetes and impaired glucose tolerance and plasma glucose levels in the U.S. population aged 20–74. *Diabetes* 36:523–534, 1987.

3. Harris MI: Undiagnosed NIDDM: Clinical and public health issues. *Diabetes Care* 16:642–652, 1993.
4. Ray NF, Wills S, Thamer M: *Direct and Indirect Costs of Diabetes in the United States in 1992.* The American Diabetes Association Report. Washington, DC, Medical Technology and Practice Pattern Institute, December 1993.
5. Harris MI: Epidemiological correlates of NIDDM in Hispanics, whites, and blacks in the U.S. population. *Diabetes Care* 14:639–648, 1991.
6. National Diabetes Data Group: Classification and diagnosis of diabetes mellitus and other categories of glucose intolerance. *Diabetes* 28:1039–1057, 1979.
7. Eisenbarth GS: Type I diabetes mellitus: A chronic autoimmune disorder. *N Engl J Med* 314:1360–1368, 1986.
8. Kitabchi AE, Fisher JN, Murphy MB, et al: Diabetes ketoacidosis and hyperglycemic hyperosmolar nonketotic state. In Kahn CR, Weir G (eds): *Joslin's Diabetes Mellitus Textbook,* ed 13. Philadelphia, Lea & Febiger, 1994, pp 738–770.
9. Clare-Salzer MJ, Tobin AJ, Kaufman DL: Glutamate decarboxylase: An autoantigen in IDDM. *Diabetes Care* 15:132, 1992.
10. DeFronzo RA, Bonadonna RC, Ferrannini E: Pathogenesis of NIDDM, a balanced overview. *Diabetes Care* 15:369–395, 1992.
11. Karam JH: Type II diabetes and Syndrome X: Pathogenesis and glycemic management. *Endocrinol Metab Clin North Am* 21:329–350, 1992.
12. In Raskin P (ed): *Medical Management of Non-Insulin-Dependent (Type II) Diabetes,* ed 3., Alexandria, VA, American Diabetes Association, 1994.
13. Yudkin JS, Alberti KGMM, McLarty DG, et al: Impaired glucose tolerance: Is it a risk factor for diabetes or a diagnostic ragbag? *Br Med J* 301:397–402, 1990.
14. Karam JH, Forsham PH: Pancreatic hormones and diabetes mellitus. In Greenspan FS, Baxter JD (eds): *Basic and Clinical Endocrinology.* Englewood Cliffs, NJ: Appleton and Lange, 1991, pp 571–631.
15. American Diabetes Association: Standards of medical care for patients with diabetes mellitus. *Diabetes Care* 18:8–15, 1995.
16. Kitabchi AE, Murphy MB, Sherman AR, et al: Diabetes mellitus. In Ling FW, Laube DW, Nolan TE, et al (eds): *Primary Care in Gynecology.* Baltimore, Williams & Wilkins, 1996, chap. 20.
17. O'Sullivan JB, Mahan CM: Criteria for the oral glucose tolerance test in pregnancy. *Diabetes* 13:278–285, 1964.
18. The DCCT Research Group: The effect of intensive treatment of diabetes on the development and progression of long-term complications in insulin-dependent diabetes mellitus. *N Engl J Med* 329:977–986, 1993.
19. American Diabetes Association Position Statement on Application of DCCT Results to NIDDM, Alexandria, VA: American Diabetes Association, 1993.
20. Lebovitz HE: Oral antidiabetic agents. In Kahn CR, Weir GC (eds): *Joslin's Diabetes Mellitus.* Philadelphia: Lea & Febiger, 1994, pp 508–529.

Chapter 15

Clinical and Reproductive Genetics

Jeffrey A. Kuller
Jerome Yankowitz

Medical genetics is one of the most rapidly expanding fields in medicine. As the Human Genome project continues its daunting task of mapping our entire genetic code, a gene for an inherited disorder is mapped almost each week. The obstetrician-gynecologist must maintain current knowledge of these advances to counsel patients adequately and know when to refer them to a geneticist for further evaluation. An increasing number of obstetrician-gynecologists (including the authors of this chapter) have received fellowship training and board certification in medical genetics; they may provide a resource to fellow obstetrician-gynecologists. The purpose of this chapter is to outline several common conditions encountered by the obstetrician-gynecologist. Common genetic conditions that can be diagnosed during pregnancy are listed in Table 15.1.[1] After an overview of inheritance patterns, the chapter will be organized according to the genetic screening questions, as noted in the American College of Obstetricians and Gynecologists (ACOG) prenatal record (shown in Table 15.2). This ACOG form has been adapted and modified by many centers.[2] It deals with questions concerning maternal age, family history of Down syndrome and chromosomal abnormalities, neural tube defects, congenital malformations, mental retardation, spontaneous abortions, certain Mendelian disorders, and maternal serum screening. We will conclude the chapter with an overview of future techniques of genetic diagnosis.

OVERVIEW OF PATTERNS OF SINGLE-GENE INHERITANCE

The clinician's determination of the type of inheritance for a genetic condition is potentially improved by guidelines described in Thompson and Thompson's *Genetics in Medicine.*[3]

TABLE 15.1 Common Genetic Conditions that Can Be Diagnosed by Amniocentesis and/or CVS

Chromosomal abnormalities	Ornithine transcarbamylase deficiency
Cystic fibrosis	Phenylketonuria
Tay-Sachs disease	Retinoblastoma
Hemophilia A	α_1 Antitrypsin deficiency
Hemophilia B	Congenital adrenal hyperplasia
Sickle cell anemia	Lesch-Nyhan syndrome
α-Thalassemia	Myotonic dystrophy
β-Thalassemia	Duchenne muscular dystrophy
Becker muscular dystrophy	Fragile X syndrome
Huntington disease	

Criteria for Autosomal Dominant Inheritance

1. *The phenotype appears in every generation, each affected person having an affected parent.*
   Exceptions or apparent exceptions to this rule in clinical genetics: (a) cases originating by fresh mutation in a gamete of a phenotypically normal parent; (b) apparent but not true exceptions in which the disorder is not expressed (nonpenetrant) or is expressed very mildly in a person who has inherited the responsible gene.
2. *Any child of an affected parent has a 50% risk of inheriting the trait.*
   This is true for most families, in which the other parent is phenotypically normal. Because statistically each family member is the result of an independent event, there may in a single family be wide deviation from the expected 1:1 ratio.
3. *Phenotypically normal family members do not transmit the phenotype to their children.*
   Failure of penetrance or exceptionally mild expression of a condition may lead to apparent exceptions to this rule.
4. *Males and females are equally likely to transmit the phenotype to children of either sex. In particular, male-to-male transmission can occur, and males can have unaffected daughters.*

Criteria for Autosomal Recessive Inheritance

1. An autosomal recessive phenotype, if it appears in more than one member of a kindred, typically is seen only in the sibship of the proband, not in parents, offspring, or other relatives.
2. The recurrence risk for each sib of the proband is 1 in 4.
3. The parents of the affected person may in some cases be consanguineous. This is especially likely if the gene responsible for the condition is rare in the population.
4. For most autosomal recessives, males and females are equally likely to be affected.

Criteria for X-Linked Recessive Inheritance

1. The incidence of the trait is much higher in males than in females.

TABLE 15.2 Sample Prenatal Genetic Screen*

Name ________________________ Patient # ________ Date ____________

1. Will you be 35 years or older when the baby is due? Yes____ No____
2. Have you, the baby's father, or anyone in either of your families ever had any of the following disorders?
   - Down syndrome (mongolism) Yes____ No____
   - Other chromosomal abnormality Yes____ No____
   - Neural tube defect, i.e., spina bifida (meningomyelocele or open spine), anencephaly Yes____ No____
   - Hemophilia Yes____ No____
   - Cystic fibrosis Yes____ No____

   If yes, indicate the relationship of the affected person to you or to the baby's father: ____________________
3. Do you or the baby's father have a birth defect? Yes____ No____
   If yes, indicate the relationship of the affected person to you or to the baby's father: ____________________
4. In any previous marriages, have you or the baby's father had a child, born dead or alive, with a birth defect not listed in question 2 above? Yes____ No____
   If yes what was the defect and who had it? ____________________
5. Do you or the baby's father have any close relatives with mental retardation? Yes____ No____
   If yes, indicate the relationship of the affected person to you or to the baby's father: ____________________
   Indicate the cause, if known: ____________________
6. Do you, the baby's father, or a close relative in either of your families have a birth defect, any familial disorder, or a chromosomal abnormality not listed above? Yes____ No____
   If yes, indicate the condition and the relationship of the affected person to you or to the baby's father: ____________________
7. In any previous marriages, have you or the baby's father had a stillborn child or three or more first-trimester spontaneous pregnancy losses? Yes____ No____
   If yes, indicate who and the results: ____________________
8. If you or the baby's father are of Jewish ancestry, have either of you been screened for Tay-Sachs disease? Yes____ No____
   If yes, indicate who and the results: ____________________
9. If you or the baby's father are African-American, have either of you been screened for sickle cell trait? Yes____ No____
   If yes, indicate who and the results: ____________________
10. If you or the baby's father are of Italian, Greek, or Mediterranean background, have either of you been tested for β-thalassemia? Yes____ No____
    If yes, indicate who and the results: ____________________
11. If you or the baby's father are of Philippine or Southeast Asian ancestry, have either of you been tested for α-thalassemia? ____________________
12. Excluding iron and vitamins, have you taken any medications or recreational drugs since being pregnant or since your last menstrual period? (Include nonprescription drugs.) Yes____ No____
    If yes, give name of medication and time taken during pregnancy: ____________________

*Any patient replying "yes" to questions should be offered appropriate counseling. If the patient declines further counseling or testing, this should be noted in the chart. Given that genetics is a field in a state of flux, alterations or updates to this form will be required periodically.

2. The gene responsible for the condition is transmitted from an affected man through all his daughters. Any of his daughters' sons has a 50% percent chance of inheriting it.
3. The gene is never transmitted directly from father to son, but it is transmitted by an affected male to all his daughters.
4. The gene may be transmitted through a series of carrier females; if so, the affected males in a kindred are related through females.
5. Heterozygous females are usually unaffected, but some may express the condition with variable severity.

Criteria for X-Linked Dominant Inheritance

1. Affected males with normal mates have no affected sons and no normal daughters.
2. Both male and female offspring of carriers have a 50% risk of inheriting the phenotype. This is the same as the autosomal dominant pedigree pattern.
3. For rare phenotypes, affected females are about twice as common as affected males, but affected females typically have milder (though variable) expression of the phenotype.

In addition, the terms *penetrance* and *expressivity* are characteristics of gene expression that are frequently confused but have quite distinct meanings. *Penetrance* is the probability that a gene will have any phenotypic expression at all; it is an all-or-none concept. *Expressivity* is the degree of expression of the phenotype. When the manifestation of a phenotype differs in people who have the same genotype, the phenotype is said to have *variable expressivity*. Even within a family, a disorder may vary in its clinical expression.[3]

INCREASED PARENTAL AGE

It is well known that the risk of chromosome abnormalities in the fetus increases continuously with increasing maternal age.[4] The reason for the association between advanced maternal age and fetal chromosome abnormalities is thought to be due to the increased risk of nondisjunction in the ovum. The traditional age at which a woman is considered to be at *high risk* for chromosome abnormalities is 35 years at the expected time of delivery. This cutoff age is somewhat arbitrary; it has been used because at the age of 35 the risk of delivering a baby with Down syndrome is similar to the generally accepted risk of miscarriage associated with amniocentesis (Table 15.3).

Trisomy 21 (Down syndrome) is the most common chromosome abnormality in liveborns, comprising approximately one-half of all cases. Mental retardation, which ranges from mild to severe, is universally present. Approximately 50% of children with Down syndrome are born with a congenital heart defect.[4] Other chromosome abnormalities that are increased with advanced maternal age include trisomy 18, trisomy 13, 47,XXY (Klinefelter syndrome), 47,XYY, and 47,XXX. Trisomy 18 and trisomy 13 conceptuses are often stillborn or die shortly after birth. Turner syndrome (45,X) and structural chromosome abnormalities such as deletions, translocations, and inversions are not associated with increased maternal age.

TABLE 15.3 Age-Related Risk of Down Syndrome or Any Chromosomal Abnormality (Liveborn)*

Age	Down Syndrome	Total Risk
20	1/667	1/526
21	1/667	1/526
22	1/429	1/500
23	1/429	1/500
24	1/250	1/476
25	1/250	1/476
26	1/1176	1/476
27	1/1111	1/455
28	1/1053	1/435
29	1/1000	1/417
30	1/952	1/384
31	1/909	1/385
32	1/796	1/322
33	1/625	1/317
34	1/500	1/260
35	1/385	1/204
36	1/294	1/164
37	1/227	1/130
38	1/175	1/03
39	1/137	1/82
40	1/106	1/65
41	1/82	1/51
42	1/64	1/40
43	1/50	1/32
44	1/38	1/25
45	1/30	1/20
46	1/23	1/15
47	1/18	1/12
48	1/14	1/10
49	1/1	1/7

*Risks are at the time of delivery of a liveborn neonate only.

It has been demonstrated that nondisjunction of chromosomes can occur in both egg and sperm. A few studies have shown a slightly increased risk of chromosome abnormalities in pregnancies in which the father is over the age of 55. Other reports have failed to confirm these findings. Thus, if such a risk is present, it is likely to be small.[5] Advanced paternal age does not appear to predispose the offspring to new autosomal dominant mutations; an example of an autosomal dominant condition associated with increased paternal age is achondroplasia. However, the large number of different autosomal conditions that can arise from these new mutations does not allow for any specific prenatal diagnosis.

FAMILY HISTORY OF DOWN SYNDROME

Consideration of a family history of Down syndrome leads to evaluation of two potentially different recurrence risks. The first, and more common, situation is that of the woman who has previously delivered a child with an extra chromosome 21. The second, and less common situation, is the delivery of a child with translocation trisomy 21. Down syndrome occurs as trisomy 21 in approximately 95% of all cases. When a woman has delivered a child with trisomy 21, the recurrence risk is 1–2%.[6] Recent evidence points to low-level parental mosaicism as a contributor to this risk.[7] A similar risk involves women who have had a child or fetus with trisomy 18 or 13, although this conclusion is based on fewer affected pregnancies.[6] If parents have previously had a child with trisomy 21, their risk of chromosome abnormalities in future pregnancies includes not only Down syndrome but also other aneuploid conditions. Prenatal diagnosis by chorionic villus sampling (CVS) or amniocentesis should be offered to all women who have had a pregnancy with a documented trisomic fetus due to this 1–2% recurrence risk. By the age of 35 years, the risk of aneuploidy is equivalent to the mother's age-related risk.

If a woman has delivered a child with translocation trisomy 21, the recurrence risk will depend on whether the translocation was inherited or de novo. If it was inherited from one of the parents who carries a balanced rearrangement in the chromosomes (and thus passed it on to the child in an unbalanced form), the recurrence risk is substantial. Generally, the risk of transmission of an unbalanced chromosomal rearrangement is higher if the mother rather than the father is the balanced carrier. If the conceptus carried a de novo translocation trisomy 21, the recurrence rate is 1% or less.

Because the majority of children with Down syndrome are delivered to women less than 35 years of age with no family history of aneuploidy, serum screening has been targeted to this population. *Maternal serum analyte screening* or *triple screening* refers to the use of alpha-fetoprotein (AFP), unconjugated estriol (μE_3), and human chorionic gonadotropin (hCG) to assign a risk of Down syndrome and other chromosomal aneuploid conditions. In 1984, it was shown that maternal serum AFP levels are lower in pregnancies affected by Down syndrome. In 1987, it was found that maternal serum hCG is two times higher on average in the presence of a fetus with Down syndrome. In 1988, maternal serum μE_3 was found to be 25% lower in a pregnancy complicated by Down syndrome. This multiple-marker screening detects 63% of Down syndrome overall. It can detect 48% of Down syndrome in women younger than 35 years (with a false-positive rate of 5%) and 87% in women older than 35 years (with a false-positive rate of 25%).[8] All three serum markers have been found to be lowered in trisomy 18 (without open defects).

The patient should be counseled that a positive test does not indicate the presence of a fetal chromosomal abnormality but merely establishes a higher risk for this condition. Of great importance is that the physician and the patient understand that screening should be offered without regard to the patient's feelings concerning pregnancy termination. Much of the information obtained from the serum screening or other prenatal diagnosis may be potentially valuable in planning additional testing prior to delivery, as well as the need for special services at the time of delivery or throughout pregnancy.

PREVIOUS CHILD WITH A NEURAL TUBE DEFECT

Neural tube defects follow a multifactorial pattern of recurrence. They are one of the most common congenital malformations; the incidence varies worldwide, with the

TABLE 15.4 Recurrence Risks for Multifactorial Disorders

No. of Siblings	Percent
None	
Neither parent	0.04–0.5
One parent	1.0–20.0
Both parents	29.8–35.4
One	
Neither parent	1.0–15.0
One parent	10.0–38.0
Both parents	35.3–41.6
Two	
Neither parent	8.1–13.0
One parent	17.3–24.5
Both parents	39.6–45.7

Source: Adapted from various sources, including Ref. 3.

highest incidence in Wales and Ireland. These defects are due to failure of the neural axis to close at 4 weeks of development, or about 6 weeks after the last menstrual period. If the neural tube fails to close at the cranial end of the neural tube, anencephaly results. If the failure to close is slightly lower caudad in the neural tube, an encephalocele can result. Encephaloceles are often associated with mental retardation without paralysis, especially if gray matter is contained within the encephalocele. Spina bifida occurs with defects lower in the neural axis. Mental retardation is unusual; paralysis, incontinence, anesthesia, and positional abnormalities are more common. Anencephaly is an open lesion 99% of the time and spina bifida 85–90% of the time. Spina bifida is slightly more common in females; this female predominance increases to 2:1 in anencephalics. Recurrence risk follows the usual multifactorial pattern, and therefore is dependent on the number of relatives affected and how closely related they are to the fetus (Table 15.4).[1,9,10]

There is wide support for a role for folate metabolism in the etiology of neural tube defects. Also, maternal antiepileptic medications, including valproic acid and carbamazapine, increase the risk of a neural tube defect; this risk is 1–2% for valproic acid and 1% for carbamazapine. This increased risk from these seizure medications may be due to their effect on folate metabolism. Folic acid is now recommended for both initial prevention and prevention of recurrence of neural tube defects by the Centers for Disease Control and Prevention, the U.S. Public Health Service, and the ACOG. All women of reproductive age should consume 0.4 mg of folic acid per day prior to pregnancy and throughout the first trimester. When there has been a previous offspring with a neural tube defect, the woman should increase this dose to 4.0 mg/day under a physician's guidance.[11,12]

Screening for neural tube defects involves maternal serum AFP testing. Open fetal defects typically cause an increase of fetal AFP in the amniotic fluid and therefore in the maternal circulation. In a California statewide program, 1 in 18 amniocenteses for elevated maternal serum AFP resulted in discovery of a neural tube defect.[9,10] The term *false-positive* is erroneously applied to cases of elevated maternal serum AFP in the absence of a neural tube defect. This elevation is a marker for other complications of pregnancy, including fetal-to-maternal hemorrhage, increased risk of preterm labor, premature rupture of membranes, preeclampsia, fetal death, and abruption, as well as other congenital abnormalities.[10]

HEMOPHILIA

Approximately 1 to 2 in 10,000 males suffer from hemophilia; the majority of cases result from hemophilia A (classic hemophilia), which is due to a deficiency of factor VIII. Approximately 20% of the total hemophiliac population is due to a deficiency of factor IX resulting in hemophilia B (Christmas disease). Hemophilias A and B are clinically similar and can be distinguished only by specific assays for the deficient coagulation factor. The genes for hemophilias A and B are on the X chromosome, causing males to be affected and females to be carriers.[13]

The female carrier of hemophilia A or B usually does not demonstrate any bleeding manifestations. Occasionally, carriers may have unusually low levels of factor VIII or IX, presumably due to an unusually large proportion of the normal X chromosome undergoing inactivation. These individuals may have menorrhagia and occasionally hemarthroses. Pregnancy and delivery, however, are generally free of serious hemorrhagic complications.

Any woman whose father has hemophilia or who has had an affected son and another affected maternal relative is an obligate carrier of the gene; she therefore has a 50% chance of having an affected son. A woman may or may not be a carrier if she has only one affected relative. Confirmation of the diagnosis in the affected individual(s) is imperative for accurate risk determination and testing. The probability of carrier status is obtained through pedigree analysis and Bayesian calculations that include a family and medical history. Carriers of hemophilia A or B have, on average, approximately 50% of the normal levels of factor VIII or factor IX, respectively. Coagulant assays can establish an odds ratio for carrier status, but there may still be uncertainty regarding carrier status because of the overlap of factor levels in carriers and noncarriers.

If DNA analysis of the affected male identifies a mutation or inversion, it can be accurately determined if female relatives are carriers or noncarriers. However, carrier diagnosis is often not possible because of the high incidence of new mutations in the hemophilia gene. For many families, linkage using restriction fragment length polymorphism (RFLP) analysis is employed to track the affected factor VIII or factor IX gene within the family.

Women who are known hemophilia carriers by DNA analysis have the options of CVS or amniocentesis for accurate prenatal diagnosis. Fetal blood sampling to measure either factor VIII or factor IX is offered to women for whom DNA analysis is either not available or not informative.[13] A detailed ultrasound examination is available for possible hemophilia carriers for fetal sex determination. If the fetus is identified as female, invasive prenatal testing can be avoided.

Standard obstetric indications for cesarean delivery should be used in a pregnancy potentially complicated by fetal hemophilia. Elective use of procedures that may entail fetal trauma, such as fetal scalp sampling and use of forceps or a vacuum extractor, should generally be avoided.

MUSCULAR DYSTROPHY

Duchenne and Becker muscular dystrophies are X-linked disorders of dystrophin structure and function occurring in 1/3300 live male births. Duchenne muscular dystrophy (DMD) is an X-linked recessive disease manifested by progressive muscular wasting beginning at 4–5 years of age and death usually in the second or third decade. DMD is the most common X-linked lethal disease in humans. One-third of DMD cases are caused by a new mutation.[14] Patients with Becker muscular dystrophy are more mildly affected.

The gene for Duchenne and Becker muscular dystrophies is located on the short arm of the X chromosome between Xp21 and Xp22. The gene codes for a large protein called *dystrophin*.[15,16] DMD is the consequence of dystrophin deficiency in skeletal muscle and is disease specific.[17]

Prenatal diagnosis of DMD enables the reproductive option of pregnancy termination of affected males. Cloning of the entire dystrophin gene has enabled the development of molecular genetic diagnosis.[18] Multiplex polymerase chain reaction (PCR) and Southern blot analysis for direct identification of gene deletions can provide successful prenatal diagnosis and carrier detection in 65% of cases.

When a deletion cannot be identified in an affected patient, RFLP analysis provides indirect evidence of carrier status.[19] However, the DMD gene is so large (more than 2 million base pairs long) that there is a 12% crossover rate within the gene itself at each meiosis.[20] When recombination occurs in nondeletion patients, definitive prenatal diagnosis may not be possible using RFLP analysis.

CYSTIC FIBROSIS

Cystic fibrosis is the most common fatal autosomal recessive disorder among Caucasian children, with an incidence of 1 in 2000. It is characterized by deficiency in exocrine pancreatic function, leading to malabsorption and chronic lung disease with infection and declining pulmonary function. Fertility among both males and females is often markedly reduced. The gene is located at chromosome 7q31. In the Caucasian population, 70% of the mutations are due to deletion of a phenylalanine residing at position 508 (referred to as the ΔF508 mutation). Dozens of other mutations have also been identified. Most laboratories screen patients using a battery of 6–12 of the most common cystic fibrosis mutations. These common mutations account for 75–80% of all cystic fibrosis mutations. The inability to identify all mutations has presented a problem for accomplishing population carrier detection. Controversy exists over whether individuals in the general population should be offered screening because of the concomitant need for extensive education and counseling. Thus, the American College of Medical Genetics, the ACOG, and the American Academy of Pediatrics do not currently recommend screening for patients without a family history of cystic fibrosis.

SICKLE CELL ANEMIA

Sickle cell anemia is a unique genetic disorder in that every patient with sickle cell anemia has the same mutation of the β-globin gene. Sickle cell disease is characterized by lifelong hemolytic anema, an increased propensity to infection, and repeated vasocclusive episodes. Patients with sickle cell trait are usually asymptomatic. The risk of developing sickle cell anemia is one in four (25%) if both parents have sickle cell trait. Hemoglobin electrophoresis is the recommended test for individuals at risk for sickle cell anemia. A sickle prep test, although excellent for mass screening, cannot distinguish between the heterozygote and homozygote or determine the presence of hemoglobin C. Accurate prenatal diagnosis of sickle cell anemia is available by CVS or amniocentesis.

α-THALASSEMIA

Decreased production of one or more of the globin chains results in the thalassemias. There are two α-globin gene loci located on chromosome 16. A mutation of the α-globin gene can affect either one or both α genes, resulting in any one of four α-thalassemia states: silent carrier (three functional α genes), α-thalassemia trait (two functional α genes), hemoglobin H disease (one functional α gene), and hemoglobin Bart's hydrops fetalis syndrome (no functional α genes). Silent carriers are asymptomatic, whereas patients with α-thalassemia trait may have mild anemia and microcytosis. Hemoglobin H disease is associated with mild to moderate hemolytic anemia and splenomegaly. Infants with Bart's hydrops are usually stillborn between 20 and 40 weeks' gestation.

α-Thalassemia is common in Southeast Asian, South Chinese, and Filipino populations. Approximately 30% of African-Americans are silent carriers, and 3% have α-thalassemia trait. The a-thalassemia trait in African-Americans is usually due to a deletion of a single α gene on *both* number 16 chromosomes (trans). Therefore, Bart's hydrops is generally not seen in fetuses of African-American α-thalassemia carriers. This is in contrast to the usual Asian genotype, in which there is a deletion of both α genes on *one* chromosome (cis). Specific mutations have been identified for the various Asian ethnic groups, most differing from normal by only one amino acid.

A complete blood count with red blood cell indices is recommended as a screening test for the thalassemias. Carriers for thalassemia characteristically demonstrate low red blood cell indices. If the complete blood count demonstrates both low red blood cell indices and a decreased hematocrit, the patient should be evaluated for iron deficiency. If iron deficiency is ruled out, hemoglobin electrophoresis should be performed. A normal hemoglobin A_2 level is suggestive of a-thalassemia trait. Hemoglobin A_2 is elevated in most β-thalassemia heterozygotes to a level between 3.5% and 7%. Asian couples who have α-thalassemia trait have a one in four (25%) risk of having a fetus with Bart's hydrops. Prenatal diagnosis of α-thalassemia is performed by DNA analysis of cultured cells obtained from CVS or amniocentesis.[21]

β-THALASSEMIA

A mutation in the β-globin gene, located on chromosome 11, can cause absent or decreased synthesis of β-globin chains. Although more than 90 different mutations have been identified, all of them result in a rather similar clinical picture.[22] Individuals from the Mediterranean basin (Italy, Greece, Sardinia), Southeast Asia, India, Africa, and Indonesia may have as much as a 1% chance of carrying the gene for β-thalassemia.[21] A person with β-thalassemia trait has one normal and one altered β-globin gene. Patients with β-thalassemia trait are asymptomatic and rarely manifest mild anemia. If both parents have β-thalassemia trait, they have a one in four (25%) chance of having a child with β-thalassemia major.

β-Thalassemia major is characterized by severe anemia requiring frequent transfusions. Accumulation of iron from transfusion and deposition in tissues leads to progressive hepatic, cardiac, and endocrine dysfunction. Unless iron overload is controlled by chelation therapy, patients generally die in the second or third decade of life secondary to cardiac failure.[23]

Screening for β-thalassemia is similar to that for α-thalassemia. If the red blood cell indices are low in the face of normal iron studies, β-thalassemia is differentiated from α-thalassemia by hemoglobin electrophoresis showing an elevated hemoglobin A_2 level. Prenatal diagnosis of β-thalassemia is offered if both members of a couple are carriers (giving them a one in four [25%] risk). Direct detection of the β-globin gene mutation in cultured cells from CVS or amniocentesis can determine if the couple carries an affected fetus.

TAY-SACHS DISEASE

Tay-Sachs disease is an autosomal recessive neurodegenerative disorder occurring in 1/3600 children of two distinct patient populations, Ashkenazi Jews and French Canadians. Deficiency of the enzyme hexosaminidase A results in the accumulation of the GM_2 ganglioside, mainly in neural tissues. This accumulation typically results in progressive neurologic deterioration and death by the age of 3 years. Heterozygote frequency is 1/30 for Ashkenazi Jews and French Canadians. Importantly, the disorder can occur in patients of non-Jewish and French Canadian background, as the heterozygote frequency is 1/150 to 1/300 in the general population. Most individuals of Jewish descent in the United States are either of Ashkenazi background or are uncertain whether or not they are of Ashkenazi descent. For this reason, screening should be offered to all Jewish patients.

Carrier detection is easily accomplished by testing serum for decreased hexosaminidase A levels. Pregnancy and the use of oral contraceptives diminish the serum level of the enzyme, so in these cases it is prudent to assess the hexosaminidase level using leukocytes in addition to serum. CVS or amniocentesis for assay of hexosaminidase A can be performed to test the fetus at risk.

FAMILY HISTORY OF CONGENITAL MALFORMATIONS

Serious congenital abnormalities occur in approximately 2% of all newborns. These abnormalities can be due to chromosomal disorders (about 20% of congenital abnormalities), Mendelian disorders (10% of abnormalities), or multifactorial disorders (about 35% of abnormalities). The last include isolated neural tube defects, cardiac defects, cleft lip and/or cleft palate, clubfoot, hypospadias, omphalocele, and many renal abnormalities.[24] About 30% of congenital anomalies are of unknown etiology. For any multifactorial problem, there is a 2–5% recurrence risk (as outlined in the discussion of neural tube defects). Many children with a congenital malformation should be evaluated by a geneticist skilled in dysmorphology. The difference between an apparently isolated malformation (such as a cleft lip) as a multifactorial disorder and a Mendelian disorder with a markedly higher recurrence risk must be analyzed.

EVALUATION OF MENTAL RETARDATION (INCLUDING FRAGILE X SYNDROME)

The evaluation of a patient who presents prior to or during pregnancy with a family history of mental retardation requires careful pedigree analysis, medical record review to document the phenotype of the affected relative(s), and clinical evaluation and/or laboratory investigation of the patient and, when possible, the affected relative(s). Genetic conditions associated with mental retardation include inborn errors of metabolism, hereditary degenerative disorders, central nervous system defects, some malformation syndromes, and intrauterine exposures (including alcohol) and infections. When a patient presents with a family history of a relative with a specific diagnosis (i.e. Down syndrome or fragile X syndrome), appropriate genetic counseling, carrier testing, and/or prenatal diagnosis can be initiated. The most common nongenetic cause of mental retardation is fetal alcohol syndrome.

Down syndrome is the single most common genetic cause of mental retardation, but it is rarely inherited. Fragile X syndrome is the most common inherited cause of mental retardation, with an estimated frequency of 1 in 1100–1500 males and 1 in 2000–3000 females.[25] Fragile X syndrome is inherited as an X-linked dominant condition with incomplete penetrance. Affected males have normal growth but relatively large heads, connective tissue abnormalities, and developmental and behavioral abnormalities. Physical features such as long face, prominent forehead, large ears, and macroorchidism become more apparent after puberty. Many are hyperactive and have speech characterized by perseveration repetition. Autistic behavior is also seen in some affected patients. Clinically affected females may have similar features, but the expression is generally milder than in affected males.

The fragile X gene was isolated in 1991 and contains a region of unstable DNA with a trinucleotide repeat sequence.[25] Amplifications of the trinucleotide repeat sequence are associated with clinical expression of fragile X syndrome. Small amplifications of the gene represent premutations which are not usually associated with clinical expression of the fragile X phenotype and are found in normal transmitting males and many carrier females. Larger amplifications represent full mutations and are found in clinically affected males and some carrier females.[26] Fragile X syndrome testing should be considered in males and females with developmental delay or mental retardation of unknown etiology, especially if there is a family history of mental retardation. Prenatal diagnosis of fragile X syndrome by amniocentesis. CVS is a less ideal means of testing because of the possibility of obtaining inconclusive molecular results. Women identified by molecular DNA techniques as being carriers of a premutation or full mutation of the fragile X gene are candidates for prenatal diagnosis.

Careful pedigree analysis may also suggest the possibility of a familial chromosome rearrangement (translocation or inversion). For example, if the patient reports that affected relatives have birth defects, growth delay, or dysmorphic features associated with mental retardation, or if there is a family history of unexplained miscarriage and/or intrauterine or neonatal deaths, a chromosome analysis of the patient and her partner may be indicated to rule out a balanced rearrangement. Routine screening by chromosome analysis and fragile X carrier testing of all patients with a family history of mental retardation may be cost prohibitive. Ideally, it is preferable to arrange cytogenetic testing and/or fragile X syndrome testing of the affected relative. The results, positive or negative, may have important implications, not only for the patient but for other relatives as well.

RECURRENT PREGNANCY LOSS

It is known that chromosome abnormalities cause at least 50% of first trimester abortions. Autosomal trisomies form the largest group of cytogenetically abnormal, spontaneous abortions. Monosomy X (Turner syndrome in liveborns) is the single most common chromosome abnormality in spontaneous abortions. Structural chromosomal rearrangements (translocations and inversions) are an uncommon cause of miscarriage, accounting for approximately 1.5% of all abortuses. Though this represents only a small proportion of sporadic abortions, structural chromosomal abnormalities represent an important etiology of recurrent pregnancy loss because those abnormalities are often inherited.

The most common parental structural chromosomal rearrangement is a translocation. While parents with balanced translocations are typically phenotypically normal, offspring may demonstrate unbalanced rearrangements such as duplications or deletions. In a summary of reports of recurrent pregnancy wastage, 3% of parents had chromosomal abnormalities (six times the rate in the general population).[27] Thus, parental karyotype analysis is an important component of the evaluation of the couple with recurrent pregnancy loss.

FAMILY HISTORY OF CHROMOSOMAL REARRANGEMENT

When a parent carries a balanced chromosomal rearrangement, the risk of having an abnormal fetus at the time of amniocentesis depends on which parent carries the rearrangement, the type of the rearrangement, and how the rearrangement was originally ascertained. For female carriers of a Robertsonian translocation (involving acrocentric [the short arm of the chromosome has no known significant genetic material] chromosomes 13, 14, 15, 21, and 22) the risk of an unbalanced offspring is 10–15% and is 2–4% for male carriers.[28] Reciprocal translocations ascertained in a parent through an unbalanced child or relative have approximately a 20% risk of future unbalanced progeny. If the reciprocal translocation is ascertained due to repeated spontaneous abortions, the risk of unbalanced offspring is 1–5%.

THE FUTURE

Couples at risk for genetic disorders who desire definitive prenatal diagnosis results presently utilize invasive fetal testing, including CVS or amniocentesis, to determine if their pregnancy is affected. Such procedures are accomplished on an established pregnancy and carry a low but distinct risk of procedurally related pregnancy loss. If an affected fetus is identified, the parents may choose to terminate the pregnancy. This can be physically difficult and emotionally traumatic.

There is currently active genetic research in several exciting areas of interest and importance to the obstetrician-gynecologist. Fetal cells in the maternal circulation provide an innovative, noninvasive approach to prenatal diagnosis.[29] Preimplantation embryo analysis is a technique of determining a genetic diagnosis prior to implantation in the uterus, thus avoiding the potential issue of pregnancy termination for an abnormal result.[30] In utero stem cell transplantation offers treatment to an affected fetus at a potentially optimal time in its development.[31] Finally, the field of cancer genetics is exploding; in the very near future, genetic testing may be available for familial breast and ovarian cancer. In the final section of this chapter, these four areas will be explored.

Fetal Cells in Maternal Circulation

There is compelling evidence of the presence of fetal cells in the maternal circulation as early as 6 weeks of gestation,[32,33] and recent advances in molecular technology have made possible the isolation and analysis of such cells. The requirements of prenatal diagnosis using this technique are as follows: (1) the fetal cells that are present must be distinguished from the more prevalent maternal cells; (2) the cells that are present must be enriched from their initial low concentrations; and (3) the fetal cells that are extracted must be analyzed by techniques that are sufficiently sensitive and specific. The diligent efforts that have gone into developing this noninvasive approach to prenatal diagnosis have now yielded preliminary success in correctly identifying both chromosomal and molecular genetic abnormalities.[34–38] Clinical studies in several centers are ongoing to determine whether this technique is sensitive and specific enough to provide noninvasive prenatal diagnosis to all pregnant women.

Until the late 1980s, genetic analysis of sufficient sophistication to positively identify a single fetal cell among thousands or millions of maternal cells was not available. However, the development of such techniques as polymerase chain reaction (PCR) and fluorescence in situ hybridization (FISH) has greatly increased the potential to successfully pursue this type of noninvasive prenatal diagnosis. Most investigations have focused on isolating cells containing Y-specific gene sequences from women carrying male fetuses, as this is a simple way of definitively proving the fetal origin of the cells. Such studies have confirmed that fetal cells are present in the maternal circulation, although, as expected, in very low concentrations.[38,39] Estimates of the ratio of fetal to maternal cells have varied widely.

A number of cells types have been investigated as candidate fetal cells for prenatal diagnosis. The optimal cell type should fulfill four criteria: (1) it should include a nucleus with DNA available for genetic analysis; (2) it should be reliably present in the maternal circulation; (3) it should be possible to differentiate it from maternal cells; and finally, (4) it must represent the current pregnancy.

Trophoblasts are an obvious candidate cell type, as they are know to invade the uterus and thus might be expected to enter the maternal circulation. A number of investigators have attempted to isolate trophoblasts from maternal circulation using a variety of monoclonal antibodies.[40–43] Although some of these investigators initially published promising results, their findings have been difficult to duplicate by others.

Lymphocytes thought to be fetal in origin have been isolated by a number of investigators.[44–46] In these studies, maternal blood was sorted for the presence of cells expressing paternal human leukocyte antigens (HLA). Lymphocytes are a well-known source of metaphases for cytogenetic analysis. However, the lymphocytes of presumably fetal origin isolated from maternal blood have not been successfully cultured or have been unresponsive to mitogens used for karyotype preparations.[47,48] Another concern with fetal lymphocytes is the possibility that they may persist in the maternal circulation for many years. Thus, the concern has been raised that isolated fetal lymphocytes could represent a previous, possibly even unrecognized pregnancy.[49]

Nucleated red blood cells (NRBCs) have been the focus of some of the most successful work in this area. Bianchi et al. first focused on these red blood cell precursors, also known as *erythroblasts*.[39] While NRBCs are very rare in peripheral adult blood, they represent a much higher percentage of the nucleated cell population in the fetus.[50] Thus, any NRBCs present in maternal blood are more likely to represent fetal cells. In addition, NRBCs have a defined half-life and thus, in contrast to fetal lymphocytes, would not be expected to persist into a later pregnancy.

A single group of investigators have also claimed to have isolated fetal granulocytes. Other investigators have not yet confirmed these findings.

Isolating the rare fetal cell from maternal blood depends on utilizing features unique to the fetal cells. The discriminating features chosen depend on the cell type that is targeted. The majority of investigators have relied on monoclonal antibodies that recognize fetal antigens. Monoclonal antibodies are used in conjunction with a variety of separation techniques that sort for the presence or absence of the antigen of interest. Investigators have used density gradients[51] and different devices, including a flow-activated cell sorter,[39,52] magnetic activated cell sorter,[51,53] and immunomagnetic beads.[43]

The optimal timing of testing maternal blood for fetal cells is not known. Bianchi et al. concluded that fetal NRBCs were unlikely to be present after 16 weeks gestation.[54] Ganshirt-Ahlert et al., however, found that NRBCs could be isolated in all three trimesters,[51] and Simpson and Elias likewise found fetal cells to be present at least through 18 weeks' gestation, with no decrease in frequency after 16 weeks.[55] It is likely that NRBCs are present in increased numbers earlier in pregnancy, as a progressive decrease in the percentage of nucleated versus nonnucleated erythrocytes occurs as the fetus matures.[50]

Preimplantation Genetic Diagnosis

Preimplantation embryo analysis is a technique of determining genetic information on a particular embryo prior to its implantation in the uterus. This form of analysis is intended to preclude the need for pregnancy termination by identifying affected fetuses prior to implantation, so that only unaffected embryos are implanted. Although largely an investigational procedure at present, the technique holds great promise for future application.

Human preimplantation embryo analysis has been accomplished by Handyside and colleagues for sex determination in cases of X-linked disorders, where male fetuses (who may receive an affected X chromosome from their carrier mothers) are at risk to be affected.[56] Female fetuses (who may receive an affected X chromosome from their carrier mothers but who have an additional normal X chromosome from their fathers) are not at risk.

Preimplantation embryo analysis is performed in conjunction with in vitro fertilization programs. The mother is treated with gonadotropins for superovulation, and oocytes are harvested by standard methods using sonographically guided transvaginal aspiration. Semen is obtained by noncoital ejaculation. Embryos may also be harvested by uterine lavage, although there may be an increased risk of tubal pregnancy; the yield of this latter method is also improved by ovulation induction rather than spontaneous ovulation.[57]

Embryo biopsy may be performed by three different techniques. The first and earliest technique involves analysis of the first polar body of the egg prior to fertilization.[58] Because the mother is presumed to be a carrier and not affected with the condition in question, she will have two alleles for the gene involved—one which is normal and one which is abnormal or mutant. Analysis of the genetic status of the first polar body can indirectly identify the status of the oocyte. This is because, if the polar body carries the mutant allele, then the oocyte should be unaffected. However, if the polar body is normal, then the oocyte would carry the mutant allele and would not be used in fertilization. This technique cannot be used for sex determination of embryos because both polar body and oocyte will contain an X chromosome. One of the major disadvantages of polar biopsy is that it is technically difficult.

The second technique, and the one most often described, involves biopsy of the embryo at the four- to eight-cell stage after fertilization.[59,60] Harvested oocytes and sperm are incubated together in the standard fashion for in vitro fertilization, and the culture is observed until cell division to a four- to eight-cell stage has occurred. At this point, the embryos are removed to separate cultures. Under micromanipulation, zona drilling is performed. In this technique, a dilute acid solution is utilized to form a hole in the surrounding zona pellucida, and a micropipette is inserted through the hole. A single blastomere is aspirated, washed, and separately analyzed, while the residual embryo remains in culture. If the analysis reveals that the embryo is not affected with the condition in question, then this embryo can be transferred to the uterus for potential implantation.

The third technique involves biopsy of the trophoectoderm.[58,61] In this technique, the embryo is incubated until the blastocyst stage (approximately 4 days). At this time, cells will separate into the inner cell mass, destined to become the body of the embryo, and the outer cell mass or trophoectoderm, destined to become the placenta. The trophoectoderm is biopsied, with the removal of 10–15 cells; this does not appear to affect future placental growth. As in the second technique, the zona pellucida is drilled with diluted acid solution, and the spontaneous herniation of cells through the hole is aspirated with a micropipette. Such a technique has the distinct advantage of obtaining a large number of cells, which makes analysis easier.

Because of the very small number of cells obtained by embryo biopsy and the limited time available before the embryo must be transferred to the uterus if it is to implant, standard culture methods for chromosomal analysis are impossible. The tissue thus requires analysis by PCR. PCR, a technique for amplifying a very small amount of DNA, has been successfully used in the study of DNA obtained from single or very few cells.

None of the reported infants who have been delivered after embryo biopsy have had any physical anomalies which could have been attributed to embryo biopsy.[56,62,63] Of the infants born, all have been of the previously diagnosed sex. Grifo et al. have reported a case of cystic fibrosis in which the preimplantation diagnosis of a carrier but unaffected embryo was made. However, on late first trimester CVS, the fetus was in fact determined to be affected. This error was attributed to a problem of interpretation of the PCR results.[62] Single-cell PCR techniques, such as those used for preimplantation analysis, may be contaminated readily by even the most minute amounts of stray DNA. Thus, false-positive or false-negative results may arise with PCR unless extremely stringent measures are taken to minimize all possible contamination.

Stem Cell Therapy

Several human genetic defects manifest severe signs and symptoms very early in child development. Many of these disorders are hematopoietic in origin, such as β-thalassemia and Chediak-Higashi syndrome, while others are enzymatic deficiencies resulting in tissue deposition of toxic compounds. Several of these disorders, such as Hurler syndrome and other mucopolysaccaridoses, as well as adrenal and metachromatic leukodystrophies (ALD, MLD) have been successfully corrected by allogeneic bone marrow transplantation.[64,65] However, in many disorders, suitable donors are unavailable or the disease progression is rapid enough that by the time the child is diagnosed, the disease process has already caused substantial end organ damage. This is especially true for disorders such as late infantile MLD, ALD, and severe combined immunodeficiency disorder (SCID).

In utero stem cell transplantation has several theoretical advantages. First, the normal hematopoietic stem cells (sources include bone marrow, cord blood, and fetal liver) are infused intraperitoneally into the fetus early in the course of the disease before significant target organ damage occurs. The use of CVS and molecular techniques gives a reliable means to diagnose genetic disorders early in gestation, allowing the potential for this option. Second, stem cells are now relatively easy to obtain from a variety of sources and can be purified, concentrated, and administered as small-volume infusions. Finally, fetal or neonatal blood can be analyzed and stem cells can be isolated from the fetus or young infant to determine the efficacy of treatment, the degree of chimerism achieved, and the need for additional infusions. With in utero stem cell transplantation, there is no preparative fetal therapy to avoid rejection.

Evidence to date suggests that while the preimmune fetus will allow engraftment, there is still a substantial risk of graft-versus-host disease to the fetus, leading to substantial morbidity and an increased risk of fetal loss. The limited clinical experience to date of 13 in utero transplants was reported at the 1993 meeting of the American Society of Hematology by Cowan and Golbus at the University of California–San Francisco.[66] Most of the children treated had confirmed evidence of a genetic disorder (thalassemia—5, SCID—2, MLD—2, other—4) and received stem cells from a variety of sources, including haploidentical parental marrow (n = 6), fetal liver (n = 6), fetal thymus (n = 4), or sibling marrow (n = 1). Only four children had documented engraftment, and there were two fetal losses. However, the presence in four patients of engraftment is encouraging, though these data remain too early for detection of clinical benefit. Much work still needs to be done in this area, but the possibilities are exciting and suggest that this will become a viable therapeutic option in years to come.[66–70]

Genetic Testing for Breast and Ovarian Cancer Predisposition

The identification of the gene associated with early-onset breast and ovarian cancer, known as *BRCA1,* has potentially important implications for the presymptomatic assessment and monitoring of the heritable cancer risks in certain individuals and families. This gene appears to be responsible for about 5% of breast cancer cases. The isolation of the breast-ovarian cancer susceptibility gene *BRCA1*[71] and the future isolation of other breast cancer predisposition genes, such as *BRCA2,*[72] raise important questions regarding genetic testing in high-risk families, as well as the more far-reaching question of general population screening.

Current data from multiple breast cancer families, used to locate the *BRCA1* locus, indicate that women who have inherited a mutant *BRCA1* allele have a risk of breast cancer exceeding 50% before age 50 years and exceeding 80% by age 70 years.[73,74] A second breast cancer predisposition locus, *BRCA2,* has recently been mapped to human chromosome 13q12–13.[72]

Direction detection of *BRCA1* mutations is likely to be available soon. Initial studies suggest that interest in genetic testing for breast and ovarian cancer susceptibility is likely to be very high.[75] At present, the beneficial effect of DNA testing is in women with a positive family history of breast cancer. For this reason, it is recommended that testing be considered in such women, on an investigational basis, as soon as it is available. Such a test could potentially reduce anxiety and prevent unnecessary prophylactic surgery in women found not to carry a germ-line *BRCA1* mutation. It could also identify those women who would comply with and therefore benefit most from currently recommended monitoring procedures.[76] Adult women from families in which *BRCA1* and *BRCA2* is segregating and who do not themselves carry the altered gene should be counseled that they still face the same risks of sporadic breast and ovarian cancer found in the general population and should be encouraged to follow age-appropriate surveillance measures.

Until we know more precisely the probability that a particular mutation will result in cancer, the efficacy and safety of follow-up interventions, and the reliability of the test, mass screening for *BRCA1* mutations is not currently recommended. The importance of education for those patients at high risk, for health professionals, and for the lay public cannot be overstated.

REFERENCES

1. Kuller JA, Yankowitz J: Genetics for the obstetrician/gynecologist. *Primary Care Update Ob/Gyn* 2:71–76, 1995.
2. Yankowitz J: Genetic screening. *Postgrad Obstet Gynecol* 14:1–7, 1994.
3. Thompson M, McInnes R, Willard H: *Thompson and Thompson Genetics in Medicine,* ed 5. Philadelphia, WB Saunders, 1991, pp 1–500.
4. Hook EB: Rates of chromosome abnormalities at different maternal ages. *Obstet Gynecol* 58:282–285, 1981.
5. Matsunaga E, Tonomura A, Oishi H, et al: Reexamination of paternal age effect in Down's syndrome. *Hum Genet* 40:259–268, 1978.
6. Stene J, Stene E, Mikkelsen M: Risk for chromosome abnormality at amniocentesis following a child with a non-inherited chromosome aberration. *Prenatol Diagn* 4(Spec. Iss.):81–95, 1984.

7. Pangalos CG, Talbot CC, Lewis JG, et al: DNA polymorphism analysis in families with recurrence of free trisomy 21. *Am J Hum Genet* 51:1015–1027, 1992.
8. Haddow JE, Palomaki GE, Knight GJ, et al: Prenatal screening for Down's syndrome with use of maternal serum markers. *N Engl J Med* 327:588–593, 1992.
9. Crandall BF: Prenatal screening for the detection of neural tube defects. In Simpson JL, Elias S (eds): *Essentials of Prenatal Diagnosis.* New York, Churchill Livingstone, 1993, p 253.
10. Milunsky A: Maternal serum screening for neural tube and other defects. In Milunsky A (ed): *Genetic Disorders and the Fetus,* ed 3. Baltimore, Johns Hopkins University Press, 1992, pp 507–563, 880.
11. Centers for Disease Control and Prevention: Recommendations for use of folic acid to reduce number of spina bifida cases and other neural tube defects. *JAMA* 269:1233–1238, 1993.
12. Werler MM, Shapiro S, Mitchell AA: Periconceptional folic acid exposure and risk of occurrent neural tube defects. *JAMA* 269:1257–1261, 1993.
13. Kazazian HH: The molecular basis of hemophilia A and the present status of carrier and antenatal diagnosis of the disease. *Thromb Haemost* 70:60–62, 1993.
14. Moser H: Duchenne muscular dystrophy: Pathogenetic aspects and genetic prevention. *Hum Genet* 66:17–40, 1984.
15. Monaco AP, Neve RL, Colletti-Feener CA, et al: Isolation of candidate cDNAs for portions of the Duchenne muscular dystrophy gene. *Nature* 323:646–650, 1986.
16. Hoffman EP, Brown RH, Kunkel LM: Dystrophin: The protein product of the Duchenne muscular dystrophy locus. *Cell* 51:919–928, 1987.
17. Hoffman EP, Fischbck KH, Brown RH, et al: Characterization of dystrophin in muscle-biopsy specimens from patients with Duchenne's or Becker's muscular dystrophy. *N Engl J Med* 318:1363–1368, 1988.
18. Koenig M, Hoffman EP, Bertelson CJ, et al: Complete cloning of the Duchenne muscular dystrophy (DMD) cDNA and preliminary genomic organization of the DMD gene in normal and affected individuals. *Cell* 50:509–517, 1987.
19. Katayama S, Montano M, Slotnick N, et al: Prenatal diagnosis and carrier detection of Duchenne muscular dystrophy by restriction fragment length polymorphism analysis with pERT 87 deoxyribonucleic acid probes. *Am J Obstet Gynecol* 158:548–555, 1988.
20. Abbs S, Roberts G, Mathew CG, et al: Accurate assessment of intragenic recombination frequency within the Duchenne muscular dystrophy gene. *Genomics* 7:602–606, 1990.
21. Kazazian HH: The thalassemia syndromes: Molecular basis and prenatal diagnosis in 1990. *Semin Hematol* 27:209–228, 1990.
22. Forget BG: The pathophysiology and molecular genetics of beta thalassemia. *Mt Sinai J Med* 60:95–103, 1993.
23. Weatherall DJ, Clegg JB, Higgs DR, et al: The hemoglobinopathies. In Scriver CR, Beaudet AL, Sly WS, et al (eds): *The Metabolic Basis of Inherited Disease,* ed 6. New York, McGraw-Hill, 1989, pp 2281–2339.
24. Fanaroff AA, Martin RJ, Miller MJ: Identification and management of high-risk problems in the neonate. In Creasy RK, Resnik R (eds): *Maternal-Fetal Medicine: Principles and Practice,* ed 2. Philadelphia, WB Saunders, 1989, p 1150.
25. Rousseau F, Heitz D, Biancalana V, et al: Direct diagnosis by DNA analysis of the fragile X syndrome of mental retardation. *N Engl J Med* 325:1673–1681, 1991.
26. Tarleton JC, Saul RA: Molecular genetic advances in fragile X syndrome. *J Pediatr* 122:169–185, 1993.
27. Tharapel AT, Tharapel SA, Bannerman RM: Recurrent pregnancy losses and parental chromosome abnormalities: A review. *Br J Obstet Gynaecol* 92:899–914, 1985.
28. Boué A, Gallano P: A collaborative study of the segregation of inherited chromosome structural rearrangements in 1356 prenatal diagnoses. *Prenatol Diagn* 4(Spec. Iss.):45–67, 1984.
29. Norton ME, Bianchi DW: Prenatal diagnosis using fetal cells in the maternal circulation. In Kuller JA, Chescheir NC, Cefalo RC (eds): *Prenatal Diagnosis and Reproductive Genetics.* St Louis, Mosby 1996.

30. Fries MH: Preimplantation embryo analysis. In Kuller JA, Chescheir NC, Cefalo RC (eds): *Prenatal Diagnosis and Reproductive Genetics*. St Louis, Mosby, 1996.

31. Wiley JM; Stem cell transplantation for the treatment of genetic disease. In Kuller JA, Chescheir NC, Cefalo RC (eds): *Prenatal Diagnosis and Reproductive Genetics*. St Louis, Mosby, 1996.

32. Liou JD, Pao CC, Hor JJ, et al: Fetal cells in the maternal circulation during first trimester in pregnancies. *Hum Genet* 92:309–311, 1993.

33. Lo YM, Patel P, Baigent CN, et al: Prenatal determination of fetal RhD status by analysis of peripheral blood of rhesus negative mothers. *Lancet* 341:1147–1148, 1993.

34. Bianchi DW, Mahr A, Zickwolf GK, et al: Detection of fetal cells with 47,XY,+21 karyotype in maternal peripheral blood. *Hum Genet* 90:368–370, 1992.

35. Cacheux V, Milesi-Fluet C, Druart L, et al: Detection of 47,XYY trophoblast fetal cells in maternal blood by fluorescence in situ hybridization after using immunomagnetic lymphocyte depletion and flow cytometric sorting. *Fetal Diagn Ther* 7:190–194, 1992.

36. Camaschella C, Alfarano A, Gottardi E, et al: Prenatal diagnosis of fetal hemoglobin Lepore-Boston disease on maternal peripheral blood. *Blood* 75:2102–2106, 1990.

37. Ganshirt-Ahlert D, Borjesson-Stoll M, Burschyk M: Detection of fetal trisomies 21 and 18 from maternal blood using triple density gradient and magnetic cell sorting. *Am J Reprod Immunol* 30:194–197, 1993.

38. Price J, Elias S, Wachtel SS, et al: Prenatal diagnosis using fetal cells isolated from maternal blood by multiparameter flow cytometry. *Am J Obstet Gynecol* 165:1731–1737, 1991.

39. Bianchi DW, Flint AF, Pizzimenti MF, et al: Isolation of fetal DNA from nucleated erythrocytes in maternal blood. *Proc Natl Acad Sci USA* 87:3279–3283, 1990.

40. Bruch JF, Metezeau P, Garcia-Fonknechten N, et al: Trophoblast-like cells sorted from peripheral maternal blood using flow cytometry: A multiparametric study involving transmission electron microscopy and fetal DNA amplification. *Prenatol Diagn* 11:787–798, 1991.

41. Covone AE, Johnson PM, Mutton D: Trophoblast cells in peripheral blood from pregnant women. *Lancet* 2:841–843, 1984.

42. Covone AE, Kozma R, Johnson PM, et al: Analysis of peripheral maternal blood samples for the presence of placental-derived cells using Y-specific probes and McAb H315. *Prenatol Diagn* 8:591–607, 1988.

43. Mueller UW, Hawes CS, Wright AE, et al: Isolation of fetal trophoblast cells from peripheral blood of pregnant women. *Lancet* 336:197–200, 1990.

44. Herzenberg LA, Bianchi DW, Schroder J, et al: Fetal cells in the blood of pregnant women: Detection and enrichment by fluorescence-activated cell sorting. *Proc Natl Acad Sci USA* 76:1453–1455, 1979.

45. Iverson GM, Bianchi DW, Cann HM, et al: Detection and isolation of fetal cells from maternal blood using the fluorescence-activated cell sorter (FACS). *Prenatol Diagn* 1:61–73, 1981.

46. Yeoh SC, Sargent IL, Redman CWG: Detection of fetal cells in maternal blood. *Prenatol Diagn* 11:117–123, 1991.

47. Youssef M, Shulman LP, Tharapel AT: Failure to document fetal cells in maternal circulation using the Selypes-Lorencz "air-culture" cytogenetic technique. *Hum Genet* 85:133–134, 1990.

48. Zilliacus R, de la Chapelle A, Schroder J, et al: Transplacental passage of fetal blood cells. *Scand J Haematol* 15:333–338, 1975.

49. Bianchi DW, Sylvester S, Zickwolf GK, et al: Fetal stem cells persist in maternal blood for decades postpartum. *Am J Hum Genet* 53(Suppl):A251, 1993.

50. De Waele M, Foulon W, Renmans W: Hematologic values and lymphocyte subsets in fetal blood. *Am J Clin Pathol* 89:742–746, 1988.

51. Ganshirt-Ahlert D, Burschyk M, Garritsen HSP: Magnetic cell sorting and the transferring receptor as potential means of prenatal diagnosis from maternal blood. *Am J Obstet Gynecol* 166:1350–1355, 1992.

52. Wachtel S, Elias S, Price J: Fetal cells in the maternal circulation: Isolation by multi-

parameter flow cytometry and confirmation by polymerase chain reaction. *Hum Reprod* 6:1466–1469, 1991.

53. Miltenyi S, Muller W, Weichel W, et al: High gradient magnetic cell separation with MACS. *Cytometry* 11:231–238, 1990.

54. Bianchi DW, Stewart JE, Garber MF, et al: Possible effect of gestational age on the detection of fetal nucleated erythrocytes in maternal blood. *Prenatol Diagn* 11:523–528, 1991.

55. Simpson JL, Elias S: Isolating fetal cells from maternal blood: Advances in prenatal diagnosis through molecular technology. *JAMA* 270:2357–2361, 1993.

56. Handyside AH, Kontogianni EH, Hardy K, et al: Pregnancies from biopsied human preimplantation embryos sexed by Y-specific DNA amplification. *Nature* 344:768–770, 1990.

57. Buster JE, Bustillo M, Rodi IA, et al: Biologic and morphologic development of donated human ova recovered by nonsurgical uterine lavage. *Am J Obstet Gynecol* 153:211–217, 1985.

58. Verlinsky Y: Biopsy of human gametes: In Verlinsky Y, Kuliev A (eds): *Preimplantation Genetics*. New York: Plenum Press, 1991, pp 39–47.

59. Monk M, Handyside AH: Sexing of preimplantation mouse embryos by measurement of X-linked gene dosage in a single blastomere. *J Reprod Fertil* 82:365–368, 1988.

60. Wilton LJ, Shaw JM, Tounson AO: Successful single-cell biopsy and cryopreservation of preimplantation mouse embryos. *Fertil Steril* 51:513–517, 1989.

61. Simpson JL, Carson SA: Preimplantation genetic analysis. *N Engl J Med* 327:951–953, 1992.

62. Grifo J, Tang YX, Alikani M, et al: First babies born in the USA after preimplantation genetic diagnosis of sex linked diseases. *Am J Hum Genet* 53(Suppl):7, 1993.

63. Handyside AH, Lesko JG, Tarin JJ, et al: Birth of a normal girl after in vitro fertilization and preimplantation diagnostic testing for cystic fibrosis. *N Engl J Med* 327:905–909, 1992.

64. Krivit W, Shapiro EG: Bone marrow transplantation for storage diseases. In Forman SJ, Blume KG, Thomas ED (eds): *Bone Marrow Transplantation*. Boston, Blackwell, 1993, pp 883–892.

65. Storb R, Etzioni R, Anasetti C, et al: Cyclophosphamide combined with antithymocyte globulin in preparation for allogeneic marrow transplants in patients with aplastic anemia. *Blood* 80(Suppl 1):669a, 1992.

66. Cowan MJ, Golbus M: In utero hematopoietic stem cell transplants for inherited diseases. *Am J Pediatr Hematol Oncol* 16:35–42, 1994.

67. Flake AW, Zanjani ED: In utero transplantation of hematopoietic stem cells. *Crit Rev Oncol Hematol* 15:35–48, 1993.

68. Van-Zant G, Thompson BP, Chen-J: Differentiation of chimeric bone marrow in vivo reveals genotype-restricted contributions to hematopoiesis. *Exp Hematol* 19:941–949, 1991.

69. Zanjani ED, Ascensao JL, Flake AW, et al: The fetus as an optimal donor and recipient of hemopoietic stem cells. *Bone Marrow Transplant* 10:107–114, 1992.

70. Zanjani ED, Ascensao JL, Tavassoli M: Liver-derived fetal hematopoietic stem cells selectively and preferentially home to the fetal bone marrow. *Blood* 81:399–404, 1993.

71. Miki Y, Swensen J, Shattuck-Eidens D, et al: Isolation of BRCA1, the 17q-linked breast and ovarian cancer susceptibility gene. *Science* 266:66–71, 1994.

72. Wooster R, Neuhausen SL, Mangion J, et al: Localization of a breast cancer susceptibility gene, BRCA2, to chromosome 13q12–13. *Science* 265:2088–2090, 1994.

73. Hall JM, Lee MK, Newman B, et al: Linkage of early-onset familial breast cancer to chromosome 17q21. *Science* 250:1684–1689, 1990.

74. Easton DF, Bishop T, Ford D, et al: The Breast Cancer Linkage Consortium. Genetic linkage analysis in familial breast and ovarian cancer: Results from 214 families. *Am J Hum Genet* 52:678–701, 1993.

75. Lerman C, Daly M, Masny A, et al: Attitudes about genetic testing for breast-ovarian cancer susceptibility. *J Clin Oncol* 12:843–850, 1994.

76. Lerman C, Croyle R: Psychological issues in genetic testing for breast cancer susceptibility. *Arch Intern Med* 154:609–616, 1994.

Chapter 16

A Kaleidoscopic Look at Statistics

Alan D. Weinberg

The information imparted in this chapter assumes that the reader has some knowledge of statistics. This chapter should be viewed as both a review and a reference. Consider this as more or less an outline of statistical procedures for the layman or nonbiostatistician. The reader is encouraged to seek many other texts as references and to go beyond some of the topics discussed in this chapter. The attempt is to review some of the basic hypothesis test procedures covered in an introductory statistics course, as well as a few more advanced topics that are omnipresent in the literature, and perhaps just a few steps beyond.

One purpose of this chapter is to increase the clinician's ability to read a scientific journal and develop fundamental knowledge of why certain statistical tools are utilized and how they are interpreted. It is not the intention to give advice as to how to go about analyzing data. To be as comprehensive as one chapter will allow in describing what takes many years to understand, I have included the various formulas that correspond to statistical tests. The purpose is to make it easy to read and interpret published material.

Note: *p*-values are given in the examples throughout the chapter but explained toward the end.

Finally, the author would like to thank Andy Ianuzzi for his artwork.

THE NORMAL DISTRIBUTION

Much of statistics is based on the intriguing mathematical concept of probability. One of the most well-known ways probability events may occur is described by the normal distribution.

Let's take a look at the formula of the normal distribution:

$$f(x) = \frac{1}{\sqrt{2\pi}\sigma} e^{-\frac{(x-\mu)^2}{2\sigma^2}} \tag{16.1}$$

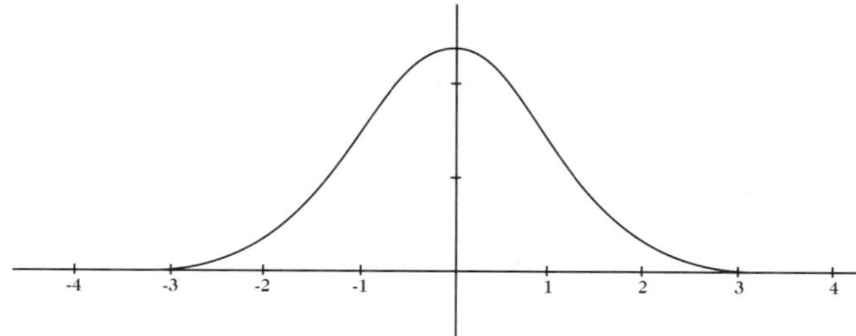

Here the variable of interest (age, weight, IQ, blood pressure, etc.) is x, $\pi = 3.14$; e, from the exponential function, is a constant equal to 2.71828; μ is the population mean; σ^2 is our population variance. You can substitute y for $f(x)$ if you prefer. We use the sample mean $\bar{x}$ and sample variance s^2 to make inferential decisions concerning a particular population. Let us discuss these sample statistics in more detail before we get back to the normal distribution.

The measure of variation or spread of the data can best be explained by the *sample variance:*

$$s^2 = \frac{\Sigma(x_i - \bar{x})^2}{n - 1} \tag{16.2}$$

This is our best estimate of the population variance σ^2.

Take a good look at it. It is really an average of the squared deviations, i.e., the distance between an individual measurement (x_i) and the sample mean, except that we divide by $n - 1$ in place of n. This $n - 1$ is the number of *degrees of freedom.* The square root of this variance, s, is referred to as the *standard deviation.* It is interesting to note that a normal distribution is approximately six standard deviations wide—three on each side of the mean.

This rather complicated function (16.1) describes the familiar bell curve. Many refer to it as the *Gaussian* curve—a correct title but a bit of a misnomer. This formidable-looking mathematical equation was published in 1733 by Abraham De Moivre (1667–1754). Carl Friedrich Gauss (1777–1855) is only credited with extending the work.

A few words about its characteristics: As mentioned, it is bell-shaped, symmetric about its mean, and its mean = median = mode. Assume that its total area is equal to 100% or 1. That will become important in a short while. Approximately 95% of the curve falls within two standard deviations of the mean.

The normal distribution is a probability distribution. It is completely determined by μ and σ. Therefore, there are different distributions (shapes) for different values of μ and σ. Life would be so simple if there were one formula that described any pattern of data that exemplifies normally distributed data. There is.

Given *any* normal distribution with mean = μ and variance = σ^2, we can use the following formula—the *z-score, z-value,* or *z-transformation*—to convert or *standardize* this distribution to the *standard normal distribution,* where $\mu = 0$ and $\sigma = 1$:

$$z = \frac{x - \mu}{\sigma} \tag{16.3}$$

z is the standard normal variable. It is also the distance, in standard deviations, between the variable of interest (x) and the mean.

Consider the following: An individual measurement is x_i. Knowing the mean and variance of the population from which this individual came will enable us to transform this x-value into a corresponding and equivalent z-score.

If we ask "What is the *probability* that a given x value is less than a certain value k?" a lesson we learned from freshman calculus will help us see the connection between mathematics, probability, and statistics. By integrating the normal equation from $-\infty$ to k, we obtain the area under the curve which is mathematically equivalent to the probability of the event occurring (the "event" that $x < k$).

$$P(x < k) = \int_{-\infty}^{k} \frac{1}{\sqrt{2\pi}\sigma} e^{-\frac{(x-\mu)^2}{2\sigma^2}}\,dx \tag{16.4a}$$

Remember all those integration problems you encountered in freshman calculus? Here is one very good reason for having solved them.

Alternatively, we can take x, μ, and σ, convert x to its corresponding z value, and integrate the following:

$$P(z < k') = \int_{-\infty}^{k'} \frac{1}{\sqrt{2\pi}} e^{-\frac{(z)^2}{2}}\,dz \tag{16.4b}$$

Therefore, the result of this integration is equivalent to answering the question "What is the probability that a given z-score is less than k'?" Fortunately, statisticians do not have to go through the arduous task of performing this integration. There are tables which give us the exact probability for a given z-value, i.e., the area under the standard normal curve.

Example 1:

An individual measurement yields a z-score of 2.

If we are interested in the probability that a certain sample mean falls two standard deviations to the right of the mean, we could either (1) integrate the above equation from $-\infty$ to 2 or (2) find a table of z-values in any statistics text. The area under the curve from $-\infty$ to 2 is 0.9772. It is this same table, generated from a foundation incorporating laws of probability, that enables us to make inferential decisions based on samples.

$$P(z < 2) = \int_{-\infty}^{2} \frac{1}{\sqrt{2\pi}} e^{-\frac{(z)^2}{2}}\,dz = 0.9772$$

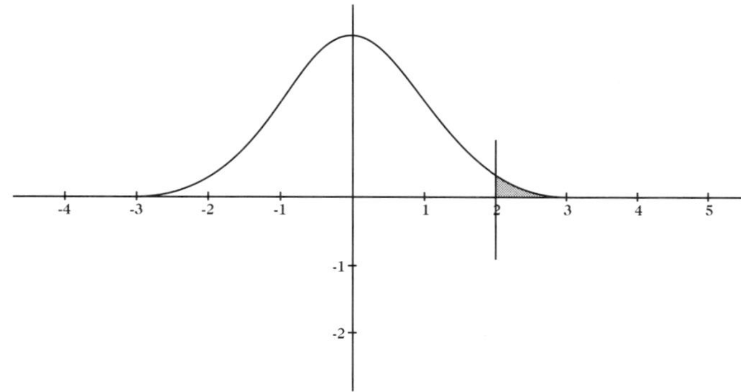

A few definitions and corresponding notation may be in order now.

DEFINITIONS

population—[*N*] the largest collection of entities for which there is an interest at a particular time, i.e., the universe.

sample—[*n*] part of a population, a subset: $x1, x2, x3, x4 \ldots xn$.

statistic—a descriptive measure computed from the data of a *sample*. It is represented by lowercase *Latin* letters such as x, s, b, p, and d.

parameter—a descriptive measure computed from the data of a *population*—It is represented by lowercase *Greek* letters such as μ, σ, β, π, and δ.

THE CENTRAL LIMIT THEOREM

With this glorious theorem, we can use normal distribution theory for much of our statistical analyses. It offers us the following: Given a population from any distribution, normal or not, with mean μ and variance σ^2, the sampling distribution of x (i.e., the distribution of all sample means of size n from this population) will be *normally distributed*, with mean μ and variance σ^2/n (when the sample size is large: $n > 30$).

That's incredible! Since we are in the business of analyzing *samples*, not *individuals*, who cares about the distribution of individuals in a population as long as we can rest assured that the distribution of all possible sample means is normal?

A sample of size 30 is usually used as a cutoff point. Sampling distributions of the mean based on sample sizes of 30 or more are considered normally distributed by virtue of the central limit theorem.

An analogous standardizing equation to (16.3) for a sample mean is

$$z = \frac{\bar{x} - \mu}{\sigma / \sqrt{n}} \tag{16.5}$$

Here $\bar{x}$ is the sample mean, μ is the hypothesized population mean, and n is the sample size. The denominator is considered the *standard error* of the mean.

THE STUDENT'S t DISTRIBUTION

Now that you are familiar with the z or normal distribution, another probability distribution, almost as common and equally important, will be introduced.

A brewer named W.S. Gossett (1876–1937) came up with a distribution in 1908, similar in shape and function to the normal distribution, for data where σ^2 is *unknown*, sample sizes are less than 30, and therefore the sample variance,

$$s^2 = \frac{\Sigma(x_i - \bar{x})^2}{n - 1} \tag{16.2}$$

must be substituted for σ^2. His anonymous paper (he signed it "by Student"—he was afraid his competitors might have the same idea) announced the birth of the now omnipresent and most useful t-distribution. (Not exactly, but I thought the above tale sure sounds good.) Actually, Gosset was an employee of the Guinness brewery in Dublin, where he interpreted data and planned barley experiments. He published his findings under the pseudonym "Student" because Guinness employees were forbidden to publish. In the real world of statistics, most often σ is not known and therefore the standard normal distribution (normal theory—use of the normal distribution and associated z table) cannot be utilized. The t statistic is the appropriate substitute for small samples ($n < 30$).

HYPOTHESIS TESTING

In the examples that follow, the classical hypothesis test approach to statistical inference will be followed. That is, the following steps will be taken with gross simplification:

1. Establish certain assumptions concerning the normality of the data, the randomness of sampling techniques, and so on.
2. Establish a null (Ho) and alternate hypothesis (Ha) about the population or populations in question.
3. Calculate the test statistic.
4. Establish a rejection region based on the type I error or level of uncertainty.
5. Decision: Reject or fail to reject the null hypothesis based on an α level (usually 0.05).
6. Conclusion: A summary statement based on the outcome of step 4.

With the advent of computer technology, the readily available p-value summarizes the last four steps (see the section on the p-value).

One-Sample Test of Means (One Sample t-Test)

Objective: To test a sample mean against a hypothesized parameter μ under the null, the following test statistic is used:

$$t = \frac{\bar{x} - \mu}{s/\sqrt{n}} \tag{16.6}$$

The formula is quite similar to (16.5) except that *s*, the standard deviation, replaces σ. We refer our calculated test statistic to a *t*-distribution table with corresponding values of degrees of freedom $(n - 1)$ and compare it to a *t*-critical value.

The hypothesis is

$$Ho: \mu = a$$
$$Ha: \mu \neq a$$

where *a* is some hypothesized population mean value from which this sample presumably came.

Example 2

Suppose that the chest circumference of presumably normal newborn baby girls is normally distributed, with $\mu = 13.0$ in. A group of 25 newborn girls from a population group living in a remote region and thought perhaps to constitute a genetic isolate are studied and found to have an average chest circumference of 12.6 in. and a standard deviation of 0.7 in. Is this evidence that the group of 25 come from a population with parameter values different from the value $\mu = 13.0$?

The test statistic is

$$t = \frac{\bar{x} - \mu}{s/\sqrt{n}} = (12.6 - 13.0) / (0.7/5) = -2.857 \quad \text{vs.} \quad t_{crit} = -2.0639$$

Conclusion: Since $|-2.857| > |-2.0639|$, we can claim that the mean chest circumference of the genetic isolate is different from the population norm with 95% confidence. The *p*-value, generated from a computer, is 0.0087.

Two-Sample Test of Means (Two-Sample *t*-Test)

Objective: The comparison of two groups.

One can generalize the above formula to two independent groups and then employ the following two-sample *t*-test:

$$t = \frac{(\bar{x}_1 - \bar{x}_2) - (\mu_1 - \mu_2)}{\sqrt{s_p^2\left(\frac{1}{n_1} + \frac{1}{n_2}\right)}} \qquad (16.7)$$

s_p^2 is the pooled variance, a weighted average of the two sample variances:

$$s_p^2 = \frac{(n_1 - 1)s_1^2 + (n_2 - 1)s_2^2}{n_1 + n_2 - 2} \qquad (16.7a)$$

This is the classic test when comparing two groups, i.e., two treatment groups (drug vs. placebo, treatment vs. control, etc.).

The hypothesis is

$$Ho: \mu_1 = \mu_2$$
$$Ha: \mu_1 \neq \mu_2$$

Example 3

Suppose you want to compare the birth weights of two groups of neonates to whether there is a difference. The following information is given:

Group	x (g)	s	n
Group 1	3330	400	90
Group 2	3480	450	250

The test statistic yields $t = -2.7898$ vs. $t_{crit} = 1.96$, $df = 338$. Therefore, we can claim a difference in the birth weight means between the two groups with 95% confidence. The p-value, generated from a computer, is 0.0056.

Cochran's Caveat

One important assumption here is that the variances of the two groups, although unknown, are *assumed equal*. Statisticians believe that two treatment groups might differ in the way they react to the treatment (their group means would illustrate this) but should vary about the same. An F-test of homogeneity can test whether we can assume equality of variances. If we reject this proposal, a more conservative t-test (it is harder to reject the null hypothesis of no difference; see Cochran in the Bibliography) should be utilized. This variation on the two-sample t-test theme is a bit more tedious with a hand calculator. SAS output gives both t-test results, but the point here is that if one can't assume equality of variances, Cochran's test* may be used and reported.

CONFIDENCE INTERVALS

It is useful to know how confidence intervals (or *confidence limits*) are derived.

Derivation: Construction of a 95% Confidence Interval

1. Consider the standard normal distribution and the statement:

$$P\{-1.96 < z < 1.96\} = 0.95 \quad \text{(one could verify this)}$$

2. Substitute for z:

$$P\left\{-1.96 < z = \frac{\bar{x} - \mu}{\sigma/\sqrt{n}} < 1.96\right\} = 0.95$$

3. Multiply all three items within the braces by the standard error.
4. Subtract $\bar{x}$ from all three items.
5. Finally, multiplying across by (-1) and reversing the order of the inequalities yields a *95% confidence interval* for an unknown μ, given $\bar{x}$, s:

*The Welch approximation or Saaterwait approximation accomplish the same goal.

$$P\left\{\bar{x} - 1.96\frac{\sigma}{\sqrt{n}} < \mu < \bar{x} + 1.96\frac{\sigma}{\sqrt{n}}\right\} = 0.95 \qquad (16.8a)$$

or for any α,

$$P\left\{\bar{x} - Z_{crit}\frac{\sigma}{\sqrt{n}} < \mu < \bar{x} + Z_{crit}\frac{\sigma}{\sqrt{n}}\right\} = 1 - \alpha \qquad (16.8b)$$

There are many variations on this theme for the myriad statistical designs, but many confidence intervals, in general, have the following property:

CI: [estimator + (reliability coefficient) × (standard error)]

I recommend *Daniel's Practical Interpretation:*

We are 100 $(1 - \alpha)$ % confident that the single computed interval, $\bar{x} + Z_{\text{crit}}\frac{\sigma}{\sqrt{n}}$, $\bar{x} - Z_{\text{crit}}\frac{\sigma}{\sqrt{n}}$, contains the population mean (μ).

A few comments are in order here. The sample standard deviation *s* may be substituted for σ and the *t* distribution for the normal distribution. Confidence intervals may replace hypothesis testing for the purposes of inferential decision making.

$$P\left\{\bar{x} - t_{crit}\frac{s}{\sqrt{n}} < \mu < \bar{x} + t_{crit}\frac{s}{\sqrt{n}}\right\} = 1 - \alpha \qquad (16.8c)$$

Other examples include confidence limits for a one-sample proportion:

$$P\left\{\hat{p} - Z_{crit}\sqrt{\frac{\hat{p}\hat{q}}{n}} \leq \pi \leq \hat{p} + Z_{crit}\sqrt{\frac{\hat{p}\hat{q}}{n}}\right\} = 1 - \alpha \qquad (16.8d)$$

$$P\left\{\hat{p} - Z_{crit}\sqrt{\frac{\hat{p}\hat{q}}{n}} - \frac{1}{2n} \leq \pi \leq \hat{p} + Z_{crit}\sqrt{\frac{\hat{p}\hat{q}}{n}} + \frac{1}{2n}\right\} = 1 - \alpha^{*} \qquad (16.8e)$$

Paired *t*-Tests

In situations in which pairs of observations are made (e.g., before and after an intervention), a paired *t*-test should be used on the difference scores ($d_i = x_{\text{before}} - x_{\text{after}}$). When analyzing identical twins, littermates, or before-after studies on the same individual or just *matching* individuals on certain factors such as age, race, or socioeconomic factors, the paired *t* is the appropriate statistical test. Inferences will be made on the average mean difference between the paired individuals. This should reduce some of the extraneous variance in the data and also increase power. (Note: here the two groups are *not* independent.)

Example 4

Alahuhta et al. (see the Bibliography) evaluated the influence of extradural block for elective cesarean section on various hemodynamic variables, including maternal diastolic arterial pressures, during two different stages of the study. The following

*With continuity correction.

are the lowest values of this variable at the two stages (see Daniel, p. 240, in the Bibliography).

The subjects were eight parturients in gestational weeks 38–42 with uncomplicated singleton pregnancies undergoing elective cesarean section under extradural anesthesia. The objective was to determine if the block modified fetal myocardial function.

Stage 1:	70	87	72	70	73	66	63	57
Stage 2:	79	87	73	77	80	64	64	60
d_i:	9	0	1	7	7	−2	1	3

The mean difference $d = 3.25$, with $s_d = 3.955$

The hypothesis is

$$Ho: \quad \delta = 0$$

$$Ha: \quad \delta \neq 0$$

The test statistic is

$$t = \frac{\bar{d} - \delta}{s_d / \sqrt{n}} = t = \frac{3.25}{3.955 / \sqrt{8}} = 2.3242 \tag{16.9}$$

since $2.3242 < 2.3646$ (t_{crit} $df = n - 1 = 7$), classically we cannot claim a difference ($p = 0.0531$).

CHI-SQUARE STATISTICS

When discrete data in the form of contingency tables are examined and the question is whether two variables are independent or associated, chi-square analysis is chosen. Classic examples include drug–response and disease–exposure.

The hypothesis is

H_o: The two variables of interest are independent

H_a: The two variables of interest are associated.

The test statistic for any $r \times c$ table is [r = number of rows, c = number of columns]:

$$\chi^2 = \sum_{i=1}^{k} \left[\frac{(O_i - E_i)^2}{E_i} \right] \tag{16.10}$$

where O_i is the observed frequency (the actual data) and E_i is the expected frequencies computed by [(row total)(column total) / n] (n = sample size). The symbol k is the number of cells in the table, which equals $r \times c$.

The calculated test statistic is then compared to a chi-square critical value (table) with $(r - 1)(c - 1)$ degrees of freedom.

Given Table 1 with the following symbolic notation:

	a	b	
	c	d	

A short formula used exclusively for this 2 × 2 *contingency table* is

$$\chi^2 = \frac{n(ad - bc)^2}{(a + c)(b + d)(a + d)(c + d)} \tag{16.11}$$

This observed value is compared to a chi-square critical value (table) with one degree of freedom (3.84) for purposes of hypothesis testing. *p*-Values may be computed.

There is some controversy as to whether a correction factor needs to be utilized here. We are using a continuous distribution to approximate a discrete one. Some statisticians swear by the *continuity correction* (or *Yates correction*); others discourage its use. The literature is fraught with discussions pro and con. The chi-square equation for a 2 × 2 with continuity correction is:

$$\chi^2 = \frac{n(|ad - bc| - n/2)^2}{(a + c)(b + d)(a + d)(c + d)} \tag{16.12}$$

where $n/2$ is the correction factor.

This is a more conservative test; therefore, its use makes it harder to reject the null hypothesis.

Example 5

In a recent study of employment-related stress and preterm delivery (PTD) (see Hickey in the Bibliography), the association between women working during pregnancy and PTD was explored univariately. Other variables were also considered (age, marital status, etc.). Consider the following 2 × 2 table:

	PTD	
Worked During Pregnancy	**Yes**	**No**
No	67	406
Yes	64	403

Test whether there is an association between a women's working during pregnancy and PTD.

The test statistic calculated value is

$$\chi^2 = 0.004$$

which, compared to 3.84, is not significant. We conclude that there is not enough evidence to claim an association between women's working during pregnancy and PTD. ($p = 0.851$).

FISHER'S EXACT TEST

There is another controversial chi-square caveat for the 2 × 2 contingency table. If the numbers are small, i.e., the expected frequencies [(row total × column total) /*n*] are below 5, the chi-square statistic may not be a valid test.

An alternative procedure, the *Fisher's Exact Test* (1935) is considerably more complicated unless you have a computer. It gives the exact probability of the 2 × 2 table occurring, given that the marginals are fixed. It is mathematically equivalent to the *hypergeometric* probability distribution. Many believe that the Fisher's exact test is appropriate only when both marginal totals are fixed by the experiment (see Daniel, p. 537, in the Bibliography). Here again, statisticians differ on its worthiness. So if you see it in the literature, realize it's the ersatz chi-square test when individual cell values are small.

THE ODDS RATIO

The chi-squared analysis determines whether there is an association between two discrete or dichotomous variables, but it says absolutely nothing about the *strength* of the association betwen the variables. The odds ratio does. It is easy to compute for the 2×2:

$$ad/bc \tag{16.13}$$

The odds ratio approximates how much more likely (or unlikely) it is for the outcome to be present among those with factor $x = 1$ than among those with factor $x = 0$, for example, {1 = smoker; 0 = nonsmoker} {1 = male; 0 = female} {1 = treatment; 0 = control} (see Hosmer and Lemeshow in the Bibliography).

The odds ratio compares the odds of the yes proportion from one group to the odds of the yes proportion of group 2 (see Stokes).

McNEMAR'S TEST

In a retrospective study, with each case matched to one control, a special type of chi-square test known as *McNemar's test* (1947) should be used. The proper unit of analysis is the matched pair rather than the individual subject.

For the 2×2 in Table 2:

	a	*b*
	c	*d*

The McNemar test statistic for matched pairs for a 2×2 with continuity correction is

$$\chi^2 = \frac{(|b - c| - 1)**2}{b + c} \tag{16.14}$$

which is compared to one degree of freedom. The odds ratio is simply *b*/*c*.

REGRESSION

Recall, your eighth-grade algebra class? One evening your teacher gave you a number of homework problems, each with two sets of points; call them ($x1$, $y1$) and ($x2$, $y2$). You had to come up with the slope and the equation of the straight line, $y = mx + b$, where y was the value of a point on the vertical axis, x was the value of a point on the horizontal axis, m was the slope of the line, and b was the y-intercept, the point where the line crosses the y-axis.

It's a bit more complicated in statistics, where we may have numerous points scattered around an imaginary line. Charles Darwin's first cousin, Sir Francis Galton (1822–1911), an explorer, meteorolgist, and anthroplogist, paved the way for analysis known as *linear regression,* a statistical tool that utilizes the linear relationship between two or more variables. Galton observed the heights of fathers versus their sons.

Statisticians have replaced the *m*'s and *b*'s in our eighth-grade version of the equation, switched the order, and added an error term, to yield the following straight-line regression equation model:

$$y = \beta_o + \beta_1 x_1 + \epsilon \tag{16.15}$$

sometimes referred to as *simple linear regression.*

The x variable is called the *independent, explanatory,* or *predictor variable* (also *covariate*), and the y variable is called the *dependent, outcome,* or *response variable.* β_1 represents the slope of the hypothesized equation, β_o the y-intercept, and ϵ the error term, i.e., part of the variability of y not explained by its relationship with x. These are population parameters, considered the *coefficients* of the equation. Formulas to compute estimates of β_1, β_o appear in the Appendix, and the operation can easily be done with a hand calculator or, better yet, a computer. The formulas are derived from the concept that a hypothesized regression equation is sought that will minimize the spread or scatter of data that invariably will surround this line. The method (using a bit of calculus) is known as the *method of least squares.* The objective is to find the straight-line equation, or *least squares regression equation,* which best exemplifies the data and comes closest to removing as much of the scatter surrounding this line as possible. These calculations will generate a sample estimate of the straight-line equation:

$$\hat{y} = \hat{b}_o + \hat{b}_1 x_1 \tag{16.15a}$$

Example 6

Greene and Touchstone (see the Bibliography) conducted a study relating birthweight to the estriol level of pregnant women. Here is a partial list of the data:

Subject	Estriol (y) (mg/24 h)	Birthweight (g/100) (x)
1	7	25
2	9	25
3	9	25
.	.	.
.	.	.
.	.	.
31	24	43

The least squares estimate of the regression equation is calculated to be $y = 21.52 + 0.608x_1$.

Once calculated, the significance of the slope can be tested by a simple t-test.

The hypothesis is

$$Ho: \quad \beta_i = 0$$
$$Ha: \quad \beta i \neq 0$$
$$t = \frac{\hat{b}_1 - \beta_1}{s_b \Big/ \sqrt{n}} \tag{16.16}$$

Notationally, $\hat{b}_1$ is the sample slope estimate (0.608), β_1 is the hypothesized population value under the null (0), and s_b is the standard error of the slope estimate. We have already discussed n.

Rejection of this hypothesis, (i.e., $p < 0.05$) leads to the conclusion that the slope of the proposed linear equation is other than zero; hence, a relationship exists between x and y. Failing to reject the null hypothesis ($p > 0.05$) is synonymous with being unable to accept a slope other than zero, which implies that y does not change as x grows larger, yielding the conclusion that birthweight has no effect on an increase in estriol or that there is no straight-line relationship.

Once it is assumed that the straight-line relationship between the two variables is valid, we can predict the expected birthweight for a pregnant women with a particular estriol level.

Example 7

What is the expected mean birthweight if a pregnant women has an estriol level of 14 mg/24 h?

$y = 21.52 + 0.608(14) = 30.032 \times 100$ g $= 3003.2$ g, as demonstrated in Rosner (see the Bibliography).

Confidence limits around this prediction are obtainable, with some difficulty, from a hand calculator. The reader is referred to Neter, Wasserman and Kutner (in the Bibliography) for these formulas.

We can generalize this to *multiple linear regression*, where we consider more than one *independent* or *prognostic variable* (or *covariate*) in the prediction equation.

$$y = \beta_o + \beta_1 x_1 + \beta_2 x_2 + \ldots \beta_n x_n \tag{16.17}$$

The dependent variable y is just a combination of the product of each independent x variable and its corresponding beta slope coefficient.

This is very difficult to do by hand or calculator, as it involves matrix algebra. Computer programs are the method of choice here. Various software packages offer *stepwise regression* techniques, which automate the process, allowing certain variables into the linear model while not accepting others. As each variable is allowed into the equation, a statistical F test is performed to determine whether this new variable adds any additional information to the predictive capability of the equation. Another way of stating this is that a variable will be accepted into this "model" if it appreciably lowers the variability of the data around the regression line, i.e., helps explain more of the variance than if it were left out of the equation. It is of interest to note that one may even enter dichotomous variables (*indicator* or *dummy variables*) into the model that take on only the values 0 and 1 (e.g., sex, race, socioeconomic status, smoking status).

I believe that this computerized stepwise procedure should not be tried at home. Many other factors, assumptions, and statistical techniques go into model building, i.e., residual diagnostics, satisfying the assumption of *homoscedasticity*, (equality of variances along the y axis), transformation of variables (i.e., logarithmic, inverse, square-root, arc-sine), plotting, etc. Just the push of a button does not suffice here.

CORRELATION

Correlation measures the strength of the linear relationship between two variables and is measured between -1 and 1. An r of $+1$ describes a perfect straight-line fit and a positive slope, almost an impossibility in the biological world. A zero (0) is indicative of no linear relationship.

ANOVA

When more than two groups are being compared and the variable of interest is continuous, our two-sample t-test is obviously no longer useful. *Analysis of variance (ANOVA)* is the appropriate procedure.

The hypothesis is

$$Ho: \quad \mu 1 = \mu 2 = \ldots \mu n$$

Ha: at least one group mean is different.

An F test statistic is computed upon completion of the following ANOVA table:

ANOVA Table 2

Source	*d.f.*	*SS*	*MS*	*F*
Treatments	___	___	___	___
Error	___	___	___	
Total	___	___		

Rejection of the null hypothesis (via the F-test) is just the beginning of further analysis. The investigator may use other analyses to explore the possibility of differences between two particular groups, combinations of groups, or possibly all treatments vs. a placebo or control group (see Dunnett in the Bibliography). This brings us to the area of multiple testing or multiple comparisons. Multiple comparison tests that protect against the inflation of an alpha type I error include the Scheffe, Bonferroni, Tukey, and Dunnett tests.

Bonferroni derived the following formula when multiple testing is considered. The overall alpha level is $\alpha^* < 1 - (1 - \alpha)^{**}k$. If three tests are performed, the probability of rejecting one or more of the tests *incorrectly* is

$$\alpha^* < 1 - (1 - 0.05)^{**}3 = \alpha^* < 1 - (0.95)^{**}3 = \alpha^* < 0.143.$$

The probability of falsely rejecting at least one true null hypothesis is 0.143, which is unacceptable when we usually only tolerate 0.05. Hence multiple testing inflates our type I error rate and must be avoided or corrected for by one of the above-mentioned tests.

Once again, the reader may want to explore test books devoted to the design of clinical experiments.

There are many variations on the ANOVA theme. Entire texts are written regarding these methods. Included among these are repeated measures ANOVA, analysis of covariance (ANCOVA), two-way ANOVA, and blocking and stratification techniques, to name only a few.

P-VALUES

A *p*-value for a hypothesis test is the probability of obtaining, when *HO* is true, a value of the test statistic as extreme as or more extreme (in the appropriate direction) than the one actually computed (see Daniel, p. 200, in the Bibliography). How is it calculated?

Example 8

Consider a *z*-test statistic result of 2.84 for normally distributed data regarding the difference between two independent groups. The *p*-value answers the following question: If the null hypothesis were true ($\mu 1 = \mu 2$), what is the probability of obtaining a mean value of their differences large enough to yield a *z*-value ≥ 2.84 (i.e., a *z*-value 2.84 standard deviations away from the standard normal mean of zero)? Integrating the normal probability distribution (i.e., finding the area under the curve) of values as extreme as or more extreme than the test statistic ($\pm$ 2.84) or obtaining the corresponding probability from the *z*-table gives us a *p*-value of <0.04. The chances are 4 in 100 of obtaining a *z*-value that large if there were no differences between the two groups.

A few other ways of describing the same phenomena follow:

1. A *p*-value of <0.05 means that an observed effect has less than 5 chances out of 100 of having occurred by chance.
2. A small *p*-value is considered a rare event for the population.
3. The *p*-value is really a measure of surprise; the smaller the *p*-value, the more surprising the result if the null hypothesis is true (James Ware, Harvard School of Public Health).
4. If we are comparing two treatments, the smaller the *p*-value (<0.05), the less likelihood there is of a treatment difference having arisen by chance (see Pocock in the Bibliography).

The *p*-value should be considered only a guide to interpretation, but it is nevertheless important (see the Cox and Schlesselman works in the Bibliography).

This *p*-value, so easily obtained by our high-speed computers, replaces the more formal, classical approach to the hypothesis testing one may have learned in an introductory statistics course. We no longer classically "reject" or "fail to reject" the null by hypothesis testing. We look for the size of the *p*-value, usually comparing it to 0.05. In general for hypothesis tests, the larger the value of the test statistic, the smaller the p-value, and the stronger the evidence and the claim that the null hypothesis is not true.

STATISTICAL SIGNIFICANCE

One must be careful about the rigid analogy between <0.05 and statistical significance. As Pocock suggests, 0.05 is merely a guideline.

Clinical Significant

According to Joseph Fleiss, when considering the comparison of two proportions, "Given at least some information, the investigator can, using his or her imagination and expertise, come up with an estimate of a difference between two proportions that is scientifically or clinically important. Given no information, the investigator has no basis for designing the study intelligently and would be hard put to justify designing it at all (Fleiss, p. 34; see Bibliography).

One-Tailed vs. Two-Tailed Tests

The choice here depends in part on the hypothesis. When it relates to a difference in either direction, a *two-tailed test* is employed; when it relates to a difference in one direction only, a *one-tailed test* is appropriate. The two-tailed test is more conservative and is recommended so that the investigator considers the possibility of an outcome in the opposite direction anticipated.

LOGISTIC REGRESSION

This is a widely used technique that is a generalization of multiple regression—and a very useful and interesting one. Here the major difference is that the dependent or outcome variable y is dichotomous or binary. That is, this variable can take on only two values, 1 or 0, yes or no, success or failure (e.g., death or life, disease or no disease, rejection or no rejection, infection or no infection, relapse or no relapse). A scatter plot might take on the following appearance if y = disease (1,0) and x = age:

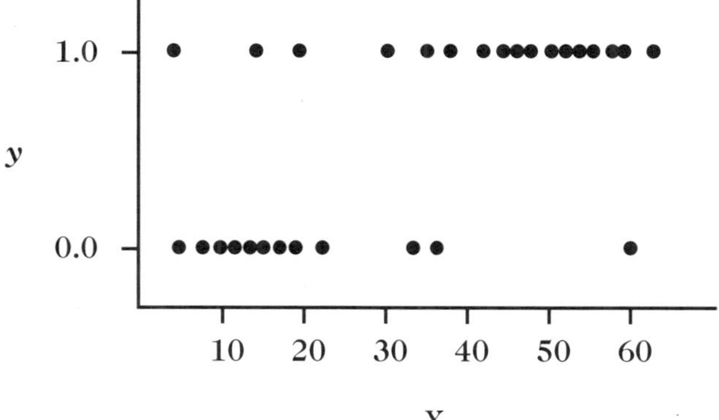

Not much quantitative inference can be derived from this graph, nor can we employ multiple regression techniques just yet.

Taking a look at the proportions of the event vs. age, we have the following depiction:

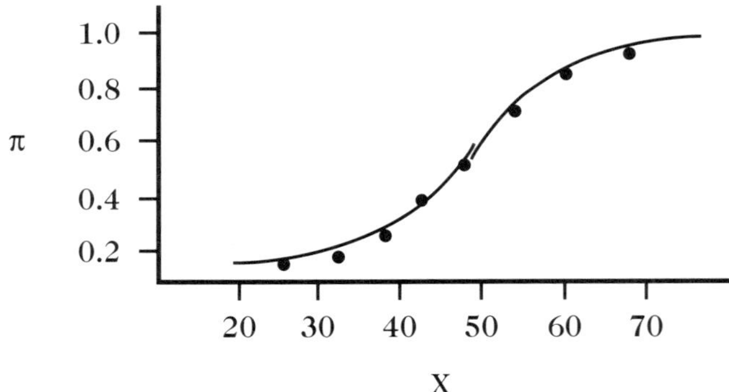

A mathematical equation, the *sigmoid curve,* describes this relationship very well:

$$\pi = \frac{e^x}{1 + e^x} \tag{16.18}$$

Generalizing it to the multivariable domain gives us

$$\pi = \frac{e^{(\beta_o + \beta_1 x_1 + \beta_2 x_2 + \ldots \beta_n x_n)}}{1 + e^{(\beta_o + \beta_1 x_1 + \beta_2 x_2 + \ldots \beta_n x_n)}} \tag{16.19}$$

The x covariates are independent predictor variables that may be continuous or discrete (e.g., age, blood pressure, weight, gender, (0, 1). Do you see what's coming?

With a bit of high school algebra, some mathematical juggling, and the fact that $\ln(e) = 1$* we may derive the following important relationship (the *logistic regression equation* or *logit model*)

$$\ln\left[\frac{\pi}{1 - \pi}\right] = \beta_o + \beta_1 x_1 + \beta_2 x_2 + \ldots \beta_n x_n \tag{16.20}$$

which, you may have noticed, is linear. This is incredibly important (epidemiologically) for the following reasons: It is a fact that $\pi/(1 - \pi)$ = the odds of the event occurring (e.g., the odds of death after surgery, the odds of relapse). The right side of the equation is a similar multivariable set of linear covariates (predictors) we encountered in multiple regression (eq. 16.17). The left side of the equation, the log-odds of the event occurring, replaces the continuous dependent variable y in linear regression. We now have a linear model we can work with. We may use multiple regression techniques to build logistic models. A graph of a linear predictor equation might look like the following:

*ln = natural logarithm.

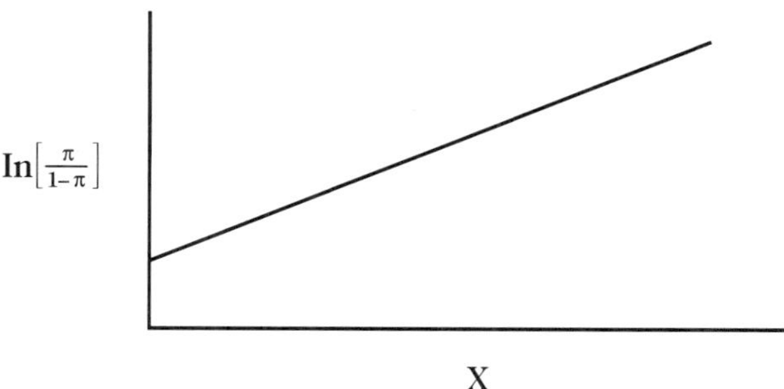

Once we have a best-fit model, we can make the following claim: For example, if age, weight, or blood pressure were included in our logistic model, we could claim that age has a significant effect on the outcome, after adjustment for the other covariates. So, that high school algebra has given us the following model and interpretation: The log-odds of the event is related linearly to the summation of the product of the *x* variables and their coefficients. With this statistical apparatus, we are able to model risk factor predictive equations.

Techniques similar to those discussed in multiple regression (computer programs in SAS, SPSS, etc.) may then be used to discern which variables should be included in the logit model and assumed to be risk factors, linear predictors, explanatory variables, and so on. These programs estimate the beta-coefficient parameters ($\beta_0, \beta_1, \beta_2, \ldots \beta_n$) by an estimating procedure known as *maximum likelihood,* which is a sophisticated technique involving calculus.

Once we are satisfied with the linear fit, i.e., the significance of a set of predictors (independent variables), we can plug the beta coefficients and patient independent variable values into our sigmoid curve equation to predict the probability of the event occurring for a given patient with his/her risk variables.

One goal of logistic regression is to estimate statistically the effects of each variable, adjusted for all other variables in the model. Each estimated coefficient provides an estimate of the log odds, adjusting for all other variables, included in the model (see Hosmer and Lemeshow in the Bibliography).

Odds ratios are easily obtained. Exponentiating the beta coefficient, i.e., raising the exponential function (e) to the power of beta ($e^{\beta i}$), yields the odds of the event occurring for the given risk factor, again, after adjusting for the other variables in the model.

When testing the significance of a coefficient of a variable in any model, the following question should be considered: Does the model which includes the variable in question tell us more about the outcome (or response) variable than does a model that does not include that variable?

SURVIVAL ANALYSIS

Here the dependent variable of interest is the time from some initial observation until the occurrence of an event (death, relapse, etc.). The time from initial observation until failure is called *survival time.*

Kaplan-Meier Product Limit Method

At time t_i let

d_i = number of deaths occurring within the ith interval
n_i = number of patients alive and under observation at the beginning of the interval

The probability of dying during the interval (estimated) is

$$\hat{q}_i = \frac{d_i}{n_i}$$

The probability of surviving through the interval (estimated) is

$$\hat{p}_i = 1 - \hat{q}_i = 1 - \frac{d_i}{n_i} = \frac{(n_i - d_i)}{n_i}$$

If the probability of survival at each interval is *independent* of the probability of survival at all other intervals, then

$$\hat{S}(j) = \prod_{t=1}^{j} \hat{p}_i = (\hat{p}_1) \times (\hat{p}_2) \times (\hat{p}_3) \times \ldots (\hat{p}_j)^*$$

Taking this idea one step further, Kaplan and Meier (see Bibliography) proposed *that each death* occupy an *interval* by itself. Graphing the probability of survival at each interval would yield a Kaplan-Meier product limit estimate curve similar to the one below.

Nonparametric Method of Estimating Survival Functions

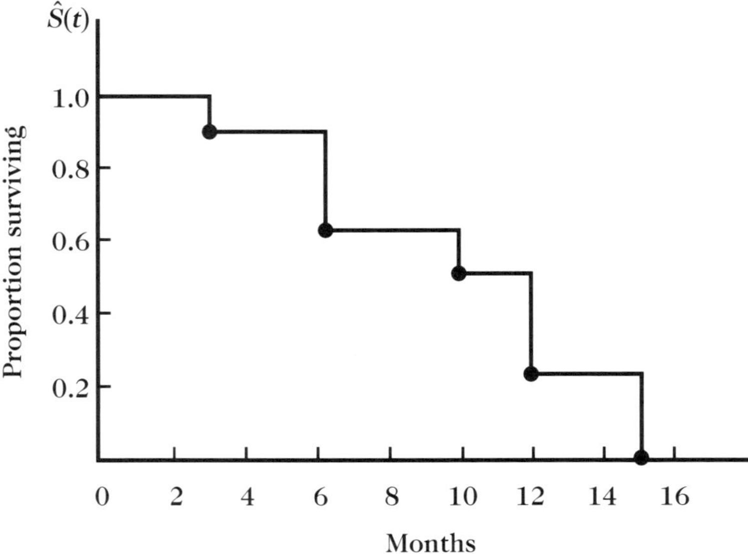

*Here we invoke probability's *law of independence*. The same law that *claims* that the probability of rolling two 6's or craps in a game of die is = (1/6) × (1/6) = 1/36.

An important aspect of this type of analysis is the idea of *censoring*. Certain subjects may not experience the event of interest by the end of the study, i.e., they may still be alive or "free" from the event (relapse, rejection, etc.). Perhaps they are lost to follow-up or have removed themselves from the study. Their exact survival times will not be known, but by censoring the observation at the time of last follow-up, they can be included in the analysis (included in the denominator, if you will) up to their censoring time.

A variety of tests may be used to compare two or more survival curves or distributions in the attempt to discern whether survival differs between the two treatment groups—to find a "statistically significant" difference. They include the *log-rank, Wilcoxon,* and Gehan *tests* to name a few. The log-rank is very common and is utilized when each event is weighed with the same importance.

An important concept in survival analysis is the *hazard function*, also known as the *instantaneous rate of failure* or the *force of mortality*. It is defined as the instantaneous probability of failure at a particular time T given the individual has survived until time T.

Covariate Adjustment

1. Differences may exist between treatment groups (intervention and control) at entry in terms of other covariates, (e.g., age, sex, race, prior medical history, smoking habits, diet).
2. Both the *Cox model* (Sir David Cox) and the *multiphase hazard model (UAB)* adjust for these variables in the *multivariable* domain. This enables us to look at the effect of *each* factor, adjusted for all of the other factors.
3. The hazard rate may be incorporated as a linear function of several covariates:

$$\lambda\,(x_1, x_2, x_3 \ldots x_n) = e^{\beta_1 x_1 = \beta_2 x_2 + \ldots \beta_n x_n)}$$

Once again, the hypothesis test

$$\text{Ho:} \quad \beta_i = 0$$

$$\text{Ha:} \quad \beta_i \neq 0$$

tests whether the covariate is a significant prognostic factor, i.e., is effective after having adjusted for the other factors.

NONPARAMETRIC TESTS

When data cannot be assumed to originate from a normal distribution and when sample sizes are small, there is an array of statistical tests that may be utilized. Some of the more popular *nonparametric* tests, along with their parametric analogs, are listed below.

Parametric test	Nonparametric test
Two-sample *t*-test	Wilcoxon rank sum or Mann-Whitney *U* test
Paired *t*-test	Wilcoxon signed-rank test (1945), sign test
Correlation	Spearman's rho
ANOVA	Kruskal-Wallis*
ANOVA—blocked design	Friedman test*

*See the Bibliography

Nonparametric tests rank order the data and then calculate test statistics based on the ranks and not the actual raw data.

CONCLUSION

There are endless designs and alternative tests which help fill a statistical library. There has been no mention of kappa, log-linear models, autocorrelated data, the Mantal-Haenzel statistic, interater reliability, and many others, I encourage the further exploration by the reader of other text material.

BIBLIOGRAPHY

Agresti A: *Categorical Data Analysis.* New York: Wiley, 1990.

Alahuhta S, Rasanen J, Jouppila R, Joupilla P, et al: Uteroplacental and fetal haemodynamics during extradural anaesthesia for caesarean section. *Br J Anaesth* 66:319–323, 1991.

Anderson SA, Auquier WW, Hauck D, et al: *Statistical Methods for Comparative Studies: Techniques for Bias Reduction.* New York: Wiley, 1980.

Blackstone EH, Naftel DC, Turner ME Jr: The decomposition of time-varying hazard into phases, each incorporating a separate stream of concomitant information. *J Am Stat Assoc* 395: 615–624, 1986.

Cochran WG: Approximate significance levels of the Behrens-Fisher test. *Biometrics* 20:191–195, 1964.

Colton T: *Statistics in Medicine.* Boston: Little, Brown, 1974.

Cox DR: Regression models and life tables (with discussion). *Journal of the Royal Statistical Society, B,* 34:187–220, 1972.

Daniel WW: *Biostatistics: A Foundation for Analysis in the Health Sciences,* ed 6. New York: Wiley, 1987.

Dawson-Saunders B, Trapp RG: *Basic and Clinical Biostatistics.* Norwalk, CT, Appleton and Lange, 1990.

DeMoivre A: *The Doctrine of Chances.* 1756. Reprint, ed 3. New York: Chelsea, 1967.

Dowdy S, Wearden S: *Statistics for Research,* ed 2. New York: Wiley, 1985, p. 629.

Dunnett, CW: A multiple comparisons procedure for comparing several treatments with a control. *J Am Stat Assoc* 50:1096–1121, 1955.

Fleiss JL: 1981. *Statistical Methods for Rates and Proportions,* ed 2. New York: Wiley, 1981.

Fleiss JL: *The Design and Analysis of Clinical Experiments.* New York: Wiley, 1986.

Friedman M: The use of ranks to avoid the assumption of normality implicit in the analysis of variance. *J Am Stat Assoc* 32:675–701, 1937.

Gauss CF: *Theory of Motion of the Heavenly Bodies Moving About the Sun in Conic Sections.* 1809 Reprint New York: Dover, 1963.

Gosset WS: ("Student"), "The Probable Error of a Mean," *Biometrika* 6:1–25, 1908.

Greene J, Touchstone J: Urinary tract estriol: An index of placental function. *Am J Obstet Gynecol* 85(1):1–9, 1963.

Hickey CA: Employment-related stress and preterm delivery: A contextual examination. *Public Health Rep* 410–418, 1995.

Hosmer DW and Lemeshow, S: *Applied Logistic Regression.* New York: Wiley, 1989.

Kaplan EL, Meier P: Nonparametric estimation from incomplete observations. *J Am Stat Assoc* 53:457, 1958.

Kruskal WH, Wallis WA: Use of ranks on one-criterion variance analysis. *J Am Stat Assoc* 47:583–621, 1952.

Lee ET: *Statistical Methods for Survival Data Analysis,* ed 2. New York: Wiley, 1992.

McCullagh P, Nelder JA: *Generalized Linear Models.* London: Chapman and Hall, 1983.

McNemar Q: Note on the sampling error of the difference between correlated proportions or percentages. *Psychometrika* 12:153–157, 1947.

Miller RG Jr: *Survival Analysis.* New York: Wiley, 1981.

Neter J, Wasserman W, Kutner MH: *Applied Linear Regression Models,* ed 2. Homewood, IL: Richard D. Irwin, 1983.

Pagano M, Gauvreau K: *Principles of Biostatistics.* Belmont, CA, Duxbury, 1993.

Remington RD, Schork MA: *Statistics with Applications to the Biological and Health Sciences,* ed 2. Englewood Cliffs, NJ: Prentice-Hall, 1985.

Rosner B: 1955, *Fundamentals of Biostatistics,* 4th edition, Belmont, CA, Duxbury Press.

Schlesselman, J: 1982, *Case-Control Studies,* New York, Oxford University Press.

Snedecor GW, Cochran WG: *Statistical Methods,* ed 6. Ames: Iowa State University Press, 1937.

Stigler S: *The History of Statistics.* Cambridge, MA: Harvard University Press, 1986.

Stokes M, Davis C, and Koch G: *Categorical Data Analysis Using the SAS System,* Cary, NC:SAS Institute Inc., 1995.

Strait PT: *A First Course in Probability and Statistics with Applications.* San Diego: Harcourt Brace Jovanovich, 1983.

Summary of Vital Statistics 1990: The City of New York. New York City Department of Health, 1990.

Welch BL: The significance of the difference between two means when the population variances are unequal. *Biometrika* 29:350, 1937.

APPENDIX

$$\hat{b}_1 = \sum (x_i - \hat{x})(y_i - \hat{y}) / \sum (x_i - \hat{x})^2$$

$$\hat{b}_o = \bar{y} - \hat{b}_1\bar{x}$$

Index